Acute and Critical Care Medicine at a Glance

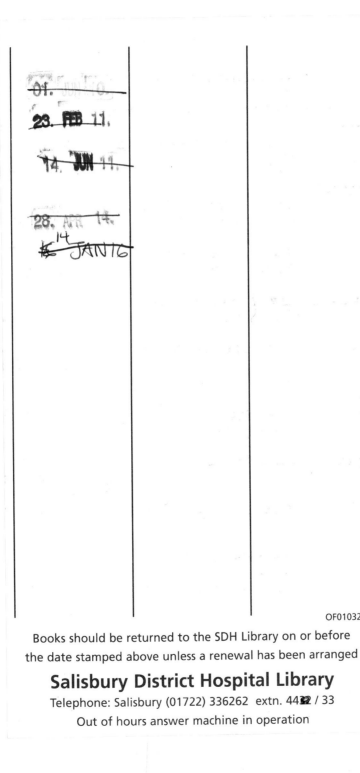

Dedication
To Clare, Helen, Marc and Niall

Acute and Critical Care Medicine at a Glance

Richard Leach

MD, FRCP
Consultant Physician and Honorary Senior Lecturer
Department of Respiratory and Critical Care Medicine
Guy's and St Thomas' Hospital Trust and King's College, London

Second edition

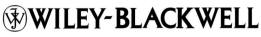

WILEY-BLACKWELL

A John Wiley & Sons, Ltd., Publication

This edition first published 2009, © 2009 by Richard Leach
Previous edition 2004

Blackwell Publishing was acquired by John Wiley & Sons in February 2007. Blackwell's publishing program has been merged with Wiley's global Scientific, Technical and Medical business to form Wiley-Blackwell.

Registered office: John Wiley & Sons Ltd, The Atrium, Southern Gate, Chichester, West Sussex, PO19 8SQ, UK

Editorial offices: 9600 Garsington Road, Oxford, OX4 2DQ, UK
The Atrium, Southern Gate, Chichester, West Sussex, PO19 8SQ, UK
111 River Street, Hoboken, NJ 07030-5774, USA

For details of our global editorial offices, for customer services and for information about how to apply for permission to reuse the copyright material in this book please see our website at www.wiley.com/wiley-blackwell

The right of the author to be identified as the author of this work has been asserted in accordance with the Copyright, Designs and Patents Act 1988.

Wiley also publishes its books in a variety of electronic formats. Some content that appears in print may not be available in electronic books.

Designations used by companies to distinguish their products are often claimed as trademarks. All brand names and product names used in this book are trade names, service marks, trademarks or registered trademarks of their respective owners. The publisher is not associated with any product or vendor mentioned in this book. This publication is designed to provide accurate and authoritative information in regard to the subject matter covered. It is sold on the understanding that the publisher is not engaged in rendering professional services. If professional advice or other expert assistance is required, the services of a competent professional should be sought.

Library of Congress Cataloging-in-Publication Data

Leach, Richard, MD.
    Acute and critical care medicine at a glance / Richard Leach. – 2nd ed.
        p.   ;   cm. – (At a glance series)
    Rev. ed. of: Critical care medicine at a glance. 2004.
    Includes index.
    ISBN 978-1-4051-6139-8
    1. Critical care medicine–Handbooks, manuals, etc.   I. Leach, Richard, MD. Critical care medicine at a glance.   II. Title.   III. Series: At a glance series (Oxford, England)
    [DNLM: 1. Critical Care–methods–Handbooks.   2. Acute Disease–therapy–Handbooks.
WX 39 L434a 2009]
    RC86.8.L43 2009
    616.02′8–dc22
    2008055876

ISBN: 9781405161398

A catalogue record for this book is available from the British Library.

Set in 9/11.5 pt Times by SNP Best-set Typesetter Ltd., Hong Kong
Printed and bound in Singapore by Fabulous Printers Pte Ltd.

1   2009

Contents

Preface 6
Acknowledgements 7
Units, symbols and abbreviations 8

Part 1 General
1 Recognizing the unwell patient 12
2 Admission and ongoing management of the acutely unwell patient 14
3 Monitoring in acute and critical care medicine 16
4 Oxygen transport 18
5 Cardiopulmonary resuscitation 20
6 Shock 22
7 Circulatory assessment 24
8 Fluid management 26
9 Fluid choice: specific situations 28
10 Inotropes and vasopressors 29
11 Failure of oxygenation and respiratory failure 30
12 Oxygenation and oxygen therapy 32
13 Airways obstruction and management 34
14 Non-invasive ventilation 36
15 Endotracheal intubation 38
16 Mechanical ventilation 40
17 Respiratory management, weaning and tracheostomy 42
18 Arterial blood gases and acid–base balance 44
19 Analgesia, sedation and paralysis 46
20 Enteral and parenteral nutrition 48
21 Hypothermia and hyperthermia 50
22 SIRS, sepsis, severe sepsis and septic shock 52
23 Hospital-acquired (nosocomial) infections 54
24 End of life issues 56

Part 2 Medical
Cardiac
25 Acute coronary syndromes I: clinical pathophysiology 58
26 Acute coronary syndromes II: investigations and management 60
27 Arrhythmias 62
28 Heart failure and pulmonary oedema 64
29 Cardiac emergencies 66
30 Deep venous thrombosis and pulmonary embolism 68

Respiratory
31 Community-acquired pneumonia 70
32 Hospital-acquired (nosocomial) pneumonia 72
33 Asthma 74
34 Chronic obstructive pulmonary disease 76
35 Acute respiratory distress syndrome 78
36 Pneumothorax and air leaks 80
37 Respiratory emergencies 82

Renal and metabolic
38 Acute kidney injury: pathophysiology and clinical aspects 84
39 Acute kidney injury: management and renal replacement therapy 86
40 Diabetic emergencies 88
41 Endocrine emergencies 90

Gastrointestinal
42 Gastrointestinal haemorrhage 92
43 Acute liver failure 94
44 Acute pancreatitis 96

Neurological
45 Acute confusional state, coma and status epilepticus 98
46 Neurological emergencies: cerebrovascular accidents 100
47 Neurological emergencies: infective 101
48 Neuromuscular conditions 102

Other systems
49 Coagulation disorders and transfusion 104
50 Drug overdose and poisoning 106
51 The immune compromised patient 108

Part 3 Surgical
52 Trauma 110
53 Head injury 112
54 Chest trauma 114
55 Acute abdominal emergencies 116
56 Obstetric emergencies 118
57 Burns, toxic inhalation and electrical injuries 120

Part 4 Self-assessment
Case studies and questions 122
Case studies answers 125

Appendices
Appendix I: Classification of antiarrhythmic drugs 132
Appendix II: Acute injury network staging system 2008 for acute kidney injury 132
Appendix III: Rockall risk-scoring system for GI bleeds 133
Appendix IV: Child–Pugh grading 133
Appendix V: Typical criteria for liver transplantation 133

Index 135

Preface

Acute and critical care medicine encompasses the clinical, diagnostic and therapeutic skills required to manage acutely ill patients in a variety of settings including intensive care, high dependency, surgical recovery, coronary care and emergency departments. These disciplines have developed rapidly over the past 30 years and are an integral part of most medical, anaesthetic and surgical specialties. Medical students, junior doctors, nursing and paramedical staff are increasingly expected to develop the skills necessary to recognize and manage acutely ill patients, and most will be familiar with the apprehension that precedes such training. Unfortunately, most current texts relating to acute or critical care medicine are unavoidably extensive. It is the aim of *Acute and Critical Care Medicine at a Glance* to provide a brief, rapidly informative text, easily assimilated prior to starting a new job, that will prepare the newcomer for those aspects of these specialties with which they may not be familiar. These include assessment of the acutely unwell patient, monitoring, emergency resuscitation, oxygenation, circulatory support, methods of ventilation and management of a wide variety of medical and surgical emergencies.

As with other volumes in the 'At a Glance' series, it is based around a two-page spread for each main topic, with figures and text complementing each other to give an overview of a topic at a glance. Although primarily designed as an introduction to acute and critical care medicine, it should be a useful undergraduate revision aid. However, such a brief text cannot hope to provide a complete guide to clinical practice and postgraduate students are advised that additional reference to more detailed textbooks will aid deeper and wider understanding of the subject. On the advice of our readers, the second edition includes new chapters on fluid management, oxygenation, non-invasive ventilation, recognition of the seriously ill patient and hospital-acquired infections; and previous chapters have been extensively updated to include recent guidelines and innovations. As with many new specialties, certain aspects of acute and critical care medicine remain controversial. Where controversy exists I have attempted to highlight differences of opinion and with the help of many colleagues and reviewers to provide a balanced perspective although on occasions this has proven difficult. Nevertheless, errors and omissions may have occurred and these are entirely our responsibility.

Many colleagues, junior doctors and medical students have advised and commented on the content of *Acute and Critical Care Medicine at a Glance*. I would particularly like to thank my medical colleagues on the acute medical, high dependency and intensive care units at Guy's, St Thomas' and Johns Hopkins Hospitals and the Anaesthetic Department at St Thomas' Hospital. Special thanks are due to the Senior Nurses at Guy's and St Thomas' Hospitals and Mrs Clare Leach for their advice on the many aspects of nursing care so essential in acute and critical care medicine. Finally, I would like to thank all the staff at Wiley-Blackwell, especially Karen Moore, who have cajoled and assisted me in producing this updated volume.

Richard Leach

Acknowledgements

List of contributors

Ms Clare Meadows, Ms Janet Nicholls, Ms Helen Dickie, Mr Tony Convery. Senior Nursing Staff on the High Dependency and Intensive Care Units. Guy's and St Thomas' Hospital Trust, London

Dr David Treacher: Oxygen transport and shock
Dr Michael Gilles: Cardiopulmonary resuscitation
Dr Duncan Wyncoll: Fluid management, acute pancreatitis and overdose
Dr Rosalind Tilley: Airways management and endotracheal intubation
Dr Angela McLuckie: SIRS, sepsis, severe sepsis and septic shock
Consultant Intensivists, Guy's and St Thomas' Hospital Trust, London

Dr Marlies Ostermann: Acute kidney injury
Consultant Renal Physician and Intensivist,
Guy's and St Thomas' Hospital Trust, London

Dr Richard Beale: Enteral and parenteral nutrition
Clinical Director of Perioperative, Critical Care and Pain services,
Guy's and St Thomas' Hospital Trust, London

Dr Nicholas Hart: Non-invasive ventilation and respiratory management
Consultant Respiratory Physician, Lane Fox Unit,
Guy's and St Thomas' Hospital Trust, London

Dr Craig Davidson: Oxygenation and oxygen therapy
Consultant Respiratory Physician and Director, Lane Fox Unit,
Guy's and St Thomas' Hospital Trust, London

Mr Jonathan Lucas: Trauma and chest trauma
Consultant Orthopaedic and Spinal Surgeon
Guy's and St Thomas' Hospital Trust, London

Professor Jeremy Ward: Acute coronary syndromes, deep venous thrombosis and pulmonary embolism
Head of Department of Physiology and Professor of Respiratory Cell Physiology, Kings College, London

Professor James T. Sylvester: Asthma
Professor of Pulmonary and Critical Care Medicine
The Johns Hopkins Medical Institutions, Baltimore, MD USA

Professor Charles M. Wiener: Asthma and COPD
Professor of Medicine and Physiology
Johns Hopkins School of Medicine, Baltimore MD USA

Ms Catherine McKenzie, Senior Pharmacist, Guy's and St Thomas' Hospital Trust, London

Figures

Some figures in this book are taken from:
Norwitz, E. & Schorge, J. (2006) *Obstetrics and Gynecology at a Glance*, 2nd edition. Blackwell Publishing Ltd, Oxford.
O'Callaghan, C. (2006) *The Renal System at a Glance*, 2nd edition. Blackwell Publishing Ltd, Oxford.
Ward, J.P.T. *et al.* (2006) *The Respiratory System at a Glance*, 2nd edition. Blackwell Publishing Ltd, Oxford.

Units, symbols and abbreviations

Units

The medical profession and scientific community generally use SI (Système International) units.

Pressure conversion. SI unit of pressure: 1 pascal (Pa) = $1\,N/m^2$. As this is small, in medicine the kPa (= 10^3Pa) is more commonly used. Note that millimetres of mercury (mmHg) are still the commonest unit for expressing arterial and venous blood pressures, and low pressures – e.g. central venous pressure and intrapleural pressure – are sometimes expressed as centimetres of H_2O (cmH_2O). Blood gas partial pressures are reported by some laboratories in kPa and by some in mmHg, so you need to be familiar with both systems.

1 kPa = 7.5 mmHg = $10.2\,cmH_2O$
1 mmHg = 1 torr = 0.133 kPa = $1.36\,cmH_2O$
1 cmH_2O = 0.098 kPa = 0.74 mmHg
1 standard atmosphere ($\approx$ 1 bar) = 101.3 kPa = 760 mmHg = $1033\,cmH_2O$

Contents are still commonly expressed per 100 mL (dL^{-1}), and these need to be multiplied by 10 to give the more standard SI unit per litre. Contents are also increasingly being expressed as mmol/L.

For haemoglobin: 1 g/dL = 10 g/L = 0.062 mmol/L
For ideal gases (including oxygen and nitrogen): 1 mmol = 22.4 mL standard temperature and pressure dry (STPD)
For non-ideal gases, such as nitrous oxide and carbon dioxide: 1 mmol = 22.25 mL STPD

Symbols

Symbols used in respiratory and cardiovascular physiology are shown in Table 1.

Typical inspired, alveolar and blood gas values in healthy young adults are shown in Table 2. Ranges are given for arterial blood gas values. Mean arterial Po_2 falls with age, and by 60 years is about 11 kPa/82 mmHg. Typical values for lung volumes and other lung function tests are given in Table 3 and *The Respiratory System at a Glance*. Ranges for many values are affected by age, sex and height, as well as by the method of measurement, and hence it is necessary to refer to appropriate nomograms.

Table 1 Standard respiratory symbols

Primary symbols
F = fractional concentration of gas
C = content of a gas in blood
V = volume of a gas
P = pressure or partial pressure
S = saturation of haemoglobin with oxygen
Q = volume of blood
A dot over a letter means a time derivative, e.g. $\dot{V}$ = ventilation (L/min) $\dot{Q}$ = blood flow (L/min)

Secondary symbols
Gas
I = inspired gas
E = expired gas
A = alveolar gas
D = dead space gas
T = tidal
B = barometric
ET = end-tidal

Blood
a = arterial
v = venous
c = capillary

A dash means mixed or mean, e.g. $\bar{v}$ = mixed venous
A′ after a symbol means end, e.g. c′ = end-capillary

Tertiary symbols
O_2 = oxygen
CO_2 = carbon dioxide
CO = carbon monoxide

Examples
Vo_2 = oxygen consumption
P_Aco_2 = alveolar partial pressure of carbon dioxide

Table 2 Inspired, alveolar and blood gas values

Inspired Po_2 (dry, sea level)	21 kPa	159 mmHg
Alveolar Po_2	13.3 kPa	100 mmHg
Arterial Po_2	12.5 (11.2–13.9) kPa	94 (84–104) mmHg
A–a Po_2 gradient	<2 kPa	<15 mmHg (greater in elderly)
Oxygen saturation	>97%	
Oxygen content	20 mL/dL	
Inspired Pco_2	0.03 kPa	0.2 mmHg
Alveolar Pco_2	5.3 (4.7–6.1) kPa	40 (35–45) mmHg
Arterial Pco_2	5.3 (4.7–6.1) kPa	40 (35–45) mmHg
Arterial CO_2 content	48 ml/dL	
Arterial $[H^+]$/pH	36–44nmol/L/7.44–7.36	
Resting mixed venous Po_2	5.3 kPa	40 mmHg
Resting mixed venous O_2 content	15 mL/dL	
Resting mixed venous O_2 saturation	75%	
Resting mixed venous Pco_2	6.1 kPa	46 mmHg
Resting mixed venous CO_2 content	52 mL/dL	
Arterial $[HCO_3^-]$	24 (21–27) mM	

Table 3 Typical lung volumes for an adult male

Tidal volume (V_T) (at rest)	500 mL
Vital capacity (VC)	5500 mL
Inspiratory capacity (IC)	3800 mL
Expiratory reserve volume (ERV)	1200 mL
Total lung capacity (TLC)	6000 mL
Functional residual capacity (FRC)	2200 mL
Residual volume (RV)	1000 mL

Abbreviations

±	with or without
~	about
A–a gradient	$P_{(A-a)}O_2$ gradient, the difference between alveolar and arterial Po_2
AA	amino acids
ABC	airways, breathing, circulation
ABG	arterial blood gas
ABI	acute bowel ischaemia
AC	activated charcoal
ACE	angiotensin-converting enzyme
ACH	acetylcholine
AChR	acetylcholine receptor
ACT	activated clotting time
ACTH	adrenocorticotrophic hormone
ADH	antidiuretic hormone
AF	atrial flutter; atrial fibrillation
AFE	amniotic fluid embolism
AG	anion gap
AIDS	acquired immunodeficiency syndrome
ALF	acute liver failure
ALI	acute lung injury
ALS	advanced life support
ANA	antinuclear antibodies
ANCA	antineutrophil cytoplasmic antibodies
AP	action potential
AP	anteroposterior
APACHE	acute physiology and chronic health evaluation
APH	antepartum haemorrhage
APTT	activated partial thromboplastin time
ARDS	acute respiratory distress syndrome
ARF	acute renal failure
ASD	atrial septal defect
ATLS	advanced trauma life support
ATN	acute tubular necrosis
ATP	adenosine triphosphate
ATS	American Thoracic Society
AVM	arteriovenous malformation
AVN	atrioventricular node
AXR	abdominal radiograph
BE	base excess
BIPAP	bilevel positive pressure ventilation
BIPAP-APRV	BIPAP airways pressure release ventilation
BLS	basic life support
BMR	basal metabolic rate
BP	blood pressure
BPF	bronchopleural fistula
BS	blood sugar
BSA	body surface area
BSD	brainstem death
BSFT	brainstem function test
BTS	British Thoracic Society
CA	coronary artery
cAMP	cyclic adenosine monophosphate
C_aO_2	oxygen content in arterial blood
CAP	community-acquired pneumonia
CBF	cerebral blood flow
CBV	cerebral blood volume
CCB	calcium channel blocker
CCF	congestive cardiac failure
CCM	critical care medicine
CE	cardiac enzymes
CHF	chronic heart failure
CIDP	chronic inflammatory demyelinating polyneuropathy
CK-MB	creatine kinase-MB
CLD	chronic liver disease
CMV	controlled mechanical ventilation
CMV	cytomegalovirus
CN	cyanide
CNS	central nervous system
CO	cardiac output
CO	carbon monoxide
CO_2	carbon dioxide
CO-Hb	carboxyhaemoglobin
COPD	chronic obstructive pulmonary disease
COX	cyclo-oxygenase
CPA	cardiopulmonary arrest
CPAP	continuous positive airways pressure
CPB	cardiopulmonary bypass
CPD-A	citrate, phosphate, dextrose-adenine
CPP	cerebral perfusion pressure
CPR	cardiopulmonary resuscitation
CRF	chronic renal failure
CRP	C-reactive protein
CS	caesarian section
CSF	cerebrospinal fluid
CT	computed tomography
CTT	cardiac troponin T
CVA	cerebrovascular accident
CVC	central venous catheter
C_vO_2	oxygen content in venous blood
CVP	central venous pressure
CVS	cardiovascular system
CXR	chest radiograph
D5%	5% dextrose
DBP	diastolic blood pressure
DC	direct current
DD	diastolic dysfunction
DDAVP	desmopressin acetate or arginine vasopressin
DIC	disseminated intravascular coagulation
DKA	diabetic ketoacidosis
DM	diabetes mellitus
Do_2	global oxygen delivery
DPG	2,3 diphosphoglycerate
DVT	deep venous thrombosis
ECF	extracellular fluid
ECG	electrocardiogram
ECM	external cardiac massage
ECMO	extracorporeal membrane oxygenation
EEG	electroencephalogram
EMD	electromechanical dissociation
EN	enteral nutrition
ER	emergency room
ERCP	endoscopic retrograde choledochopancreatography
ERF	established renal failure
ESR	erythrocyte sedimentation rate
ETI	endotracheal intubation
ETT	endotracheal tube

f	frequency	MDR	multidrug-resistant
FDP	fibrinogen degradation product	MG	myasthenia gravis
FEV$_1$	forced expiratory volume in 1 second	MH	malignant hyperthermia
FFP	fresh frozen plasma	MI	myocardial infarction
F_io$_2$	fraction of inspired oxygen	MILS	manual in-line cervical stabilization
FRC	functional residual capacity	MIP	maximum inspiratory pressure
FVC	forced vital capacity	MOC	myocardial oxygen consumption
FWB	fresh whole blood	MOF	multiorgan failure
GBS	Guillain–Barré syndrome	MRI	magnetic resonance imaging
GCS	Glasgow Coma Score	MRSA	methicillin-resistant *Staphylococcus aureus*
GDP	gross domestic product	MV	mechanical ventilation
GFR	glomerular filtration rate	MW	molecular weight
GH	growth hormone	NAC	N-acetylcysteine
GI	gastrointestinal	NC	narrow QRS complex
GL	gastric lavage	NDI	nephrogenic diabetes insipidus
H$_2$O	water	NG	nasogastric
HAP	hospital-acquired pneumonia	NIPPV	nasal intermittent positive pressure ventilation
Hb	haemoglobin	NIV	non-invasive ventilation
HB	heart block	NMJ	neuromuscular junction
HDU	high dependency unit	NMS	neuroleptic malignant syndrome
HE	hypertensive emergency	NO	nitric oxide
HF	heart failure	NPV	negative pressure ventilation
HHT	hereditary haemorrhagic telangiectasia	NS	normal saline
HIT	heparin-induced thrombocytopenia	NS	nutritional support
HIV	human immunodeficiency virus	NSAID	non-steroidal anti-inflammatory drug
HLA	human leucocyte antigen	NYHA	New York Heart Association
HONK	hyperosmolar non-ketotic coma	O$_2$	oxygen
HpE	hepatic encephalopathy	OCP	oral contraceptive pill
HR	heart rate	OER	oxygen extraction ratio
HRS	hepatorenal syndrome	OGD	oesophagogastroduodenoscopy
HT	hypertension	OHA	out-of-hospital arrest
HTLV1	human lymphocytic virus 1	OT	oxygen therapy
HUS	haemolytic–uraemic syndrome	$P_{(A-a)}$o$_2$	alveolar–arterial oxygen tension difference
IBD	inflammatory bowel disease	P$_{50}$	Po$_2$ at which 50% of haemoglobin is saturated
ICF	intracellular fluid	PA	pulmonary artery
ICH	intracerebral haemorrhage	$P_a$co$_2$	partial pressure of CO$_2$ in arterial blood
ICP	intracranial pressure	PAI	primary adrenal insufficiency
ICU	intensive care unit	P_ao$_2$	partial pressure of oxygen in arterial blood
IHA	in-hospital arrest	P_Ao$_2$	partial pressure of oxygen in the alveolus
IHD	ischaemic heart disease	PAOP	pulmonary artery occlusion pressure
IJV	internal jugular vein	PAWP	pulmonary artery wedge pressure
IMA	inferior mesenteric artery	Pco$_2$	partial pressure of CO$_2$
IP	intrathoracic pressure	PCP	*Pneumocystis (jirovecii) carinii* pneumonia
IPPV	intermittent positive pressure ventilation	PCT	percutaneous tracheostomy
ISF	interstitial fluid	PCV	pressure-controlled ventilation
ITP	idiopathic thrombocytopenic purpura	PCWP	pulmonary capillary wedge pressure
LA	left atrial; left atrium	PE	pulmonary embolism
LAP	left atrial pressure	PEA	pulseless electrical activity
LBBB	left bundle branch block	PEEP	positive end-expiratory pressure
LC	lung compliance	PEEP$_i$	intrinsic or auto-PEEP
LDH	lactate dehydrogenase	PEFR	peak expiratory flow rate
LMWH	low molecular weight heparin	pH	logarithmic hydrogen ion concentration in arterial blood
LRT	lower respiratory tract		
LTOD	life-threatening organ damage	PHT	pulmonary hypertension
LUS	lower uterine segment	PiCCO	pulsion continuous cardiac output monitor
LV	left ventricular; left ventricle	PIH	pregnancy-induced hypertension
LVF	left ventricular failure	P_io$_2$	partial pressure of inspired oxygen
MAP	mean arterial pressure	PIP	peak inspiratory pressure
MDMA	methylene dioxymethamphetamine	pK_A	log of the dissociation constant K_A

P_{O_2}	partial pressure of oxygen	SRI	serotonin reuptake inhibitor
POD	paracetamol overdose	SS	scoring system(s)
PP	placenta praevia	ST	surgical tracheostomy
PPH	postpartum haemorrhage	SV	spontaneous ventilation
PPI	proton pump inhibitor	SV	stroke volume
PPV	positive pressure ventilation	$S_v{O_2}$	mixed venous oxygen saturation
P_{plat}	plateau pressure	SVR	systemic vascular resistance
PRC	packed red cells	SVT	supraventricular tachycardia
PrHT	portal hypertension	SVT/AC	supraventricular tachycardia with abnormal
PS	pressure support		conduction
PSP	primary spontaneous pneumothorax	T3	triiodothyronine
PSV	pressure support ventilation	T4	thyroxine
PT	prothrombin time	TB	tuberculosis
PTCA	percutaneous coronary angioplasty	TC	time constant
PVD	peripheral vascular disease	TCA	tricyclic antidepressant
PVS	persistent vegetative state	TDB	third-degree burn
QOL	quality of life	TE	thromboembolic
Qs/Qt	shunt fraction	TID	tubulointerstitial disease
Q_T	cardiac output	TII	toxic inhalational injury
RA	right atrial; right atrium	TIPS	transjugular intrahepatic portal stent
RAD	right axis deviation	TISS	therapeutic intervention scoring system
RAP	right atrial pressure	TLC	total lung capacity
RBBB	right bundle branch block	TNF	tumour necrosis factor
RES	reticuloendothelial system	TP	traumatic pneumothorax
RF	respiratory failure	TPA	tissue plasminogen activator
RFCA	radiofrequency catheter ablation	TPN	total parenteral nutrition
RPC	retained products of conception	TS	trauma score
RR	respiratory rate	TSH	thyroid-stimulating hormone
RRT	renal replacement therapy	TT	thrombolytic therapy
RSI	rapid sequence induction	TTP	thrombotic thrombocytopenic purpura
RUQ	right upper quadrant	Tv	tidal ventilation
RV	right ventricular; right ventricle	UA	unstable angina
RV	residual volume	UAO	upper airways obstruction
RVF	right ventricular failure	UFH	unfractionated heparin
SA	stable angina	USS	ultrasound scan
SAG-M	saline, adenine, glucose-mannitol	VC	vital capacity
SAH	subarachnoid haemorrhage	VCV	volume-controlled ventilation
SAI	secondary adrenal insufficiency	VF	ventricular fibrillation
SAN	sinoatrial node	VMA	vanillyl mandelic acid
$S_a{O_2}$	saturation of oxygen in arterial blood	V_{O_2}	global oxygen consumption
SAPS	simplified acute physiology score	V/Q	ventilation/perfusion
SBO	small bowel obstruction	VSD	ventricular septal defect
SBP	spontaneous bacterial peritonitis	V_T	respiratory tidal volume *or* tidal ventilation
SDB	second-degree burn	VT	ventricular tachycardia
SE	subcutaneous emphysema	VTE	venous thromboembolism
SEMI	subendocardial myocardial infarction	VWD	Von Willebrand's disease
SEp	status epilepticus	WC	wide QRS complex
SIMV	synchronized intermittent mandatory ventilation	WCC	white cell count
SIRS	systemic inflammatory response syndrome	WoB	work of breathing
$S_j{O_2}$	cerebral oxygen saturation	WOT	withdrawal of treatment
SK	streptokinase	WPW	Wolff–Parkinson–White
SLE	systemic lupus erythematosus		
SMA	superior mesenteric artery	Na^+	sodium
SMR	standard mortality ratio (observed mortality ÷ predicted mortality)	K^+	potassium
		Ca^{2+}	calcium
SNPA	soft nasopharyngeal airway	Mg^{2+}	magnesium
S_{O_2}	haemoglobin saturation	Cl^-	chloride
SOL	space-occupying lesion	HCO_3^-	bicarbonate
SP	secondary pneumothorax		

1 Recognizing the unwell patient

(a) Patient at risk early warning scoring system: a score ≥5 indicates that a 'Patient At Risk Team' (PART) or 'Medical Emergency Team' (MET), composed of doctors and senior nurses familiar with assessment and management of acutely unwell patients, should be summoned

Score	3	2	1	0	1	2	3
Heart rate (beats/min)	–	≤40	41–50	51–100	101–110	110–129	≥130
BP (systolic; mmHg)	≤70	71–80	81–100	101–199	–	≥200	–
Respiratory rate	–	≤8	–	9–24	–	25–29	≥30
S_aO_2 (%)	≤88	89–90	91–94	≥9	–	–	–
% Oxygen	–	–	–	–	≥8L/min or 40%	–	–
Core temperature (°C)	–	≤35	35.1–35.9	36–37.4	≥37.5	≥38.5	–
Conscious level	–	–	–	Alert	Drowsy; responds to voice	Acute confusion or agitation	Responds to pain only
Urine output	≤20mls/hr for 2hrs	<1ml/kg for 2 hrs	–	>500mls in 24hrs	250–500mls in 24hrs	<250mls in 24hrs	0/mls in 24hrs

(b) Assessing the acutely ill patient

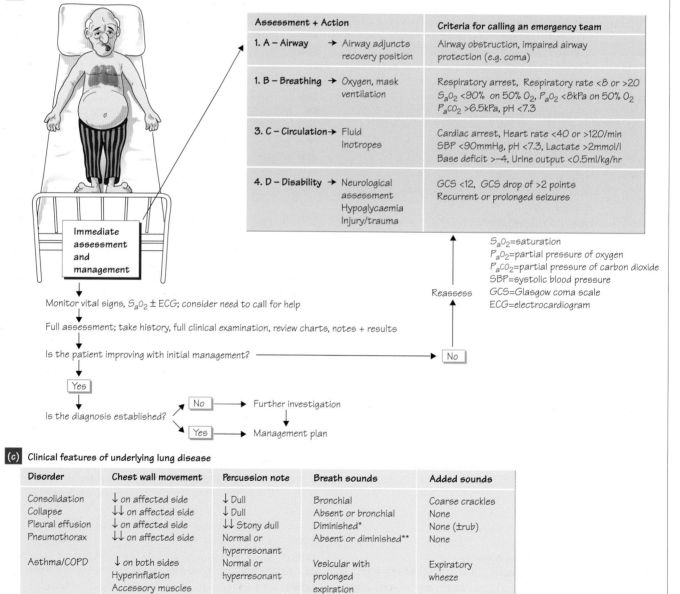

Assessment + Action		Criteria for calling an emergency team
1. A – Airway	→ Airway adjuncts recovery position	Airway obstruction, impaired airway protection (e.g. coma)
1. B – Breathing	→ Oxygen, mask ventilation	Respiratory arrest, Respiratory rate <8 or >20 S_aO_2 <90% on 50% O_2, P_aO_2 <8kPa on 50% O_2 P_aCO_2 >6.5kPa, pH <7.3
3. C – Circulation	→ Fluid Inotropes	Cardiac arrest, Heart rate <40 or >120/min SBP <90mmHg, pH <7.3, Lactate >2mmol/l Base deficit >–4, Urine output <0.5ml/kg/hr
4. D – Disability	→ Neurological assessment Hypoglycaemia Injury/trauma	GCS <12, GCS drop of >2 points Recurrent or prolonged seizures

S_aO_2=saturation
P_aO_2=partial pressure of oxygen
P_aCO_2=partial pressure of carbon dioxide
SBP=systolic blood pressure
GCS=Glasgow coma scale
ECG=electrocardiogram

Immediate assessment and management

Monitor vital signs, S_aO_2 ± ECG; consider need to call for help

Full assessment; take history, full clinical examination, review charts, notes + results

Is the patient improving with initial management? ⟶ No

Reassess

Yes

Is the diagnosis established?
No ⟶ Further investigation
Yes ⟶ Management plan

(c) Clinical features of underlying lung disease

Disorder	Chest wall movement	Percussion note	Breath sounds	Added sounds
Consolidation	↓ on affected side	↓ Dull	Bronchial	Coarse crackles
Collapse	↓↓ on affected side	↓ Dull	Absent or bronchial	None
Pleural effusion	↓ on affected side	↓↓ Stony dull	Diminished*	None (±rub)
Pneumothorax	↓↓ on affected side	Normal or hyperresonant	Absent or diminished**	None
Asthma/COPD	↓ on both sides Hyperinflation Accessory muscles	Normal or hyperresonant	Vesicular with prolonged expiration	Expiratory wheeze

 Acute and Critical Care Medicine at a Glance, 2e. By R. Leach. Published 2009 by Blackwell Publishing. ISBN 978-1-4051-6139-8.

In the acutely unwell patient, assessment of deranged physiology and immediate resuscitation precedes diagnostic considerations because incomplete history, cursory examination and limited investigation often preclude classification by primary organ dysfunction. It is this initial diagnostic uncertainty and the need for immediate physiological support that defines acute and critical care medicine.

Recognizing the acutely unwell patient

Early recognition that a patient's condition is deteriorating is essential and should initiate immediate action to correct abnormal physiology and prevent vital organ damage (e.g. brain, kidneys). Clinical severity may be obvious from the end of the bed: as in sudden, catastrophic events (e.g. pulmonary embolism); presentation with established severe illness (e.g. emergency room); or in advanced, previously unrecognized, deterioration on the ward. In these cases, organ damage may have already occurred but immediate action prevents further injury. It is failure to recognize progressive deterioration on the ward, usually manifest as worsening physiological variables, and initiate preventative action, that is a common and unacceptable cause of morbidity and mortality.

Identification of 'at risk' patients (e.g. sepsis, postoperative) allows complications to be anticipated and prevented. 'At-risk' patients must be monitored, deterioration recognized and appropriate action initiated. Simple physiological parameters including temperature, blood pressure (BP), heart rate, respiratory rate, urine output and conscious level correlate with mortality. One, two or three abnormalities correlate with 30-day mortalities of 4.4%, 9.2% and 21.3% respectively. Early warning scoring systems based on these parameters (Fig. a) promote early detection and trigger interventions aimed at preventing unnecessary cardiac arrests and critical care admissions.

Assessment of the acutely ill patient

A normal response to the question 'Are you alright?' indicates that a patient's airway is patent and that they are breathing, conscious and orientated. No response (e.g. coma) or difficulty responding (e.g. breathlessness) suggests serious illness. Immediate assessment and management of these acutely ill patients is summarized in Fig. (b). It aims to ensure patient safety and survival rather than establishing a diagnosis. Assessment starts with detection and simultaneous treatment of life-threatening emergencies. It uses the **ABC system: A** – Airway, **B** – Breathing, **C** – Circulation, in this order, as airways obstruction causes death faster than disordered breathing, which in turn causes death faster than circulatory collapse. Appropriate life-saving procedures or investigations are performed (e.g. airway clearance, tension pneumothorax decompression) during examination (i.e. before the next step). Simple monitors (e.g. saturation, BP) are used to assist assessment when safely possible.

Airway (Chapters 5, 13) Obstruction is a medical emergency and unless rapidly corrected leads to hypoxia, coma and death within minutes. Causes include aspiration (e.g. food, coins, teeth, vomit), laryngeal oedema (e.g. allergy, burns), bronchospasm and pharyngeal obstruction by the tongue when reduced tone causes it to fall backwards in obtunded patients.
• **Complete obstruction** is characterized by absent airflow (feel over the patient's mouth), accessory muscle use, intercostal recession on inspiration, paradoxical abdominal movement and absent breath sounds on chest auscultation.

• **Partial obstruction** reduces airflow despite increased respiratory effort. Breathing is often noisy, with 'stridor' suggesting laryngeal and 'snoring' nasopharyngeal obstruction.
Simple measures correct most airways obstruction. Suction removes blood, vomit and foreign bodies. Pharyngeal obstruction by the tongue (i.e. during coma) can usually be prevented by chin lift manoeuvres or insertion of an oropharyngeal (Guedel) airway (Chapter 13). Occasionally endotracheal intubation or rarely emergency cricothyroidectomy may be required.

Breathing (Chapters 5, 13) The most useful early sign that breathing is compromised is a respiratory rate <8 or >20/minute, whereas central cyanosis is usually a late sign. Examine depth and pattern of breathing, accessory muscle use, abdominal breathing and chest wall expansion. Abnormal expansion, altered percussion note (e.g. hyper-resonance), airways noise (e.g. stridor) and breath sounds may determine the cause of underlying lung disease (Fig. c). Saturation (S_aO_2), measured by pulse oximetry, and inspired oxygen concentration (F_iO_2) should be recorded. Arterial blood gases (ABG) provide information about ventilation as well as oxygenation (i.e. S_aO_2 may be normal but P_aCO_2 high due to poor ventilation). The S_aO_2 should be >90% in all critically ill patients. Respiratory acidosis (pH < 7.3, P_aCO_2 > 6.7 kPa) or hypoxaemia despite high flow oxygen therapy (S_aO_2 < 90%, P_aO_2 < 8 kPa) requires urgent intervention. Treatment depends on cause (e.g. COPD) and is discussed in later chapters.

Circulation (Chapters 5, 7) Assessment includes central and peripheral pulses (i.e. rate, rhythm, equality), BP, peripheral perfusion (e.g. limb temperature), urine output and conscious level. Initially BP is maintained by compensatory mechanisms (e.g. increased peripheral resistance). Cardiac output (CO) has to fall by >20% (i.e. equivalent to 1 L of rapid blood loss) before BP falls. Thready, fast pulses indicate poor CO, whereas bounding pulses suggest sepsis. Capillary refill time is usually <2 seconds and prolongation suggests poor tissue perfusion. Metabolic acidosis (base excess >−4) and raised lactate (>2 mmol/L) on ABG indicate tissue hypoxia. Hypovolaemia should be considered the primary cause of shock, unless there is obvious heart failure (i.e. resuscitate hypotensive patients with cool peripheries and tachycardia with intravenous fluids (Chapters 8, 9)).

Disability Neurological status is rapidly determined by pupil examination and conscious level assessment using simple scales (Fig. a) or the Glasgow Coma Scale (Chapters 3, 53). Hypoglycaemia, ischemia and injury (e.g. unrecognized hip fracture) must be excluded in every patient.

Full patient assessment When stability has been achieved, and assistance summoned, a thorough history and examination is required. The patient's notes, treatment, investigations and charts must be reviewed. Trends in physiological parameters are often more useful than isolated values. If the diagnosis has not been established arrange further investigations as appropriate. Document a clear management plan and communicate this to those involved.

Management of the acutely unwell patient frequently involves several teams (e.g. medicine, surgery, critical care) but should be a 'seamless' process in which co-operation, communication and patient interests are foremost. Treatment should occur in clinical areas where staffing and technical support are matched to patient needs.

2 Admission and ongoing management of the acutely unwell patient

1. Regular review of monitored trends and response to therapy
Followed by clinical examination, reassessment of the care plan (with written instructions) and adjustment of prescribing. Clearly communicate the revised plan to other caregivers

2. Respiratory care
Altered ventilation, poor secretion clearance, impaired muscle function and lung collapse (atelectasis) occur in the supine position. Respiratory care includes assisted coughing, deep breathing and alveolar recruitment techniques (e.g. CPAP), chest percussion, postural drainage, positioning (e.g. sitting up), bronchodilators, tracheal toilette, suctioning and tracheostomy care

3. Cardiovascular care
Prolonged immobility impairs autonomic vasomotor responses to sitting and standing causing profound postural hypotension. Tilt tables may be beneficial prior to mobilization

4. Gastrointestinal (GI) / nutritional care
The supine position predisposes to gastro-oesophageal reflux and aspiration pneumonia. Nursing patients 30° head-up prevents this. Early enteral feeding reduces infection, peptic ulceration and GI bleeding. Immobility is associated with gastric stasis and constipation; gastric stimulants and laxatives are essential

5. Neuromuscular
Immobility (± prolonged neuro-muscular blockade) and sedation promote muscle atrophy, joint contractures and foot drop. Physiotherapy and splints may be required

6. Comfort and reassurance
Anxiety, discomfort and pain must be recognized and relieved with reassurance, physical measures, analgesics and sedatives. In particular, endotracheal or nasogastric tubes, bladder or bowel distention, inflamed line sites, painful joints and urinary catheters often cause discomfort and may be overlooked. Fan use is controversial as dust-borne microorganisms may be disseminated. Visible clocks help patients maintain circadian rhythms (i.e. day/night patterns)

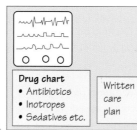

Drug chart
- Antibiotics
- Inotropes
- Sedatives etc.

Written care plan

7. Communication with the patient
Use of amnesic drugs makes repeated explanations and reassurance essential. Assist interaction with appropriate communication aids

8. Typical Doctors daily checklist
F = Feeding
L = Line care
A = Aperients
T = Thrombo-prophylaxis
H = Hydration
U = Ulcer prophylaxis
G = Glucose

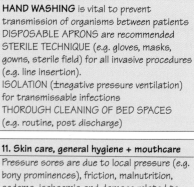

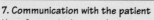

Guiding principles
- Delivery of optimal and appropriate care
- Relief of distress
- Compassion and support
- Dignity
- Information
- Care and support of relatives and care-givers

9. Venous thrombosis prophylaxis
Trauma, sepsis, surgery and immobility predispose to lower limb thrombosis. Mechanical and pharmacological prophylaxis prevent potentially life-threatening pulmonary embolism

10. Infection Control
HAND WASHING is vital to prevent transmission of organisms between patients DISPOSABLE APRONS are recommended STERILE TECHNIQUE (e.g. gloves, masks, gowns, sterile field) for all invasive procedures (e.g. line insertion). ISOLATION (±negative pressure ventilation) for transmissable infections THOROUGH CLEANING OF BED SPACES (e.g. routine, post discharge)

11. Skin care, general hygiene + mouthcare
Pressure sores are due to local pressure (e.g. bony prominences), friction, malnutrition, oedema, ischaemia and damage related to moist or soiled skin. Turn patients every two hours and protect susceptible areas. Special beds relieve pressure and assist turning. Mouthcare and general hygiene are essential

12. Fluid, electrolyte and glucose balance
Regularly assess fluid + electrolyte balance Insulin resistance + hyperglycaemia are common but maintaining normoglycaemia improves outcome

13. Dressing and wound care
Replace wound dressings as necessary. Change arterial and central venous catheter dressings every 48–72h

14. Line care
Lines must be inspected daily. Peripheral lines should be changed every 72–96hrs. Central and arterial lines are not changed routinely but risk infection after >5 days

15. Bladder care
Urinary catheters can cause painful urethral ulcers and must be stabilised. Early removal reduces urinary tract infections

16. Visiting hours
Opinions differ with regard to relatives visiting hours. Some units restrict visits (e.g. 2 periods/day), others have almost unrestricted hours

17. Communication with relatives
Family members receive information from many caregivers with different perspectives and knowledge. Critical care-teams must aim to be consistent in their assessments and honest about uncertainties. One or two physicians should act as primary contacts. All conversations must be documented. Compassionate care of relatives is always appreciated, avoids anger and is one of the best indicators of good care

 Acute and Critical Care Medicine at a Glance, 2e. By R. Leach. Published 2009 by Blackwell Publishing. ISBN 978-1-4051-6139-8.

Organization

Acute and critical care wards provide monitoring and treatment for patients with potentially reversible, life-threatening conditions that is not available on general wards. Patients should be managed and moved between areas where staffing and technical support match their severity of illness and clinical needs. Five types of ward area are described: (a) level 3: intensive care units (ICU); (b) level 2: medical/surgical high dependency units (HDU), post-operative recovery areas, emergency resuscitation rooms; (c) level 1: acute admission wards, coronary care units; (d) general wards (e) self-care wards.

Acute and critical care medicine (ACCM) encompasses the initial resuscitation, monitoring, investigation and treatment of acutely unwell or critically ill patients in levels 1–3 wards. All these patients require a high degree of monitoring and nursing support. Level 3 patients often require mechanical ventilation or have multiorgan failure. Level 2 patients may need invasive monitoring (i.e. arterial line), non-invasive ventilation, inotropic support or renal replacement therapy. Level 1 patients usually require non-invasive monitoring (e.g. ECG, saturation, BP) and close observation. There is considerable overlap between level 1 and 2 patients. Provision of level 2 and 3 care varies from ~2–5% of hospital beds in the UK to >5–10% in the USA.

Admission and discharge guidelines

Aggressive hospital treatment may be inappropriate in advanced disease and patients must be allocated to a ward appropriate to their needs and prognosis. Resuscitation status should always be documented. Admission and discharge guidelines for ICU and HDU facilitate appropriate use of resources and prevent unnecessary suffering in patients who have no prospect of recovery. Factors determining ICU/HDU admission include the primary diagnosis, severity, likely success of treatment, co-morbid illness, life expectancy, potential quality of life post-discharge and patient's (relative's) wishes. Age alone should not be a contraindication to admission and every case must be judged on its merit. If there is uncertainty the patient should be given the benefit of the doubt and active treatment continued until further information is available.

Appropriate discharge occurs when patients are physiologically stable and independent of monitoring and support. Out of hours and weekend discharges should be avoided and a detailed handover is essential. In patients with no realistic hope of recovery, and after family consultation, withdrawal of therapy may be appropriate. When feasible, organ donation should be tactfully discussed. Management must always remain positive to ensure death with dignity (Chapter 24).

General supportive care

Optimal care is delivered by a multi-skilled team of doctors, nurses, physiotherapists, technicians and other care-givers. The Figure illustrates important aspects of general management. Prolonged bed rest predisposes to respiratory (e.g. atelectasis), cardiovascular (e.g. autonomic failure), neurological (e.g. muscle wasting) and endocrine (e.g. glucose intolerance) problems, fluid and electrolyte imbalance (e.g. Na^+, K^+, Ca^{2+} depletion), constipation, infection, venous thrombosis and pressure sores. The importance of skilled nursing in the management of these patients cannot be over-emphasized. Assessment, continuous monitoring and intervention, drug administration, comfort (e.g. analgesia, toilette), reassurance, psychological support, assistance with communication, advocacy, skin care, positioning (e.g. to prevent aspiration, atelectasis, pressure sores), feeding and early detection of clinical complications (e.g. line infection) are all vital nursing roles which have a profound effect on outcome. Nurses also provide essential support for relatives, doctors, physiotherapists and other care-givers (e.g. technicians, radiologists).

Severity of Illness Scoring Systems (SISS)

SISS predict outcome and evaluate care in ICU/HDU. Two have been validated and are widely used:

- **APACHE II** (Acute Physiology and Chronic Health Evaluation): aims to measure case-mix and predict outcome in ICU patients *as a group*. It should not be used to predict individual outcome. Scoring is based on the primary disease process, physiological reserve including age and chronic health history (e.g. chronic liver, cardiovascular, respiratory, renal and immune conditions) and the severity of illness determined from the worst value in the first 24 hours of 12 acute physiological variables including rectal temperature, mean blood pressure (BP), heart rate, respiratory rate (RR), arterial P_aO_2 and pH, serum sodium, potassium and creatinine, haemocrit, white cell count and Glasgow Coma Score (GCS; Chapter 53). Predicted mortality, by diagnosis, has been calculated from large databases, which allows individual units to evaluate their performance against reference ICUs by calculating standard mortality ratio (SMR = observed mortality ÷ predicted mortality) for each diagnostic group. A high SMR (>1.5) should prompt investigation and management changes for specific conditions.
- **SAPS** (Simplified Acute Physiology Score): is similar to APACHE II with equivalent accuracy.

Pathology Specific Scoring Systems (PSSS) are often used in ACCM.

- **Trauma Score (TS)**: assesses triage status based on RR, respiratory effort, systolic BP, capillary refill and GCS. Survival is related to TS in blunt and penetrating injuries. A high score indicates the need for transfer to a trauma centre. **Revised TS:** uses only GCS, RR and systolic BP. Prognostic reliability is improved but it is less suitable for triage.
- **Abbreviated Injury Scale:** assesses multiple injuries and correlates with morbidity and mortality.
- **Other PSSS:** include the paediatric trauma score, neonatal Apgar score and GCS (Chapter 53).

Cost of ACCM

Measuring costs is complex. In ICU/HDU the most widely used system is the **Therapeutic Intervention Scoring System** (TISS), which scores the overall requirements for care, by measuring nursing activity and interventions. TISS correlates well with staff, equipment and drug costs and can also be used as an index of nurse dependency. The majority (>50%) of ICU expenditure is on labour costs, in particular constant bedside nursing. Drugs, imaging, laboratory tests and supplies account for ~40% of spending. Consequently, cost saving usually requires personnel reductions and risks lowering quality of care. Current estimates of daily ('basic') ICU costs vary from £800 to £1600 in the UK. HDU costs are ~50% and general ward care ~20% of ICU costs. In the USA ~14% of gross domestic product (GDP) is spent on healthcare with ICU/HDU costs ~7% of total expenditure. In comparison, the UK spends ~9% of GDP, with ~2–5% of total expenditure on HDU/ICU provision.

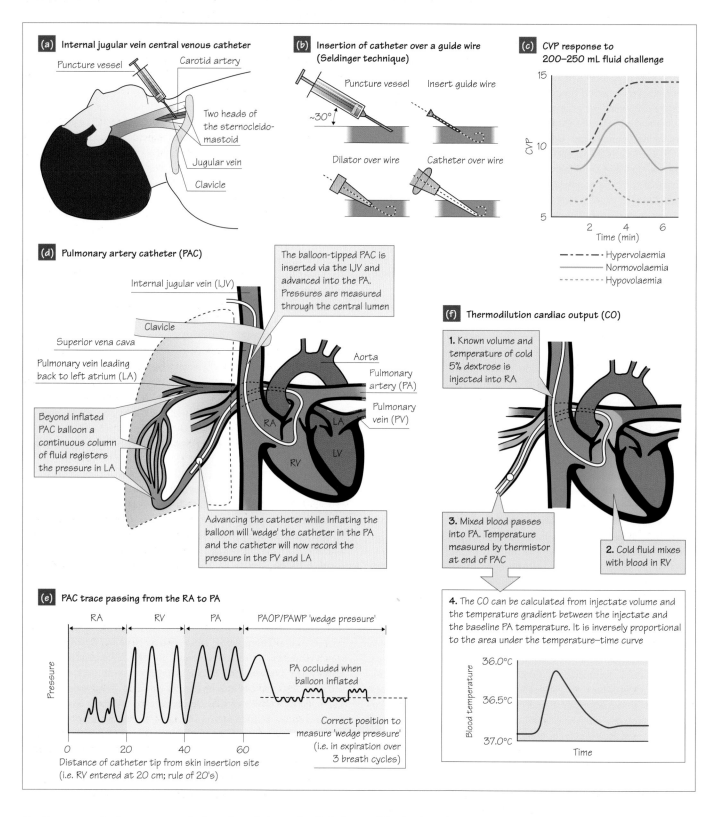

(a) Internal jugular vein central venous catheter

Puncture vessel
Carotid artery
Two heads of the sternocleido-mastoid
Jugular vein
Clavicle

(b) Insertion of catheter over a guide wire (Seldinger technique)

Puncture vessel
Insert guide wire
~30°
Dilator over wire
Catheter over wire

(c) CVP response to 200–250 mL fluid challenge

CVP

Time (min)

– · – · – Hypervolaemia
—— Normovolaemia
- - - - - Hypovolaemia

(d) Pulmonary artery catheter (PAC)

The balloon-tipped PAC is inserted via the IJV and advanced into the PA. Pressures are measured through the central lumen

Internal jugular vein (IJV)
Clavicle
Superior vena cava
Pulmonary vein leading back to left atrium (LA)
Beyond inflated PAC balloon a continuous column of fluid registers the pressure in LA

Aorta
Pulmonary artery (PA)
Pulmonary vein (PV)

RA
LA
LV
RV

Advancing the catheter while inflating the balloon will 'wedge' the catheter in the PA and the catheter will now record the pressure in the PV and LA

(f) Thermodilution cardiac output (CO)

1. Known volume and temperature of cold 5% dextrose is injected into RA

3. Mixed blood passes into PA. Temperature measured by thermistor at end of PAC

2. Cold fluid mixes with blood in RV

(e) PAC trace passing from the RA to PA

RA   RV   PA   PAOP/PAWP 'wedge pressure'

Pressure

PA occluded when balloon inflated

Correct position to measure 'wedge pressure' (i.e. in expiration over 3 breath cycles)

0   20   40   60
Distance of catheter tip from skin insertion site (i.e. RV entered at 20 cm; rule of 20's)

4. The CO can be calculated from injectate volume and the temperature gradient between the injectate and the baseline PA temperature. It is inversely proportional to the area under the temperature–time curve

36.0°C
36.5°C
37.0°C
Blood temperature
Time

Continuous monitoring ensures early detection of change in clinical parameters and accurate assessment of progress and response to therapy. The following principles apply:

- **Monitoring aids assessment** but regular clinical examination is essential. Simple physical signs like appearance (e.g. pallor), peripheral perfusion and conscious level are as important as parameters displayed on a monitor. When clinical signs and monitored parameters disagree, *assume that clinical assessment is correct*, until potential errors from monitored variables have been excluded (e.g. blocked CVP lines, incorrect calibration). **Trends:** are generally more important than single readings.

• **Use non-invasive techniques whenever possible** as invasive monitoring is associated with risks (e.g. line infection) and complications (e.g. pneumothorax). Review 'invasive techniques' regularly and replace as soon as possible. **Alarms** are a crucial safety feature (e.g. ventilator disconnection). They are set to physiological safe limits and should never be disconnected.

Haemodynamic monitoring

Blood pressure (BP) is often measured intermittently using an automated sphygmomanometer. In severely ill patients continuous intra-arterial monitoring is preferred. It should be appreciated that BP does not reflect cardiac output (CO). Thus, BP can be normal/high but CO low if peripheral vasoconstriction raises systemic vascular resistance (SVR). Conversely, vasodilated, 'septic' patients with low SVR may be hypotensive despite a high CO (Chapters 7, 22).

Central venous pressure (CVP) reflects right atrial pressure (RAP) and is measured using internal jugular (Figs a and b) or subclavian vein catheters. It is a useful means of assessing circulating blood volume and determining the rate at which fluid should be administered. However, increased venous tone can act to maintain CVP and mask volume depletion during hypovolaemia or haemorrhage. In this situation, CVP is not as important as **the response to a fluid challenge** (Fig. c). A high CVP indicates 'fluid overload', impaired myocardial contractility or high right ventricular afterload. Management depends on the cause (Chapters 6, 7, 28).

Pulmonary artery wedge/occlusion pressure (PAWP/PAOP) reflects left atrial pressure (LAP). Normally LAP is ~5–7 mmHg greater than RAP, but in ischaemic heart disease (IHD) or severe illness there is often 'disparity' between left and right ventricular function. Thus, LAP may be high despite a low RAP in left ventricular (LV) dysfunction and a small increase in RAP can cause a large increase in LAP which may precipitate pulmonary oedema (Chapter 28). In these patients, PAWP (i.e. LAP) is monitored using a pulmonary artery (PA) catheter (Figs d and e). PAWP is normally 6–12 mmHg, but may be >25–35 mmHg in LV failure (LVF). Provided the pulmonary capillary membranes are intact (i.e. not 'leaky'), a PAWP of ~15–20 mmHg ensures good LV filling and optimal function without risking pulmonary oedema. PA catheters also measure CO, mixed venous saturation and right ventricular ejection fraction (see below).

Cardiac output Thermodilution techniques for CO measurement (Fig. f; e.g. PA catheter, pulsion continuous cardiac output monitor (PiCCO)) are considered the 'gold standard', but error is at least 10%. Non- (or less) invasive techniques of CO monitoring utilize dye/lithium dilution, trans-oesophageal doppler ultrasonography, echocardiography or impedance methods.

Electrocardiogram (ECG) Rate and rhythm are displayed by standard single lead ECG monitors but ST segment changes can be monitored in patients with IHD.

Respiratory monitoring

Arterial blood gases monitor P_aO_2, P_aCO_2 and acid–base balance. Measurement aids diagnosis and allows adjustment of ventilation to achieve optimum gas exchange (Chapters 11, 16, 18).

Arterial oxygen saturation (S_aO_2) is determined by spectrophotometric analysis of the ratio of saturated to desaturated haemoglobin. Oxygenation is usually adequate if S_aO_2 is >90%. Finger and earlobe probes may be unreliable if peripheral perfusion is poor.

Mixed venous oxygen saturation (S_vO_2) is measured using fibreoptic PA catheters or PA/right atrial blood sampling and co-oximetry. It is normally >65–70%. A low S_vO_2 (<55–60%) may indicate inadequate tissue O_2 delivery even if S_aO_2 or P_aO_2 are normal (e.g. anaemia).

Lung function Alveolar–arterial Po_2 gradient and P_aO_2/F_iO_2 ratio measure gas exchange. Arterial and end-tidal CO_2 (see below) reflect alveolar ventilation (V_A). Thus, P_aCO_2 is inversely proportional to V_A ($P_aCO_2 \propto 1/V_A$). Peak expiratory flow rate (PEFR) and spirometry (e.g. FEV_1, VC) are useful for monitoring airways obstruction and lung volumes in self-ventilating patients (Chapters 33, 34). In intubated patients maximum inspiratory pressure (MIP) is normally ~100 cmH$_2$O. A MIP <25 cmH$_2$O indicates muscle weakness and that self-ventilation following extubation is unlikely.

Lung compliance (LC) reflects lung 'stiffness' or ease of inflation and is reduced in damaged lungs. It is calculated by dividing tidal ventilation (Tv; ml) by the pressure (cm/H$_2$O) required to achieve Tv. High airways pressures during ventilation indicate reduced LC.

Capnography Inspired air contains virtually no CO_2. At the end of expiration, end-tidal CO_2 concentration mirrors arterial P_aCO_2 and reflects V_A provided the distribution of ventilation is uniform.

Organ and tissue oxygenation

Global measures (e.g. S_vO_2, lactate) reflect total tissue perfusion but may be normal despite severe regional perfusion abnormalities. Raised serial lactate levels and metabolic acidosis suggest anaerobic metabolism and inadequate tissue oxygenation; although lactate may increase in the absence of hypoxia (e.g. liver failure). An S_vO_2 < 55% indicates global tissue hypoxia.

Organ specific measures include:
• **Urine flow**, which is a sensitive measure of renal perfusion (Chapter 38) provided that the kidneys are not damaged (e.g. acute tubular necrosis) or affected by drugs (e.g. diuretics). Hourly urine output is normally ~1 ml/kg.
• **Core-peripheral temperature**, the gradient between peripheral (e.g. skin temperature over the dorsum of the foot) and core temperature (e.g. rectal) is often used as an index of peripheral perfusion.
• **Gastric tonometry** which is occasionally used to detect shock-induced splanchnic ischaemia by measuring gastric luminal Pco_2 and subsequently deriving mucosal pH.
• **Neurological monitoring,** which utilizes the Glasgow Coma Score, intracranial pressure measurement and jugular venous bulb saturation (Chapter 53).

4 Oxygen transport

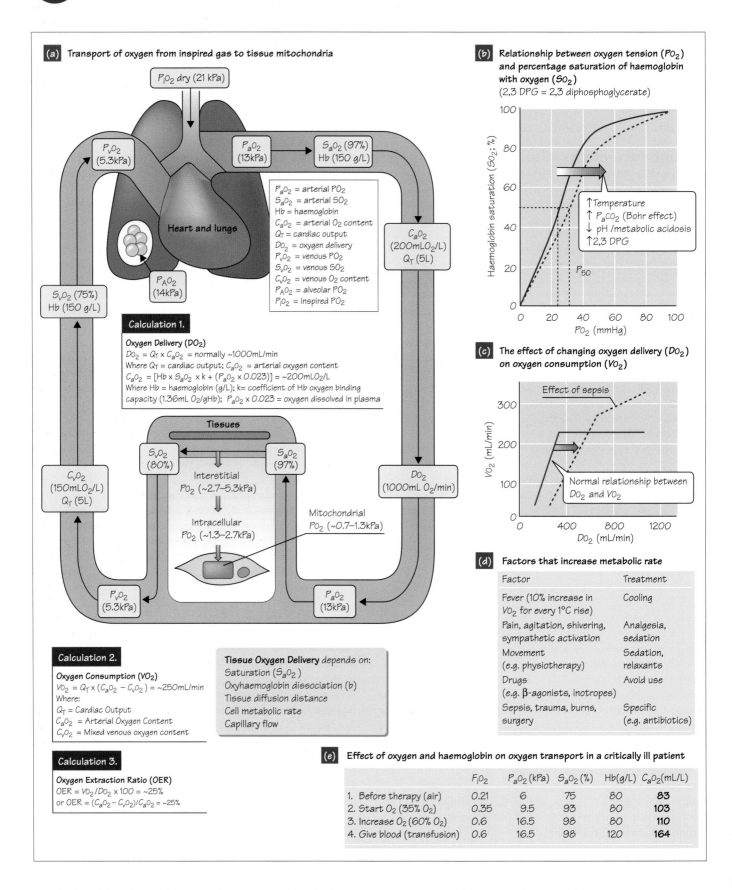

(a) Transport of oxygen from inspired gas to tissue mitochondria

P_iO_2 dry (21 kPa)

P_vO_2 (5.3kPa)

P_aO_2 (13kPa)

S_aO_2 (97%) Hb (150 g/L)

Heart and lungs

P_AO_2 (14kPa)

S_vO_2 (75%) Hb (150 g/L)

C_aO_2 (200mLO_2/L) Q_T (5L)

P_aO_2 = arterial PO_2
S_aO_2 = arterial SO_2
Hb = haemoglobin
C_aO_2 = arterial O_2 content
Q_T = cardiac output
DO_2 = oxygen delivery
P_vO_2 = venous PO_2
S_vO_2 = venous SO_2
C_vO_2 = venous O_2 content
P_AO_2 = alveolar PO_2
P_iO_2 = inspired PO_2

Calculation 1.

Oxygen Delivery (DO_2)
$DO_2 = Q_T \times C_aO_2$ = normally ~1000mL/min
Where Q_T = cardiac output; C_aO_2 = arterial oxygen content
$C_aO_2 = [Hb \times S_aO_2 \times k + (P_aO_2 \times 0.023)]$ = ~200mLO_2/L
Where Hb = haemoglobin (g/L); k= coefficient of Hb oxygen binding capacity (1.36mL O_2/gHb); $P_aO_2 \times 0.023$ = oxygen dissolved in plasma

Tissues

S_vO_2 (80%)
S_aO_2 (97%)

Interstitial PO_2 (~2.7–5.3kPa)

Intracellular PO_2 (~1.3–2.7kPa)

Mitochondrial PO_2 (~0.7–1.3kPa)

C_vO_2 (150mLO_2/L) Q_T (5L)

DO_2 (1000mL O_2/min)

P_vO_2 (5.3kPa)
P_aO_2 (13kPa)

Calculation 2.

Oxygen Consumption (VO_2)
$VO_2 = Q_T \times (C_aO_2 - C_vO_2)$ = ~250mL/min
Where:
Q_T = Cardiac Output
C_aO_2 = Arterial Oxygen Content
C_vO_2 = Mixed venous oxygen content

Tissue Oxygen Delivery depends on:
Saturation (S_aO_2)
Oxyhaemoglobin dissociation (b)
Tissue diffusion distance
Cell metabolic rate
Capillary flow

Calculation 3.

Oxygen Extraction Ratio (OER)
OER = $VO_2/DO_2 \times 100$ = ~25%
or OER = $(C_aO_2 - C_vO_2)/C_aO_2$ = ~25%

(b) Relationship between oxygen tension (PO_2) and percentage saturation of haemoglobin with oxygen (SO_2)
(2,3 DPG = 2,3 diphosphoglycerate)

Haemoglobin saturation (SO_2; %) vs *PO_2 (mmHg)*

↑Temperature
↑ P_aCO_2 (Bohr effect)
↓ pH /metabolic acidosis
↑2,3 DPG

P_{50}

(c) The effect of changing oxygen delivery (DO_2) on oxygen consumption (VO_2)

VO_2 (mL/min) vs *DO_2 (mL/min)*

Effect of sepsis

Normal relationship between DO_2 and VO_2

(d) Factors that increase metabolic rate

Factor	Treatment
Fever (10% increase in VO_2 for every 1°C rise)	Cooling
Pain, agitation, shivering, sympathetic activation	Analgesia, sedation
Movement (e.g. physiotherapy)	Sedation, relaxants
Drugs (e.g. β-agonists, inotropes)	Avoid use
Sepsis, trauma, burns, surgery	Specific (e.g. antibiotics)

(e) Effect of oxygen and haemoglobin on oxygen transport in a critically ill patient

	F_iO_2	P_aO_2 (kPa)	S_aO_2 (%)	Hb(g/L)	C_aO_2(mL/L)
1. Before therapy (air)	0.21	6	75	80	**83**
2. Start O_2 (35% O_2)	0.35	9.5	93	80	**103**
3. Increase O_2 (60% O_2)	0.6	16.5	98	80	**110**
4. Give blood (transfusion)	0.6	16.5	98	120	**164**

 Acute and Critical Care Medicine at a Glance, 2e. By R. Leach. Published 2009 by Blackwell Publishing. ISBN 978-1-4051-6139-8.

The major function of the heart, lungs and circulation is to deliver oxygen and other nutrients to body tissues and remove carbon dioxide and other waste products of metabolism. Oxygen transport is determined by:

1 Oxygen uptake by blood in the lung, which depends on blood haemoglobin (Hb) content, alveolar oxygen (P_AO_2), oxygen-haemoglobin uptake and the efficiency of lung gas exchange. It is measured as the arterial oxygen content (C_aO_2);

2 Convective oxygen transport from the lung to the tissues, which is determined (after oxygen loading in the lungs) by the magnitude and regional distribution of cardiac output (Q_T);

3 Diffusion of oxygen from the capillary blood to tissue mitochondria, governed by the capillary–mitochondrial P_O_2 gradient, capillary surface area and diffusion distance.

Oxygen delivery

Figure (a) illustrates the transport of oxygen from inspired air to tissue mitochondria.

• **Global oxygen delivery (D_O_2)** is determined from Q_T and C_aO_2 (Fig. a; Calculation 1). Most oxygen carried in blood is attached to Hb. Only a small amount is dissolved in plasma. Arterial oxygen saturation (S_aO_2) and Hb concentration are the major determinants of C_aO_2. Figure (e) illustrates the relative effects of increasing oxygen and Hb on D_O_2. Although transfusion rapidly increases D_O_2, the optimum Hb level in critically illness is ~100 g/l (10 g/dl) and is a balance between optimizing C_aO_2 and avoiding microcirculatory problem due to viscosity. Fluid administration and inotropes are used to increase Q_T and D_O_2 (Chapter 8). However, increasing D_O_2 is of limited benefit in organ ischaemia due to arterial obstruction (e.g. embolus, thrombus), whereas removal of the obstruction (e.g. embolectomy, thrombolysis) may be life-saving.

• **Tissue oxygen delivery** requires appropriate regional and microcirculatory distribution of Q_T, which is determined by a complex interaction of endothelial, receptor, metabolic and pharmacological factors. During stress or critical illness, blood flow is directed to vital organs (e.g. brain) and away from less-essential tissue beds (e.g. splanchnic, skin) which are damaged if this effect persists. For example, prolonged splanchnic ischaemia compromises bowel wall integrity causing translocation of bacteria into the circulation. Therapeutically, receptor properties of certain vasoactive agents can be used to improve individual organ oxygen delivery (i.e. dopexamine increases splanchnic blood flow).

• **Tissue factors** influence cellular oxygen status. Oxygen diffuses from the capillary to the cell and is dependent on capillary blood flow and surface area (i.e. reduced by capillary thrombosis), oxygen gradient and diffusion distance. However, increasing D_O_2 cannot compensate for cellular metabolic failure (i.e. mitochondrial dysfunction during sepsis) and some tissues (e.g. brain, kidney) are more susceptible to, and are rapidly damaged by, sustained hypoxia.

The oxyhaemoglobin dissociation curve

Figure (b) illustrates the relationship between the partial pressure of oxygen (P_O_2) in the blood and haemoglobin saturation (S_O_2). The position of the dissociation curve is affected by temperature, pH, P_ACO_2 and 2,3diphosphoglycerate (DPG) and is expressed as the P_O_2 at which haemoglobin is 50% saturated (P_{50}). This is normally 3.5 kPa (26 mmHg). Left or right shifts of the curve will alter uptake and release of oxygen by the Hb molecule. If the curve moves to the right, the S_aO_2 will be lower for a given P_O_2 (i.e. less oxygen is taken up in the lungs but more is released in the tissues). Thus, as capillary P_aCO_2 increases (i.e. rightward shift of the curve), oxygen is released from Hb, a phenomenon known as the Bohr effect.

Oxygen consumption

• **Global oxygen consumption (V_O_2)** is the sum of the oxygen consumed by individual organs and tissues and is ~250 ml/min for a 70-kg adult. It can be calculated from Q_T, S_aO_2 and S_vO_2 (Fig. a; Calculation 2) or from the inspired and mixed expired oxygen and CO_2 concentrations. The oxygen extraction ratio (OER; Fig. a; Calculation 3) determines the amount of oxygen used (V_O_2) as a percentage of that delivered (D_O_2) and is normally ~25%.

• **Metabolic rate** is increased by the factors listed in Fig. (d). It should be recognized that drugs used to increase D_O_2 (e.g. inotropes) may also increase V_O_2. Simple measures including cooling, analgesia, sedation, prevention of shivering and muscle relaxation substantially reduce V_O_2 and subsequent D_O_2 requirements

Relationship between oxygen delivery (D_O_2) and oxygen consumption (V_O_2)

Figure (c) illustrates the effect of changing D_O_2 on V_O_2 in normal and septic patients. Normally oxygen extraction from capillary blood increases as tissue V_O_2 rises or blood supply decreases. The maximum OER is about 70%. Any further increase in tissue V_O_2 or fall in oxygen supply will result in hypoxia, anaerobic metabolism and lactic acid production. In this situation D_O_2 must be improved by increasing oxygenated blood flow or relieving obstruction (e.g. thrombolysis in myocardial infarction).

In sepsis, cellular dysfunction reduces the ability of tissues to extract oxygen. This alters the relationship between D_O_2 and V_O_2 (Fig. c). In particular, V_O_2 continues to increase even at 'supranormal' levels of D_O_2. This observation encouraged the use of aggressive fluid loading and inotropic support to achieve a high D_O_2 (>600 ml/min/m²), in the belief that this strategy, sometimes termed **goal-directed therapy**, would relieve hypoxia and prevent tissue damage. However, this is not the case; microcirculatory impairment (i.e. capillary thrombi), failure of regional distribution and metabolic dysfunction are more likely than inadequate D_O_2 to cause cellular toxicity in late sepsis.

Venous blood saturation varies according to the metabolic requirements of each tissue (i.e. hepatic 30–40%, renal ~80%). In the pulmonary artery, the **mixed venous oxygen saturation** ($S_vO_2 > 65$–70%) represents oxygen not used in the tissues ($D_O_2 - V_O_2$). It is influenced by both D_O_2 and V_O_2, and provided regional blood flow and cellular oxygen utilization are normal, reflects whether global D_O_2 adequately matches global V_O_2 (Chapter 3).

5 Cardiopulmonary resuscitation

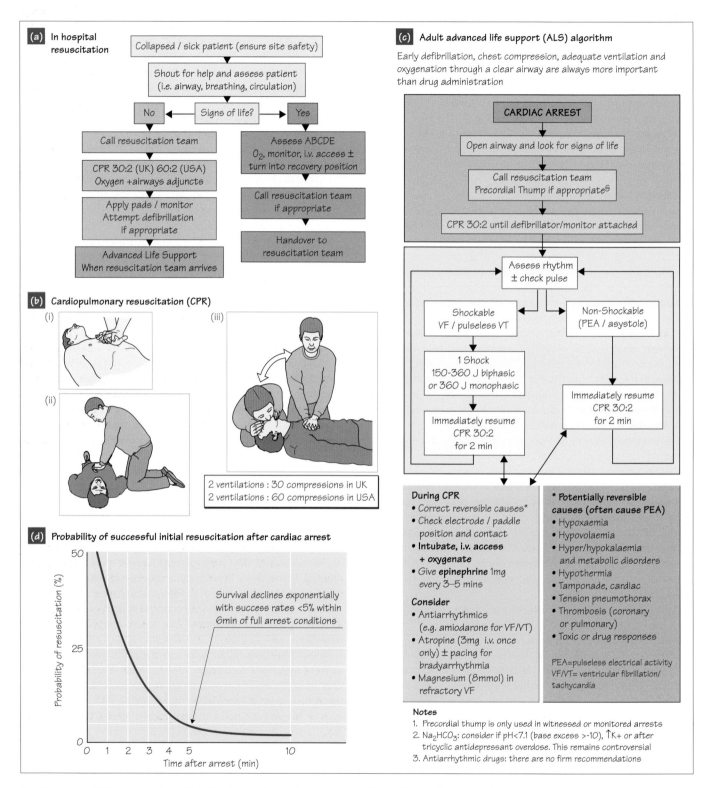

(a) In hospital resuscitation

Collapsed / sick patient (ensure site safety)

Shout for help and assess patient (i.e. airway, breathing, circulation)

Signs of life?

No → Call resuscitation team → CPR 30:2 (UK) 60:2 (USA) Oxygen +airways adjuncts → Apply pads / monitor Attempt defibrillation if appropriate → Advanced Life Support When resuscitation team arrives

Yes → Assess ABCDE O₂, monitor, i.v. access ± turn into recovery position → Call resuscitation team if appropriate → Handover to resuscitation team

(b) Cardiopulmonary resuscitation (CPR)

(i) (ii) (iii)

2 ventilations : 30 compressions in UK
2 ventilations : 60 compressions in USA

(d) Probability of successful initial resuscitation after cardiac arrest

Survival declines exponentially with success rates <5% within 6min of full arrest conditions

(Graph: Probability of resuscitation (%) vs Time after arrest (min), axis 0–50% and 0–10 min)

(c) Adult advanced life support (ALS) algorithm

Early defibrillation, chest compression, adequate ventilation and oxygenation through a clear airway are always more important than drug administration

CARDIAC ARREST

Open airway and look for signs of life

Call resuscitation team Precordial Thump if appropriate§

CPR 30:2 until defibrillator/monitor attached

Assess rhythm ± check pulse

Shockable VF / pulseless VT → 1 Shock 150-360 J biphasic or 360 J monophasic → Immediately resume CPR 30:2 for 2 min

Non-Shockable (PEA / asystole) → Immediately resume CPR 30:2 for 2 min

During CPR
- Correct reversible causes*
- Check electrode / paddle position and contact
- **Intubate, i.v. access + oxygenate**
- Give **epinephrine** 1mg every 3–5 mins

Consider
- Antiarrhythmics (e.g. amiodarone for VF/VT)
- Atropine (3mg i.v. once only) ± pacing for bradyarrhythmia
- Magnesium (8mmol) in refractory VF

* Potentially reversible causes (often cause PEA)
- Hypoxaemia
- Hypovolaemia
- Hyper/hypokalaemia and metabolic disorders
- Hypothermia
- Tamponade, cardiac
- Tension pneumothorax
- Thrombosis (coronary or pulmonary)
- Toxic or drug responses

PEA=pulseless electrical activity
VF/VT= ventricular fibrillation/tachycardia

Notes
1. Precordial thump is only used in witnessed or monitored arrests
2. Na₂HCO₃: consider if pH<7.1 (base excess >-10), ↑K+ or after tricyclic antidepressant overdose. This remains controversial
3. Antiarrhythmic drugs: there are no firm recommendations

Cardiac arrest (CA) occurs when clinically detectable cardiac output ceases. The main cause (~80%) is ischaemic heart disease (IHD). Most patients die and even in successfully resuscitated patients mortality is high (~70%). Overall survival to hospital discharge is ~10% but higher (~20%) in those with ventricular fibrillation or tachycardia (VF/VT).

Out-of-hospital arrests (OHA) are usually due to IHD-induced VF (~80%). Electrical defibrillation is the only effective treatment for VF. Delay reduces the chance of successful defibrillation by ~7–10% per minute. **In-hospital arrests** (IHA) are mainly due to pulseless electrical activity (PEA) or asystole (~60–70%) and the outcome is very poor. Progressive physiological deterioration often precedes IHA and about half present with hypoxaemic bradycardia due to a respiratory cause (e.g. pulmonary embolism (PE)). Early recognition of patients at risk may prevent CA and has led to the development of 'Patient at Risk' and 'Medical Emergency' Teams (MET).

Cardiopulmonary resuscitation

Effective cardiopulmonary resuscitation (CPR) maintains oxygen supply to vital organs (e.g. brain) whilst awaiting definitive medical treatment. It is started as soon as CA is established, interruptions minimized and defibrillation attempted as soon as possible for VF/VT.

Figure (a) shows the IHA management algorithm. Immediately summon help (i.e. CA or MET team at IHA, emergency medical services (EMS) at OHA) and exclude potential danger at the scene. Initial assessment of a collapsed or sick patient (Chapter 1) should include airway, breathing, circulation, neurological disability and exposure of the patient (**ABCDE**). Turn the patient onto their back. Open the airway using head tilt and chin lift, except after potential cervical injuries, when a 'jaw-thrust' manoeuvre is employed (Chapter 13). Clear the oropharynx of foreign bodies and vomitus. Then, whilst keeping the airway open, 'look, listen and feel' for breathing (i.e. place your cheek and ear over the patient's nose/mouth and observe chest movement) for ≤10 seconds. At the same time feel for the carotid pulse.

Start CPR (Fig. b) if no signs of life are detected (i.e. movement, pulse, breathing). Deliver chest compressions and lung ventilation in a ratio of 30:2 (UK) or 60:2 (USA).
• **Chest compressions** are performed at a rate of ~100/min. The correct hand position is found by placing the heel of one hand on the centre of the chest with the other hand on top. The compression depth is 4–5 cm and the chest should be allowed to recoil completely after each compression.
• **Ventilation** is performed with whatever equipment is available. A 'bag-valve mask' and oropharyngeal airway should be available during IHA (Chapter 13). Endotracheal intubation (ETI) should only be performed by individuals with the requisite training (Chapter 15). Following ETI, chest compressions and ventilation continue uninterrupted (i.e. no break for ventilation) at a breath rate of 10/min and tidal volume of ~500 ml. Avoid hyperventilation as this reduces cerebral blood flow. In OHA chest compressions continue uninterrupted until the EMS arrive unless a pocket mask is available or 'mouth-to-mouth' ventilation (M-MV) is feasible/acceptable. To perform M-MV pinch the nose whilst performing 'chin lift', maintain slight neck extension by gentle pressure on the forehead, take a breath and place your lips around the patient's mouth creating an airtight seal. Breath out slowly observing chest movement. Allow sufficient time for deflation between breaths.

Advanced life support

Figure (c) illustrates the adult advanced life support (ALS) algorithm. It is divided into management of '**shockable**' (VF/VT) and '**non-shockable**' (non VF/VT, PEA, asystolic) rhythms. Only CPR and defibrillation improve outcome. Therefore, interruptions to CPR should be minimal (i.e. for intubation, pulse checks) and defibrillation is attempted as soon as possible in VF/VT. A **precordial thump**, which generates a small electrical shock, is given in witnessed and monitored VF/VT arrests if a defibrillator is not immediately available. Central venous access is best but peripherally injected drugs can be flushed with saline. If venous access is impossible, some drugs (e.g. epinephrine (adrenaline), atropine) can be administered endobronchially using double doses. During CPR administer:
• **Epinephrine** 1 mg every 3–5 min (i.e. every second loop of the algorithm).
• **Atropine** 3 mg once in asystole or PEA with a heart rate <60/min.
• **Amiodarone** after a third unsuccessful defibrillation in VF/VT.
ETI is the ideal means of securing the airway during CPR but prehospital ETI by unskilled personnel has no benefit and may cause harm. Supraglottic airway devices (e.g. laryngeal mask airway) are a useful alternative for those unskilled in ETI. **Reversible causes** (Fig. c) must be detected and treated, including hypovolaemia, haemorrhage, PE, electrolyte disturbance, tension pneumothorax and cardiac tamponade.

Post-resuscitation care

Immediate post-CPR care involves stabilization, monitoring, reassessment (i.e. ABCDE) and transfer to a critical care area. Circulatory support is often required (e.g. fluids ± inotropes) and a clear airway (±adequate ventilation) prevents hypoxia and hypercapnia which may exacerbate brain injury and predispose to further CAs. Neurological assessment is necessary and sedation may be required to facilitate ongoing ventilation. Therapeutic mild hypothermia (32–34 °C) for 12–24 hours is recommended in comatose patients following out-of-hospital VF/VT arrests (± consider after other forms of CA). **Investigations** include routine blood tests, arterial blood gases, cardiac enzymes and ECG to exclude myocardial ischaemia, and chest radiograph (CXR) to exclude pneumothorax and check line (± endotracheal tube) position. Echocardiography is often helpful.

Prognosis

Poor prognostic factors include initial rhythms of asystole/PEA, CA location, delayed CPR (i.e. >5 min) or defibrillation, myoclonic jerks, poor preceding health, peri-arrest hyperglycaemia, sepsis or renal injury and prolonged CPR. Age alone does not predict outcome. Most successful CPR requires <2–3 min; after >6 min success rates are <5% (Fig. d) with the exceptions of hypothermia and near-drowning when survival may follow prolonged CPR. Absence of pupillary reflexes or motor responses to pain after 3 days predicts poor outcome with high specificity.

Neurological failure causes ~50% of deaths in CPR survivors. A third of comatose survivors have seizure activity in the first 24 hours and permanent neurological damage affects ~50% of conscious survivors. Recovery of consciousness is greatest in the first 24 hours and then declines exponentially.

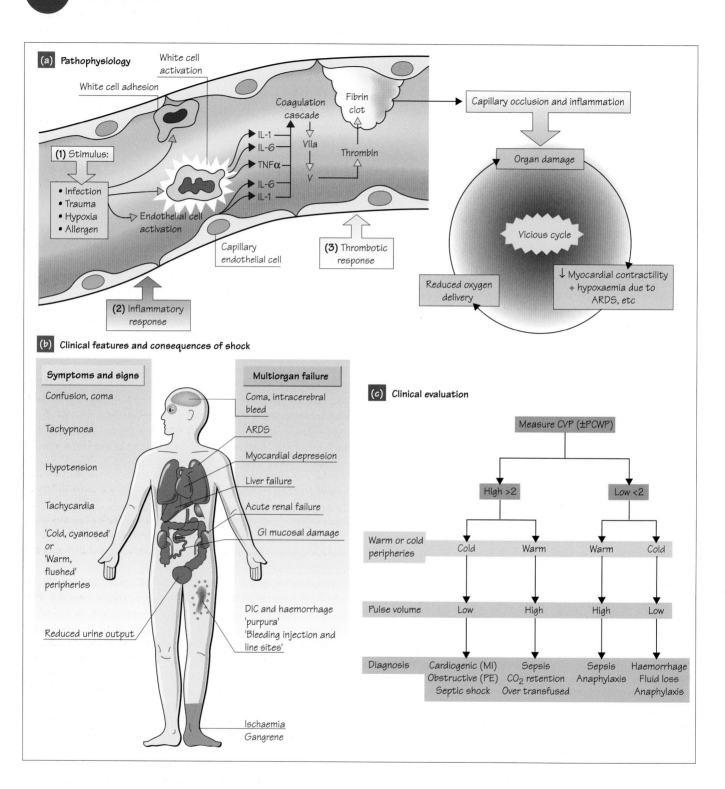

(a) Pathophysiology

White cell activation
White cell adhesion
Coagulation cascade
Fibrin clot

(1) Stimulus:
- Infection
- Trauma
- Hypoxia
- Allergen

IL-1
IL-6
TNFα
IL-6
IL-1

VIIa
V
Thrombin

Endothelial cell activation
Capillary endothelial cell
(3) Thrombotic response
(2) Inflammatory response

Capillary occlusion and inflammation
Organ damage
Vicious cycle
Reduced oxygen delivery
↓ Myocardial contractility + hypoxaemia due to ARDS, etc

(b) Clinical features and consequences of shock

Symptoms and signs
Confusion, coma
Tachypnoea
Hypotension
Tachycardia
'Cold, cyanosed' or 'Warm, flushed' peripheries
Reduced urine output

Multiorgan failure
Coma, intracerebral bleed
ARDS
Myocardial depression
Liver failure
Acute renal failure
GI mucosal damage
DIC and haemorrhage 'purpura' 'Bleeding injection and line sites'
Ischaemia Gangrene

(c) Clinical evaluation

Measure CVP (±PCWP)

	High >2		Low <2	
Warm or cold peripheries	Cold	Warm	Warm	Cold
Pulse volume	Low	High	High	Low
Diagnosis	Cardiogenic (MI) Obstructive (PE) Septic shock	Sepsis CO₂ retention Over transfused	Sepsis Anaphylaxis	Haemorrhage Fluid loss Anaphylaxis

Definition and causes

Shock describes the clinical syndrome that occurs when acute circulatory failure with inadequate or inappropriately distributed perfusion results in failure to meet tissue metabolic demands causing generalized cellular hypoxia (± lactic acidosis).

Shock can be classified into six categories but more than one form of shock may occur in an individual patient (e.g. myocardial depression may occur in late sepsis).

- **Hypovolaemic:** due to major reductions in circulating blood volume caused by haemorrhage, plasma loss (e.g. burns, pancreatitis) or extracellular fluid loss (e.g. diabetic ketoacidosis, trauma).

- **Cardiogenic:** due to severe heart failure (e.g. myocardial infarction, acute mitral regurgitation).
- **Obstructive:** caused by circulatory obstruction (e.g. pulmonary embolism, cardiac tamponade).
- **Septic/distributive:** with infection or septicaemia. Vasodilation, arteriovenous shunting and capillary damage (Fig. a) cause subsequent hypotension and maldistribution of flow.
- **Anaphylactic:** due to allergen-induced vasodilation (e.g. bee sting, peanut and other food allergies).
- **Neurogenic (spinal):** follows traumatic spinal cord lesions above T6. Interruption of sympathetic outflow causes vasodilation, hypothermia and bradycardia, which may be severe if vagal stimulation (e.g. pain, hypoxia) is unopposed.

Clinical features depend on the underlying cause (Chapters 28, 30, 52) and severity. General features include hypotension (systolic BP <100 mmHg), tachycardia (>100 beats/min), rapid respiration (>30/min), oliguria (urine output <30 ml/h) and drowsiness, confusion or agitation (Fig. b). Shock is either:
- **'Cold, clammy' shock** (e.g. hypovolaemic, cardiogenic, obstructive, late septic) with cold peripheries (skin vasoconstriction), weak pulses and evidence of low cardiac output (e.g. oliguria, peripheral cyanosis, confusion)
- **'Warm, dilated' shock** (e.g. early septic, anaphylactic) with warm peripheries (skin vasodilation), bounding pulses and a high cardiac output (i.e. flushed)

Investigations and monitoring

Investigations include routine blood tests, blood gases, lactic acid measurement, cardiac enzymes, amylase, ECG and blood crossmatching if haemorrhage is suspected. **Radiology:** includes chest radiographs. **Microbiology:** requires examination of blood, sputum, CSF and urine samples. **Monitor vital signs:** temperature, respiratory rate, S_aO_2, conscious level and urine output. **Haemodynamic assessment:** often requires intra-arterial BP measurement, echocardiography, CVP and ECG monitoring. Additional measurements (Chapter 3) are occasionally necessary (e.g. CO, SVR, PCWP, S_vO_2).

Assessment

Clinical features, CVP and SVR define the cause of shock (Fig. c). Measurement of CVP, pulmonary capillary wedge pressure (PCWP) and SVR are useful when clinical signs are difficult to interpret. For example:
- CVP is: (i) **reduced** in hypovolaemic and anaphylactic shock; (ii) **elevated** in cardiogenic and obstructive shock; (iii) **low, normal or high** in septic shock.
- SVR is: (i) **high** in cardiogenic shock with sympathetic-mediated vasoconstriction (→'cold, clammy' patient) or (ii) **low** in septic vasodilation due to release of inflammatory mediators (→'warm, dilated' patient)

Consequently, simple haemodynamic patterns may aid diagnosis:
- Hypovolaemic shock → low CVP/PCWP + low CO + high SVR
- Cardiogenic shock → high CVP/PCWP + low CO + high SVR
- Septic shock → low CVP/PCWP + high CO + low SVR

Complications

Circulatory failure and tissue hypoxia result in multi-organ failure including ARDS, acute renal failure and mucosal (e.g. peptic) ulceration (Figs a and b). A cycle of increasing 'oxygen debt' and 'shock-induced' tissue damage develops as decreased myocardial contractility and hypoxaemia further impair oxygen delivery and tissue oxygenation (Fig. a). Ischaemic damage to the intestinal mucosa causes bacterial and toxin translocation into the splanchnic circulation and further organ impairment. Eventually, 'refractory' shock develops with irreversible tissue damage and death.

Management

Early diagnosis and treatment are essential as mortality, which is high with all causes, increases if shock lasts >1 hour ('the golden hour'). Management aims to correct the underlying cause, reverse 'tissue oxygen debt' and prevent the vicious cycle of progressive organ damage. Treatment of cardiogenic, obstructive and septic shock are presented in later chapters. However, features common to all forms of shock are:
- **Identify and treat the cause** (e.g. sepsis).
- **Support.** Patients should be managed in a critical care area with appropriate monitoring and good vascular access. Hypoxaemia, which can occur in the absence of lung disease due to ventilation–perfusion mismatch, low S_vO_2 or reduced pulmonary blood flow, requires correction with supplemental oxygen. **Ventilatory support:** improves cardiac function, increases tissue oxygen delivery and reduces work of breathing, which is increased tenfold in shock (Chapters 14, 16). Indications include progressive hypoxaemia ($P_aO_2 < 8$ kPa on >40% O_2), hypercapnia ($P_aCO_2 > 7.5$ kPa), respiratory rate >35/min, reduced conscious level or exhaustion (Chapter 11).
- **Fluid resuscitation** is, with the exception of cardiogenic shock, essential in most forms of shock (e.g. haemorrhage, sepsis). Fluid is given rapidly following assessment of intravascular volume status (e.g. BP, CVP, PCWP) including the response to a fluid challenge (Chapters 7, 8). The merits of specific fluids (e.g. crystalloid, colloid) are discussed in Chapter 9 and depend on the cause of shock (Chapters 22, 52, 57). Thus, blood or blood products are most appropriate following haemorrhage or trauma. Cardiogenic shock, identified by raised CVP and PCWP, requires fluid restriction (although fluid administration may be required in right ventricular infarction!). Time course is also important; in early septic shock fluid administration is essential, but in late sepsis with ARDS, fluid restriction prevents pulmonary oedema.
- **Inotropic support** (Chapter 10) is indicated when *hypotension* (i.e. MAP < 60 mmHg) *or tissue hypoxaemia* (e.g. oliguria) persist despite adequate fluid replacement or when fluid resuscitation is contraindicated (e.g. cardiogenic shock). The type of inotropic support will depend on the cause of shock. **In septic shock** ('warm, dilated' patient), the CO is high but vasodilation and the associated low SVR cause hypotension, inadequate tissue perfusion and organ hypoxia (e.g. oliguria, confusion). In this situation, noradrenaline (norepinephrine), a peripheral vasoconstrictor, increases SVR, restoring BP and tissue perfusion. **In cardiogenic shock** ('cold, clammy' patient), the CO is low due to poor myocardial contractility and SVR is high due to sympathetic vasoconstriction. Treatment with dobutamine increases myocardial contractility and CO and reduces SVR.
- **Renal replacement therapy** (e.g. haemofiltration) may be required for anuria, hyperkalaemia, unresolving acidosis or fluid overload (Chapter 39).
- **Specific treatments** include thrombolysis (e.g. for pulmonary embolism), drainage of cardiac tamponade/pneumothorax and balloon pumps (e.g. cardiogenic shock).

7 Circulatory assessment

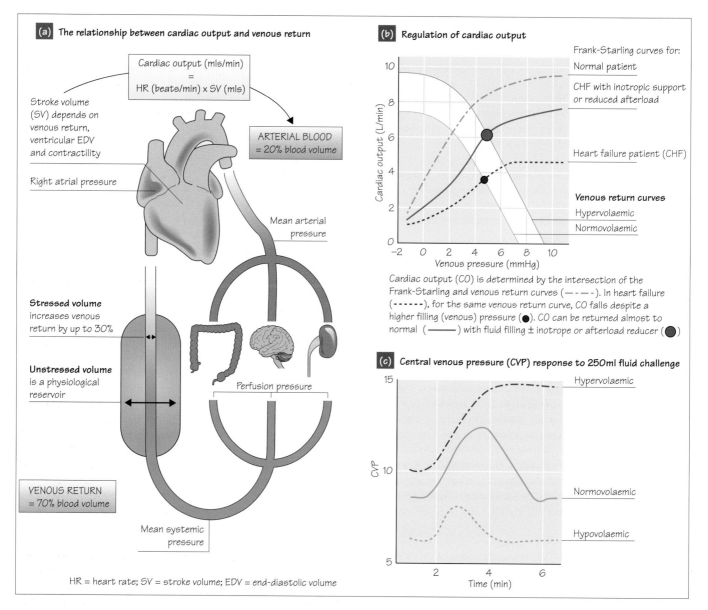

(a) The relationship between cardiac output and venous return

Cardiac output (mls/min)
=
HR (beats/min) x SV (mls)

Stroke volume (SV) depends on venous return, ventricular EDV and contractility

Right atrial pressure

ARTERIAL BLOOD = 20% blood volume

Mean arterial pressure

Stressed volume increases venous return by up to 30%

Unstressed volume is a physiological reservoir

Perfusion pressure

VENOUS RETURN = 70% blood volume

Mean systemic pressure

HR = heart rate; SV = stroke volume; EDV = end-diastolic volume

(b) Regulation of cardiac output

Frank-Starling curves for:
Normal patient
CHF with inotropic support or reduced afterload
Heart failure patient (CHF)

Venous return curves
Hypervolaemic
Normovolaemic

Cardiac output (CO) is determined by the intersection of the Frank-Starling and venous return curves (— · — · —). In heart failure (· · · · · ·), for the same venous return curve, CO falls despite a higher filling (venous) pressure (●). CO can be returned almost to normal (———) with fluid filling ± inotrope or afterload reducer (●)

(c) Central venous pressure (CVP) response to 250ml fluid challenge

Hypervolaemic
Normovolaemic
Hypovolaemic

Circulatory assessment is an essential clinical skill and when performed well is the hallmark of a good clinician. It can be particularly difficult during critical illness and depends on evaluation of both cardiac function and circuit factors (Fig. a). The main aims are to maintain cardiac output (CO) and blood pressure (BP) and ensure adequate tissue blood supply to satisfy metabolic demands.

Circulatory assessment should address:

1. Cardiac function

This includes evaluation of CO and exclusion of heart failure. CO is the product of **heart rate (HR)** and **stroke volume (SV)** [CO (ml/min) = HR (beats/min) × SV (mls)]; where SV is determined by:

• **Preload** which depends on ventricular end-diastolic volume (EDV) and is governed by the volume and pressure of blood returning to the heart (Fig. b). Loss of intravascular volume due to haemorrhage, sepsis or anaphylaxis and raised intrathoracic pressures (e.g. severe asthma) are the commonest causes of inadequate ventricular preload

• **Afterload** which describes the load, resistance or 'impedence' against which the ventricle has to work. Thus, valve stenosis, hypertension, high systemic vascular resistance (SVR), low intrathoracic pressures and ventricular dilation increase afterload

• **Myocardial contractility** or the heart's ability to perform work independently of pre- or afterload. Failure is either due to inadequate systolic ejection (systolic dysfunction) or poor diastolic filling (diastolic dysfunction).

• **Systolic dysfunction** may be due to reduced contractility (e.g. ischaemia, cardiomyopathy, sepsis) or increased impedance (e.g. hypertension, aortic stenosis). Increasing ventricular EDV (i.e. heart volume) will maintain SV (Frank–Starling relationship) provided myocardial reserve is adequate (Fig. b); otherwise SV and CO will fall and inotropic agents will be required to maintain CO and BP.

- **Diastolic dysfunction** is characterized by reduced ventricular compliance with impaired diastolic filling (i.e. a stiff ventricle) and may be due to mechanical factors (e.g. restrictive cardiomyopathy) or due to the impaired relaxation that occurs during myocardial ischaemia or severe sepsis. This results in elevated end-diastolic pressure, pulmonary venous congestion and characteristic 'flash' pulmonary oedema. Patients with advanced diabetes or hypertension secondary to renal failure are at particular risk of diastolic dysfunction and flash pulmonary oedema. In diabetes this is due to endomyocardial ischaemia caused by small vessel arteriopathy. In renal hypertension the normal blood flow from the epicardium to endomyocardium is impeded by the ventricular wall hypertrophy and subsequent endomyocardial ischaemia impairs ventricular relaxation.

CO is reduced in bradycardia and tachycardia. In tachycardia this is due to either inadequate ventricular filling time or reduced contractility. Myocardial perfusion occurs during diastole. This is shortened during tachycardia causing myocardial ischaemia and impaired contractility.

2. Circuit factors

Although frequently overlooked, circuit factors are as important as myocardial contractility in determining CO because venous return determines EDV. Arterial 'conducting' vessels contain ~20% of the blood volume, where mean arterial pressure (MAP) is determined by force of myocardial ejection and downstream impedance. The venous 'capacitance' system contains ~70% of total blood volume and acts as a physiological reservoir ('unstressed volume'). When circulatory demand increases, sympathetic tone also increases causing reservoir contraction. The resultant 'autotransfusion' ('stressed volume') can increase venous return by up to 30%. Complex neurohormonal factors control the circulatory response including systemic adrenergic, renin-aldosterone, vasopressinergic and steroid systems, which are further modulated by local factors (e.g. endothelin, nitric oxide).

Disruption of peripheral vascular regulation, usually due to reduced responsiveness to sympathetic stimulation (e.g. spinal anaesthesia, anaphylaxis, sepsis), results in circulatory failure due to venous pooling and inability to generate a 'stressed' volume. Management tends to focus inappropriately on arterial factors (i.e. SVR, 'afterload'), whereas the problem is mainly due to impaired venous return. Fluid loading to restore effective intravascular volume (Chapters 8, 9) should always proceed the use of 'vasopressor' drugs (Chapter 10)

Clinical assessment (Chapters 1, 6)

- **Inspection.** Look for features of poor perfusion and reduced CO including cool, pale limbs, peripheral cyanosis and prolonged capillary refill time (i.e. >2 seconds for colour to return to an area of skin previously subjected to pressure). Confusion and reduced urine output also indicate poor CO.
- **Auscultation.** Listen for leaking heart valves and check BP. Initially compensatory mechanisms (e.g. tachycardia, increased SVR) maintain

BP, and CO has to fall by >20%, equivalent to 1 L of acute blood loss, before BP falls. Pulse pressure narrows during arterial vasoconstriction (e.g. hypovolaemia, cardiogenic shock). During vasodilation (e.g. sepsis) diastolic BP is low.
- **Palpation.** Feel peripheral and central pulses for HR, rhythm and equality. Thready, fast pulses indicate a poor CO, whereas bounding pulses suggest sepsis.

In most patients clinical assessment is reliable, adequate and ensures successful management. However, invasive measurement of physiological variables (e.g. CO, SVR, PCWP) may be required in critically ill patients to optimize circulatory performance (Chapter 3).

Management

Management includes fluid replacement, control of bleeding and restoration of HR, CO, BP and tissue perfusion. Good venous access must be established using wide-bore peripheral and central venous cannulae. Circulatory support utilizes a hierarchy of management:

- **Diagnosis** determines treatment (e.g. fluid restriction in left heart failure vs. fluid resuscitation in hypovolaemia). Immediately life-threatening conditions such as haemorrhage, cardiac tamponade and massive pulmonary embolism must be detected and treated rapidly.
- **Rate and rhythm.** Both tachyarrhythmias (>180 beats/min) and bradycardia (e.g. vagal tone) can reduce CO. Restoring sinus rhythm and normal HR improve BP and CO. Electrolyte concentrations must be optimized ($K^+ > 4.5$ mmol/L, $Mg^{2+} > 1.2$ mmol/L) and arrhythmogenic drugs (e.g. salbutamol) withdrawn. Antiarrhythmic drugs, cardioversion or pacemakers may be required (Chapter 27).
- **Fluid therapy**: aims to optimize preload (Fig. b). In the absence of cardiac failure (i.e. raised central venous pressure (CVP), coarse bilateral basal crepitations on lung auscultation), a **'fluid challenge'** (~0.5 L over <20 min) should be given and the response assessed in terms of HR, BP and chest auscultation. The CVP response to a fluid challenge (Fig. c) is a useful measure of the patient's fluid status (i.e. hypovolaemic, hypervolaemic). A transient increase in CVP, CO and BP suggests the need for further fluid. A sustained increase in CVP indicates that the heart is operating on the flat part of the Starling curve (Fig. b) and further fluid administration risks pulmonary oedema. If there is only a transient response to the initial fluid challenge, the challenge is repeated and the patient reassessed. Aim to restore systolic BP to >100 mmHg or normal (if known). Fluid management and the selection of the appropriate fluid for replacement (e.g. crystalloid vs. colloid) are discussed in Chapters 8 and 9. In general, crystalloid solutions are used first or the fluid that is lost is replaced (e.g. blood during haemorrhage). Large volumes of maintenance fluid suggest ongoing loss and a cause should be sought. If haemorrhage is the cause (or suspected) send blood for cross-matching
- **Inotropic and vasopressor drugs:** if fluid resuscitation fails to achieve an adequate circulation or precipitates cardiac failure alternative means of improving CO and tissue perfusion including inotropic or vasopressor drugs and mechanical ventricular support devices must be considered (Chapter 10).

8 Fluid management

(a) Distribution of body water

Total body water 42 litres (~42 kg)

Extracellular space
Extracellular fluid (ECF) ~ 15–17 litres
Composition (in mmol/L): Na^+ 140, chloride 105, K^+ 3.7, phosphate 1, HCO_3 28

Intracellular space
Intracellular fluid (ICF) ~ 25 litres
Composition (in mmol/L): Na^+ 10, chloride 3, K^+ 155, phosphate 105, HCO_3 10

Vascular space
Plasma (non cellular blood) ~4 litres

Interstitial space
Interstitial fluid (ISF) ~11–13 litres

Red blood cell

Capillary endothelial cell

Negatively charged collagen impedes movement of negatively charged albumin into the ISF

Colloids (i.e proteins + haemoglobin) pull more water into the intravascular compartment

H_2O

Water distributes throughout the ICF and ECF (i.e. 5% dextrose has a large volume of distribution)

Na^+

Sodium pumped out of cells (i.e. saline has a smaller volume of distribution)

● = Albumin molecule, ● = Water molecule, ⌇ = Collagen + hyaluronic fibres, Na^+ = Sodium ion, K^+ = Potassium ion

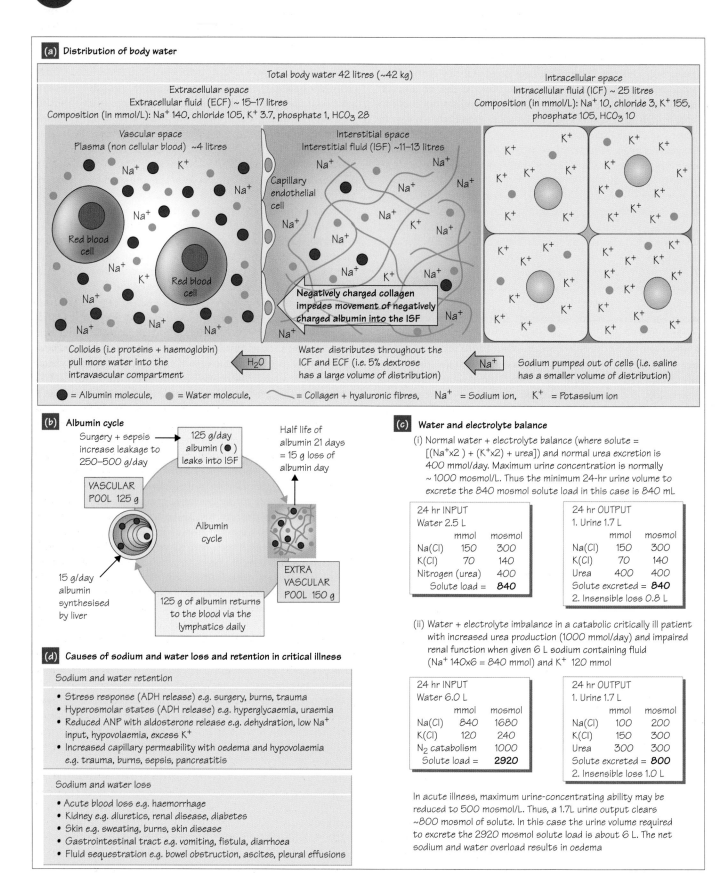

(b) Albumin cycle

Surgery + sepsis increase leakage to 250–500 g/day

125 g/day albumin (●) leaks into ISF

Half life of albumin 21 days = 15 g loss of albumin day

VASCULAR POOL 125 g

Albumin cycle

15 g/day albumin synthesised by liver

125 g of albumin returns to the blood via the lymphatics daily

EXTRA VASCULAR POOL 150 g

(c) Water and electrolyte balance

(i) Normal water + electrolyte balance (where solute = [(Na^+x2) + (K^+x2) + urea]) and normal urea excretion is 400 mmol/day. Maximum urine concentration is normally ~ 1000 mosmol/L. Thus the minimum 24-hr urine volume to excrete the 840 mosmol solute load in this case is 840 mL

24 hr INPUT Water 2.5 L		
	mmol	mosmol
Na(Cl)	150	300
K(Cl)	70	140
Nitrogen (urea)	400	
Solute load =	**840**	

24 hr OUTPUT 1. Urine 1.7 L		
	mmol	mosmol
Na(Cl)	150	300
K(Cl)	70	140
Urea	400	400
Solute excreted =	**840**	
2. Insensible loss 0.8 L		

(ii) Water + electrolyte imbalance in a catabolic critically ill patient with increased urea production (1000 mmol/day) and impaired renal function when given 6 L sodium containing fluid (Na^+ 140x6 = 840 mmol) and K^+ 120 mmol

24 hr INPUT Water 6.0 L		
	mmol	mosmol
Na(Cl)	840	1680
K(Cl)	120	240
N_2 catabolism	1000	
Solute load =	**2920**	

24 hr OUTPUT 1. Urine 1.7 L		
	mmol	mosmol
Na(Cl)	100	200
K(Cl)	150	300
Urea	300	300
Solute excreted =	**800**	
2. Insensible loss 1.0 L		

In acute illness, maximum urine-concentrating ability may be reduced to 500 mosmol/L. Thus, a 1.7L urine output clears ~800 mosmol of solute. In this case the urine volume required to excrete the 2920 mosmol solute load is about 6 L. The net sodium and water overload results in oedema

(d) Causes of sodium and water loss and retention in critical illness

Sodium and water retention

- Stress response (ADH release) e.g. surgery, burns, trauma
- Hyperosmolar states (ADH release) e.g. hyperglycaemia, uraemia
- Reduced ANP with aldosterone release e.g. dehydration, low Na^+ input, hypovolaemia, excess K^+
- Increased capillary permeability with oedema and hypovolaemia e.g. trauma, burns, sepsis, pancreatitis

Sodium and water loss

- Acute blood loss e.g. haemorrhage
- Kidney e.g. diuretics, renal disease, diabetes
- Skin e.g. sweating, burns, skin disease
- Gastrointestinal tract e.g. vomiting, fistula, diarrhoea
- Fluid sequestration e.g. bowel obstruction, ascites, pleural effusions

Water comprises 60% of body weight and totals ~42 L in a 70-kg man, of which 25 L is intracellular fluid (ICF) and 15–17 L extracellular fluid (ECF). The ECF compartment is divided into the interstitial fluid (ISF; 11–13 L) and intravascular plasma (4 L), separated by the capillary endothelium which is freely permeable to low molecular weight (MW) solutes (e.g. sodium, potassium) but increasingly impermeable to high MW solutes. Albumin permeability is partly limited by high MW but also by its negative charge which is repelled by the similarly charged interstitial space glycoproteins (e.g. collagen, hyaluronic acid) that trap water to make up the gel-like interstitial matrix (Fig. a).

Compartmental distribution of water depends on the 'osmotic pressure' exerted by small diffusible ions and the 'oncotic pressure' exerted by large non-diffusible plasma proteins.
• **Osmotic pressure** reflects the ion concentration gradients between different compartments created by cellular ion-pumps, such that sodium and chloride ions are mainly extracellular, and potassium and phosphate intracellular. For example, after a saline infusion, the rise in extracellular sodium (+chloride) elevates osmotic pressure and increases ECF volume by drawing water out of the ICF compartment.
• **Oncotic (colloid) pressure** describes the ability of 'vascular' plasma proteins to 'bind' and retain water in the circulation. Normal plasma oncotic pressure is ~3.4 kPa (26 mmHg), of which albumin accounts for ~75%, haemoglobin 20% and globulins 5%. Figure (b) illustrates the albumin cycle. Total body albumin is ~275 g (125 g intravascular, 150 g ISF). One gram of albumin binds 18 ml of water, thus intravascular albumin attracts 2.25 L (i.e. 18 ml × 125 g) of water. Normal albumin leakage from blood to ISF, and subsequent return via lymphatics, is ~125 g/day. Leakage increases by 100% after surgery and 300% during sepsis due to increased vascular permeability. The associated fall in plasma albumin reduces intravascular volume and the increase in ISF albumin causes oedema.

Fluid requirements

Normal, euvolaemic patients unable to take oral fluids require replacement of normal water and electrolyte losses. A normal adult ingests 80–150 mmol of sodium (Na^+), 40–70 mmol of potassium (K^+) and 2.5 L of water daily. When in balance most of the sodium and potassium is excreted with 400 mmol of urea 'waste' in ~1.7 L (~1 ml/kg/h or 70 ml/h) of urine. A further 0.8 L of fluid is lost as lung water vapour and sweat, termed 'insensible loss'. The urine contains a daily solute load of ~840 mosmol [($Na^+ \times 2$) + ($K^+ \times 2$) + urea] at a concentration of ~500 mosmol/L (Fig. c(i)). The kidneys can achieve a maximum urine concentration of 1000 mosmol/L. Thus, to excrete 800 mosmol, with a normal fluid intake and normal kidneys, requires a minimum urine output of 0.5 ml/kg/h or 35 ml/h.

Critically ill patients cannot maintain normal water and electrolyte balance due to stress and inflammatory responses. Stress (e.g. dehydration, hyperglycaemia) causes: (a) antidiuretic hormone (ADH) release which reduces urine output causing water and sodium retention; (b) activation of the renin-angiotensin system, due to hypotension and renal hypoperfusion, which promotes sodium conservation; and (c) catecholamine release which redistributes blood away from skin and splanchnic circulations. Inflammation increases vascular permeability and leakage of plasma proteins, electrolytes and water into ISF. This causes hypovolaemia, peripheral oedema, impaired gas exchange due to pulmonary oedema and reduced organ perfusion because most are surrounded by non-expandable capsules. In addition, fluid resuscitation, particularly with sodium containing fluids, and catabolism (i.e. increased urea production) increases solute load which may be difficult to excrete (Fig. c(ii)). Water and electrolyte homeostasis is further complicated by losses from fistula, vomiting, burns or trauma (e.g. vomit has high Cl^- concentrations).

Assessing fluid balance: hourly fluid input (e.g. resuscitation fluids, feed) and output (e.g. urine output, gastrointestinal loss, drainage) monitoring and daily measurements of serum (occasionally urinary) electrolytes and urea are essential to assess fluid balance in acutely unwell patients. Day to day trends in these parameters often guides fluid prescription. The response to '*fluid challenges*' (~500 ml over <20 min) may determine the need for volume replacement (Chapter 7). Figure (d) summarizes conditions associated with sodium and water imbalance.

Fluid choice (Chapter 9; Fig. a) is guided by the underlying condition. In general, the fluid that is lost is replaced (e.g. blood during haemorrhage, normal daily loss in euvolaemic, stable patients). In critically ill patients (e.g. sepsis, hypovolaemia) selection of replacement fluid (e.g. crystalloid, colloid) is more complex and controversial.
• **Crystalloid solutions** are water to which solutes (e.g. sodium chloride, glucose) have been added. Although inexpensive and usually isotonic, they redistribute rapidly following intravenous infusion (~1–4 hours; Fig. a) from the intravascular to other fluid compartments (e.g. ECF, ICF). Consequently large volumes are required to maintain intravascular volume, which may cause interstitial oedema. Low sodium fluids (e.g. 5% dextrose) disperse throughout the ICF and ECF (i.e. 4/42nd remain in the vascular compartment). By contrast, sodium containing fluids (e.g. normal saline) disseminate in ECF alone (i.e. cellular pumps remove ICF sodium) and therefore have a smaller volume of distribution (i.e. 4/15th remain intravascular). The use of hypertonic crystalloids (e.g. 7.5% saline) with or without colloids for initial resuscitation (i.e. to osmotically draw ICF water into the ECF) has not improved outcome in general trauma patients. However, associated small fluid resuscitation volumes and hypertonic osmotic effects may reduce cerebral oedema and benefit head trauma patients.
• **Colloid solutions** are expensive. Their large molecules cannot easily diffuse out of blood vessels and they remain intravascular longer, exerting an oncotic pressure which pulls water into, and expands the intravascular compartment. It is often quoted that four to five times as much crystalloid is required to achieve the same intravascular volume expansion as a colloid. Consequently colloids are often employed for initial resuscitation. However, in a recent study, the volume ratio of 4% albumin to saline for equivalent resuscitation was 1:1.4 and meta-analysis has shown no advantage of colloids over crystalloids. Nevertheless, albumin may be beneficial in hypoalbuminaemic (<15 g/dl) patients with severe sepsis or in ARDS patients to aid lung water clearance. Synthetic colloids include gelatin, dextran and hydroxyethyl starch. Disadvantages of colloids include allergic reactions, clotting abnormalities and renal impairment but previous concerns about increased mortality have not been substantiated.
• **Blood** is given to maintain haemoglobin concentration >80 g/L (>8 g/dl). However, young patients and those with renal disease, haemoglobinopathies or chronic anaemia may tolerate lower levels. A haemoglobin ~100 g/L (~10 g/dl) improves outcome in cardiac patients.
• **Bicarbonate** use is often controversial but replacement fluids containing 1.26% sodium bicarbonate may be used to correct metabolic acidosis (pH < 7.2) due to renal or gastrointestinal losses.

9 Fluid choice: specific situations

(a) Composition of crystalloids and colloids

Fluid	Na (mmol/L)	K (mmol/L)	Cl (mmol/L)	Osmolarity (mosmol/L)	Additions (mmol/L)
Crystalloids					
Dextrose 5%	0	0	0	278	Glucose: 278
0.9% saline	154	0	154	308	Nil
Hartmann's	131	5.4	112	275	HCO$_3$ 29; Ca 1.8
Ringer's	130	4.2	109	273	Ca 2.2

Fluid	Na (mmol/L)	K (mmol/L)	Cl (mmol/L)	Osmolarity (mosmol/L)	T^{1}/2 (hrs)	PVE
Colloids						
Gelofusin	154	0	154	279	~2	80%
Isoplex	145	4	105	284	~2	80%
5% Albumin	130–160	0	?	300	2–4h	100%
Voluven	154	0	154	308	~5	120%
10% HES	154	0	154	308	6–12	145%

T^{1}/2=Approximate effective plasma half life;
PVE=Plasma volume expansion (% of volume given);
HES=Hydroxyethyl starch
MW = molecular weight, PVD = peripheral vascular disease,
RES = reticuloendothelial system

(b) Properties of colloid solutions

Colloid MW (Da)	Properties	Disadvantages
Gelatins ~30,000	Cheap and rapidly degraded to water. Maximum volume 1.5-2.0L daily	Allergic reactions
Dextrans ~40-70,000	~30% intravascular after 24hrs. Reduces serum viscosity, so used in PVD and as DVT prophylaxis. Renal and RES clearance	Bleeding risk. Interferes with blood tests. Allergy 5%. Osmotic diuresis and renal impairment
Hydroxyethyl Starch ~50-500,000	Excellent plasma volume expansion and long intravascular times. Renal and RES clearance	Accumulates in macrophages. Bleeding risk. Possible renal impairment. Pruritus
Albumin ~68,000	Few advantages over synthetic colloids. Expensive	Infection risks. Allergic reactions

Adequate hydration is essential in every patient and is best achieved by the oral or nasogastric route. However intravenous (i.v.) fluid is often necessary in acutely unwell patients (e.g. vomiting). In the absence of normal homeostatic mechanisms, patients need **basic maintenance fluids** to replace normal daily water and electrolyte losses (see below) plus **additional resuscitation fluids** to correct losses due to underlying pathology and to maintain an adequate circulation (Fig. a,b). However, in many patients, particularly those with renal impairment, large volumes of crystalloid or colloid engenders **large solute loads** (e.g. sodium) which is difficult to excrete (Chapter 8; Fig. c) and may precipitate **hyperchloraemic acidosis (HCA)** due to high chloride (Cl$^-$) levels in some fluids (Fig. a). In these circumstances, physiologically balanced solutions (PBS) with low Cl$^-$ content (e.g. Hartmann's solution) are preferred. These cause less HCA and associated nausea, confusion and oliguria compared to other fluids (e.g. saline 0.9%).

Total fluid, crystalloid and colloid requirements are prescribed daily and adjusted if enteral feeding is not successful. Assessment takes into account pathology, extracellular fluid status (e.g. oedema), fluid losses (e.g. diarrhoea) and electrolyte concentrations. Different clinical scenarios are illustrated below:

• **Maintenance fluid** Stable, euvolaemic patients with normal renal function who cannot drink require 2–3 L (1–1.5 ml/kg/h) water, 70–150 mmol/L sodium (Na$^+$) and 40 mmol/L potassium (K$^+$) each day (Chapter 8). This equates to 1 L of saline 0.9% (Na$^+$ 154 mmol/L) and 2 L of 5% dextrose (water) with 20 mmol K$^+$ added to each litre of 5% dextrose. A simple alternative is Hartmann's solution. If there is significant hypernatraemia ($\uparrow$Na$^+$, $\uparrow$Cl$^-$) or hyponatraemia ($\downarrow$Na$^+$, $\downarrow$Cl$^-$), 5% dextrose or saline 0.9% are used respectively.

• **Post major surgery** If hypovolaemia occurs despite normal maintenance fluid (i.e. 1–1.5 ml/kg/h), increase the infusion rate to 2–3 ml/kg/h using a PBS (e.g. Hartmann's to reduce Cl$^-$ load) and support the circulation with 0.5 L Gelofusine 'fluid challenges'. Maintain haemoglobin (Hb) $\geq$8 g/dl except in unstable cardiac patients who require a Hb $\geq$10 g/dl. Large fluid requirements may indicate internal bleeding.

• **Major haemorrhage** requires urgent control of bleeding and restoration of circulating volume. Occasionally aggressive fluid resuscitation before surgery increases blood loss due to dilutional coagulopathy, acidosis and hypothermia. In these patients the priority is early surgery with restoration of circulating volume after surgery. Blood is the ideal resuscitation fluid but requires time to prepare (Chapter 49). Whilst awaiting blood, fluid replacement starts with 20–30 ml/kg Hartmann's solution, followed by 1–1.5 L Gelofusine ($\pm$1–1.5 L Voluven). Infusion rate is determined by repeated clinical assessment. Ongoing resuscitation includes plasma and platelets.

• **Sepsis and septic shock** cause interstitial, 'third space', fluid loss due to increased vascular permeability. Assessment of associated intravascular hypovolaemia is difficult and requires repeated 'fluid challenges' and close monitoring (e.g. urine output (UO), lactate). Fluid replacement follows the Surviving Sepsis Guidelines (Chapter 22) and starts immediately in hypotensive patients or if lactate is raised. Initially give 20–40 ml/kg Hartmann's in aliquots of 0.5–1 L based on clinical response. If hypotension or lactate elevation persists insert a CVP line and continue resuscitation with Gelofusine 1–1.5 L ($\pm$ Voluven 1–1.5 L) aiming for a CVP 8–12 mmHg, MAP >65 mmHg, UO >0.5 ml/kg/h and $S_v O_2$ >70%.

• **Head injury** Hyponatraemia aggravates brain oedema. A degree of hypernatraemia is beneficial and saline 0.9% is recommended for fluid resuscitation (Chapter 53). Avoid 5% dextrose except in diabetes insipidus.

10 Inotropes and vasopressors

(a) Properties of inotropic drugs

Vasoactive Agent	Receptors (▦ = main effect) or action	Midrange dose effects		
		Inotropic contractility	Chronotrope (heart rate)	Vaso-constrictor
Inoconstrictors				
Epinephrine	α, β₁, β₂	++++	+++	++
Dopamine	α, β₁, β₂	+++	++	− to ++
Inodilators				
Dobutamine	α, β₁, β₂	+++	+	− to ±
Milrinone	PDI (↑cAMP)	+++	0	− −
Enoximone	PDI (↑cAMP)	+++	0	−
Vasoconstrictor				
Norepinephrine	α, β₁	+/++	0	++++
Phenylephrine	α, β₁	+	0	++++

PDI=phosphodiesterase inhibitor;
cAMP=cyclic adenosine monophosphate;
− = vasodilation

Inotropes and vasopressors are used to provide additional haemodynamic support if optimal fluid resuscitation (Chapters 8, 9) and heart rate control are unable to correct circulatory failure. The aim is to achieve adequate tissue perfusion rather than a specific blood pressure (BP) which differs between subjects (e.g. hypertensives require higher BP). Vasoactive drugs are relatively ineffective in volume-depleted patients and an adequate circulating volume is essential. Similarly acidosis (pH < 7.1) and electrolyte derangements (e.g. hypokalaemia, hypomagnesaemia) impair inotropic drug actions and should be corrected to ensure maximal pressor effects. These agents must be administered through central lines to avoid tissue necrosis from extravasation.

Monitoring The effects of these agents in an individual case are unpredictable. The response must be closely monitored and therapy titrated to specific end points (e.g. MAP 65–70 mmHg). In general, all haemodynamically unstable patients receiving vasoactive drugs require continuous intra-arterial BP monitoring, preferably from a large artery (e.g. femoral), as smaller arteries (e.g. radial) underestimate systemic pressures in shocked patients. Volume status is most conveniently assessed with a central venous catheter but in complex cases haemodynamic monitoring of cardiac output (CO), systemic vascular resistance (SVR), left-sided filling pressures and lung water may be necessary to maintain tissue perfusion (Chapter 3).

Selection of appropriate vasopressor **therapy** requires an understanding of an agent's cardiovascular properties, knowledge of adrenergic receptor distribution and actions, and an accurate assessment of

the underlying haemodynamic disturbance. The pharmacological properties and receptor activation of individual agents is presented in Fig. a. Activation of α receptors causes peripheral vasoconstriction, β₁ receptors are chronotropic (i.e. increase heart rate) and inotropic (i.e. increase the force and velocity of myocardial contractility and consequently BP and CO), whereas β₂ **receptors** cause vasodilation and bronchodilation. A drug may activate several receptors (e.g. epinephrine (adrenaline) has α, β₁, β₂ properties) but the balance varies (i.e. dobutamine also has α, β₁, β₂ properties but β₁, β₂ effects are greater than α properties). Ideally a single drug is used but occasionally the correct balance of receptor stimulation may require drug combinations. Both vasopressin and low dose steroids (e.g. hydrocortisone 8 mg/h) may have a 'catecholamine sparing' effect particularly in septic shock.

Opinions often differ between institutions and countries as to optimal therapy in specific situations. In the absence of conclusive evidence, the controversy is likely to continue.
- **In septic shock** profound vasodilation causes hypotension despite a high CO. Current evidence supports the initial use of norepinephrine (± epinephrine), which are primarily α-vasoconstrictors, to maintain CO, BP and organ perfusion. However, prolonged sepsis may impair cardiac contractility requiring later addition of a β₁-inotropic agent to maintain CO (e.g. dobutamine).
- **In myocardial ischaemia** dobutamine β₁ properties increase cardiac contractility without raising myocardial oxygen consumption whilst β₂-vasodilator properties reduce 'afterload' and increase CO. However, norepinephrine mediated α-vasoconstriction may be required to offset hypotension induced by high dose dobutamine β₂-vasodilation.
- **In systolic heart failure** most catecholamines (e.g. dopamine, dobutamine, epinephrine) effectively support the circulation. Phosphodiesterase inhibitors (e.g. milrinone, enoximone) have a role for diastolic dysfunction and catecholamine resistance (Chapter 28).
- **'Renal protection'**: Augmentation of MAP to prevent or ameliorate renal failure can be achieved with several catecholamines (e.g. dopamine, norepinephrine). The concept that drug concentration influences receptor stimulation is controversial. In particular, there is no evidence that low-concentration 'renal dose' dopamine increases renal blood flow by stimulating dopaminergic receptors. It is no longer recommended.

Other methods of circulatory support are occasionally required. Cardiac pacemakers increase CO (Chapter 28) and ventilatory support reduces cardiorespiratory work and pulmonary oedema (Chapter 16). Intra-aortic balloon pumps are valuable in IHD, VSD and whilst awaiting heart transplantation. They are sited in the descending aorta above the renal arteries. Diastolic balloon inflation enhances coronary and systemic perfusion pressures whilst systolic deflation increases CO by reducing afterload. Complications include renal and mesenteric ischaemia, infection and aortic dissection. Left ventricular assist devices are currently being developed.

11 Failure of oxygenation and respiratory failure

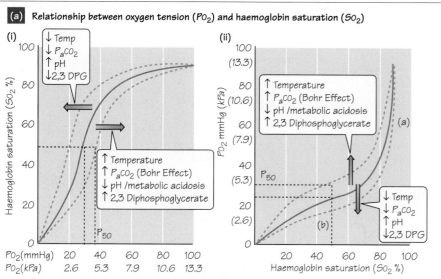

(a) Relationship between oxygen tension (PO_2) and haemoglobin saturation (SO_2)

(i)

↓ Temp
↓ P_aCO_2
↑ pH
↓2,3 DPG

↑ Temperature
↑ P_aCO_2 (Bohr Effect)
↓ pH /metabolic acidosis
↑ 2,3 Diphosphoglycerate

(ii)

↑ Temperature
↑ P_aCO_2 (Bohr Effect)
↓ pH /metabolic acidosis
↑ 2,3 Diphosphoglycerate

↓ Temp
↓ P_aCO_2
↑ pH
↓2,3 DPG

PO_2(mmHg)	20	40	60	80	100
PO_2(kPa)	2.6	5.3	7.9	10.6	13.3

Left: traditional oxyhaemoglobin curve showing effect of temperature, pH and 2,3 diphosphoglycerate.
Right: realigned to show its two key features (a) haemoglobin maintains high levels of saturation despite falling oxygen tension (i.e. pick up of oxygen in the lung is maintained despite reduced oxygen tension) (b) oxygen tension remains fairly stable as oxyhaemoglobin saturation falls (i.e. oxygen delivery to tissues maintained despite falling oxyhaemoglobin saturation)

(b) Pathophysiological mechanisms of tissue hypoxia

Arterial Hypoxaemia
1. Low inspired partial pressure of oxygen (e.g. high altitude)
2. Alveolar hypoventilation (e.g. drugs, sleep apnoea)
3. Ventilation/perfusion mismatch (e.g. patchy consolidation)
4. Right to left shunts (e.g. atrial septal defect, PAVM)

Failure of oxygen-haemoglobin transport
1. Inadequate tissue perfusion
2. Low haemoglobin concentration (e.g. anaemia)
3. Reduced oxygen dissociation (e.g. haemoglobinopathies)
4. Failure of oxygen utilisation (e.g. sepsis, cyanide poisoning)

(d) Effect of true shunt (Q_S/Q_T) and ventilation/perfusion mismatch on the arterial oxygen tension (P_aO_2) and inspired oxygen fraction (F_iO_2) relationship

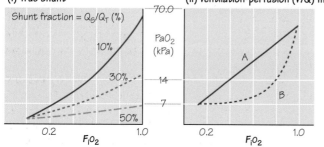

(i) True shunt

Shunt fraction = Q_S/Q_T (%)

10%
30%
50%

(ii) Ventilation-perfusion (V/Q) mismatch

70.0
PaO_2 (kPa)
A
B
14
7

Hypoxaemia caused by true right to left shunt is refractory to supplemental O_2 when 'shunt fraction' exceeds 30%

Reductions in P_aCO_2 caused by V/Q mismatch respond to O_2 but the response depends on whether there are many units with mild V/Q mismatch (A) or a few units with very low V/Q ratios (B)

(c) Alveolar oxygen tension and alveolar-arterial oxygen tension difference

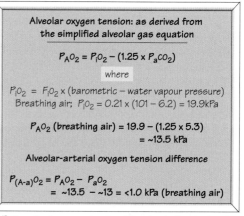

Alveolar oxygen tension: as derived from the simplified alveolar gas equation

$$P_AO_2 = P_iO_2 - (1.25 \times P_aCO_2)$$

where

$P_iO_2 = F_iO_2 \times$ (barometric − water vapour pressure)
Breathing air; $P_iO_2 = 0.21 \times (101 - 6.2) = 19.9$ kPa

P_AO_2 (breathing air) $= 19.9 - (1.25 \times 5.3)$
$= \sim 13.5$ kPa

Alveolar-arterial oxygen tension difference

$$P_{(A-a)}O_2 = P_AO_2 - P_aO_2$$
$$= \sim 13.5 - \sim 13 = <1.0 \text{ kPa (breathing air)}$$

P_AO_2 = alveolar oxygen tension, P_iO_2 = Inspired oxygen tension, F_iO_2 = fractional concentration of oxygen in inspired air, $P_{(A-a)}O_2$ = alveolar-arterial oxygen tension difference, P_aO_2 = arterial oxygen tension, P_aCO_2 = arterial CO_2 tension

(e) Calculation of shunt fraction or venous admixture (Q_S/Q_T)

$$Q_S/Q_T = (C_cO_2 - C_aO_2) / (C_cO_2 - C_vO_2)$$

Where C denotes oxygen content and c, a and v denote end capillary, arterial or venous
(end capillary and calculated alveolar oxygen tensions are assumed to be equivalent)

$$C_{c,a,v}O_2 = [(Hb \times S_aO_2 \times k) + (P_aO_2 \times 0.023)]$$

Where: Hb = haemoglobin (g/l); k= coefficient of Hb oxygen binding capacity (1.36 ml O_2/g Hb); $P_aO_2 \times 0.023$ = oxygen dissolved in plasma*

Venous admixture in a man breathing air with a Hb 100 g/L, S_aO_2 85% and S_vO_2 50% is:
$$Q_S/Q_T = ([100 \times 0.98 \times 1.36] - [100 \times 0.85 \times 1.36]) / ([100 \times 0.98 \times 1.36] - [100 \times 0.5 \times 1.36]) = (135-115) / (135-68) = 0.3 = 30\% \text{ venous admixture}$$

The 'true shunt' (i.e. corrected for partial V/Q mismatch) is calculated using 100% O_2.
In this case on 100% O_2 the S_aO_2 was 95% and S_vO_2 = 60%
$$Q_S/Q_T = ([100 \times 1 \times 1.36] - [100 \times 0.95 \times 1.36]) / ([100 \times 1 \times 1.36] - [100 \times 0.6 \times 1.36]) = (136-129) / (136-82) = 0.13 = 13\% \text{ shunt}$$

Q_S/Q_T = shunt fraction; $C_{c,a,v}O_2$ = Oxygen content (ml/L); P_aO_2 = arterial O_2 tension; S_aO_2 = arterial oxygen saturation; S_vO_2 = mixed venous oxygen saturation; Hb = haemoglobin; V/Q = ventilation/perfusion ratio; P_aCO_2 = arterial CO_2 tension; Oxygen dissolved in plasma is insignificant (i.e. not included in calculations)

Tissues require oxygen for survival; and oxygen delivery (DO_2) depends on adequate ventilation, gas exchange and circulatory distribution. **Tissue hypoxia** occurs within 4 minutes of cardiorespiratory arrest as tissue, blood and lung oxygen reserves are small. **Causes** of tissue hypoxia (Fig. b) can be classified into those resulting in: (a) arterial hypoxaemia and (b) failure of the oxygen–haemoglobin transport system without arterial hypoxaemia.

Six pathophysiological mechanisms cause arterial hypoxaemia:

1 Low inspired oxygen partial pressure (Po_2) occurs at high altitude due to the reduced barometric pressure, during fires due to O_2 combustion and following toxic fume inhalation.

2 Hypoventilation: Failure to replenish alveolar O_2 as quickly as it is removed by alveolar blood uptake.

3 Shunt refers to venous blood that bypasses lung gas-exchange and passes directly into the systemic arterial system. Increasing inspired O_2 concentration (F_iO_2) has little effect on P_aO_2 when the 'true' shunt fraction exceeds 30% (Fig. d(i)).

4 Ventilation/perfusion (V/Q) mismatch is the most frequent cause of hypoxaemia even in diseases like pulmonary fibrosis where diffusion limitation might be expected to predominate. Figure d(ii) demonstrates that desaturation due to venous admixture from many lung units with mild (Fig. d(ii):A) V/Q mismatch is readily reversed with low dose oxygen, whereas that due to a few lung units with severe (Fig. d(ii):B) V/Q mismatch (i.e. very poorly ventilated units) requires high dose oxygen. Unventilated lung units produce true shunt and the resulting hypoxaemia cannot be corrected even with 100% oxygen. Figure (e) illustrates the calculation of venous admixture due to V/Q mismatch and true shunt fraction (i.e. on 100% oxygen). High V/Q units contribute to deadspace but not hypoxaemia.

5 Impaired diffusion is rarely clinically significant but reduced capillary transit time can occasionally prevent equilibration of alveolar gas with capillary blood (e.g. high cardiac output (CO), exercise).

6 Venous saturation: Venous blood with a very low S_aO_2 returning to the right heart usually has little effect on arterial P_aO_2 but in patients with impaired gas exchange (e.g. V/Q mismatch) or low CO it may reduce P_aO_2.

Clinical features of tissue hypoxia are non-specific including altered mental state, dyspnoea, hyperventilation, arrhythmias and hypotension. Nevertheless, early recognition is required for successful therapy. **Central cyanosis** is detected when deoxygenated haemoglobin is >1.5–5 g/dl. It is an unreliable indicator of hypoxia and can be absent in hypoxic, anaemic patients but apparent in normoxic, polycythaemic subjects.

The oxygen-haemoglobin relationship is usually illustrated as in Fig. a(i) but realignment as in Fig. a(ii) demonstrates its key characteristics: (a) haemoglobin saturation remains high despite marked reductions in P_aO_2 and (b) P_aO_2 remains relatively stable as saturation declines. Temperature, pH and 2,3 diphosphoglycerate modulate this relationship. Compensatory mechanisms (e.g. rightward shift of the dissociation curve) ensure adequate tissue DO_2 in chronic hypoxia.

Monitoring oxygenation (Chapter 3)
• **Arterial Po_2** (P_aO_2) is the tension driving oxygen into tissues and **arterial So_2** (S_aO_2) reflects the level of oxygen carriage by haemoglobin molecules. **Pulse oximetry** and **blood gas analysis** measure S_aO_2

and P_aO_2 respectively. These are the principal measures used to initiate, monitor and adjust oxygen therapy. However, they can be normal when tissue hypoxia is caused by low CO, anaemia or failure of oxygen utilization. In these circumstances, **mixed venous oxygen saturation** (S_vO_2) <55–60% (normally >70%) may reflect inadequate DO_2 better (Chapter 3).
• **P_aO_2/ F_iO_2 ratio** is a convenient index of oxygen exchange that adjusts for F_iO_2.
• **Alveolar-arterial oxygen gradient** ($P_{(A-a)}O_2$) determines efficiency of gas exchange. The P_AO_2 is calculated from the simplified alveolar gas equation (Fig. c), which by incorporating P_aCO_2 eliminates hypoventilation and hypercapnia as causes of hypoxaemia (i.e. high P_ACO_2 lowers P_AO_2). The A – a gradient is increased by shunts, V/Q mismatch and diffusion impairment. It is normally ~0.2–0.4 kPa but increases with age and F_iO_2.
• **Individual organ ischaemia** is difficult to detect. Most techniques have significant limitations (e.g. gastric tonometry).

Respiratory failure (RF) may be acute, chronic or acute-on-chronic. It is due to inadequate gas exchange and is defined as an arterial oxygen (P_aO_2) <8 kPa or arterial carbon dioxide (P_aCO_2) >6 kPa. These patients must be carefully monitored (e.g. S_aO_2, respiratory rate) in an area commensurate with clinical need and treatment directed at the underlying cause:
• **Type I RF; is due to failure of oxygenation:** It occurs when blood bypasses or is not fully oxygenated in the lungs causing **hypoxaemia** (i.e. low P_aO_2). P_aCO_2 is normal or low because ventilation is unchanged or increased due to breathlessness. **Causes** (see hypoxaemia above) include V/Q mismatch (e.g. pneumonia), right to left shunts (e.g. heart defects), low F_iO_2 (e.g. altitude) and diffusion impairment (e.g. during exercise in pulmonary fibrosis). P_aO_2 is usually improved with oxygen therapy (Chapter 12) but re-expansion/recruitment of collapsed alveoli and reduction of V/Q mismatch may be equally effective (Chapters 12, 16). For example continuous positive airways pressure may improve oxygenation by recruiting collapsed lung in acute lung injury.
• **Type II RF; is due to failure of ventilation:** Hypoventilation reduces CO_2 clearance causing **hypercapnia** (high P_aCO_2) with, or occasionally, without hypoxaemia. Hypoventilation is either due to inadequate respiratory drive or ineffective ventilation. **Causes** include neuromuscular weakness (e.g. motor neurone disease), chest wall deformity (e.g. kyphoscoliosis), impaired respiratory drive (e.g. opioid overdose) and excessive work of breathing (WoB) due to primary lung disease (e.g. COPD). In critical illness, the WoB required to ventilate abnormal lungs may be >30% of total O_2 consumption (normally <5%). Ventilation is improved and WoB reduced by treating the precipitating cause, decreasing airways resistance (e.g. bronchodilation) and improving compliance (e.g. alveolar recruitment). If hypercapnia and acidosis persist, non-invasive ventilation (NIV) is often effective and widely available (Chapter 14).

Indications for intubation and mechanical ventilation in RF include a RR > 35/min, P_aO_2 < 8kPa on >50% F_iO_2; P_aCO_2 > 7.5 kPa, pH < 7.25, decreased conscious level (GCS < 8), inadequate secretion clearance, exhaustion and failure to improve within 1–4 hours with NIV.

(a) Indications for acute oxygen therapy

1. Cardiac and respiratory arrest
2. Hypoxaemia (P_aO_2 < 8kPa, S_aO_2 < 90%)
3. Hypotension (systolic BP < 100mmHg)
4. Low cardiac output
5. Metabolic acidosis (bicarbonate < 18mmol/l)
6. Respiratory distress (respiratory rate > 24/min)

(b) Oxygen prescription chart

Drug: Oxygen Circle target oxygen saturation 88–92% 92–98% (94–98%) Other Starting device/flow rate _NC 2l/min_ PRN/(Continuous) (see O_2 guidelines) Tick here if saturation not indicated* __ Signature and date _PPolly 4/8/09_ PRINT NAME Dr Pretty Polly	Time (h)	Date/time administered Initials and S_aO_2		
		4/8	5/8	
	06	RL 94%	RL 92%	
	09	RL 90%		
	14	RL 94%		
	18	RL 95%		
	22	RL 94%		

*Saturation is indicated in most cases except palliative terminal care
NC = nasal cannulae

(d) Indications for acute oxygen therapy

1. Variable performance devices

Air is entrained during breathing whilst oxygen is delivered from a reservoir (i.e. mask, reservoir bag, nasopharynx)

The F_iO_2 delivered to the lungs depends on the oxygen flow rate, the patient's inspiratory flow, respiratory rate and the amount of air entrained

e.g. Figure (i) 'Low-flow face masks', O_2 flows at ~2–10 L/min into the mask and is supplemented by air drawn into the mask. The F_iO_2 achieved depends on ventilation

Ventilation = 5 L/min
O_2 flow = 2 L/min; Air (21% O_2) flow = 3 L/min
F_iO_2 = (2+0.21 × 3)/5 × 100 = **53%**

Ventilation = 25 L/min
O_2 flow = 2 L/min; Air (21% O_2) flow = 23 L/min
F_iO_2 = (2+0.21 × 23)/25 × 100 = **27%**

These devices cannot be used if accurate control of F_iO_2 is desirable, e.g. COPD with hypercapnia

Examples of variable performance devices are 'low-flow' facemasks (see i), nasal cannulae (see ii) and non-rebreathing facemasks with reservoir bags (see iii)

2. Fixed performance devices

Are independent of the patient's pattern of breathing and inspiratory volume

Figure (iv) illustrates that a fixed O_2 flow through a Venturi valve entrains the correct proportion of air to achieve the required O_2 concentration

This system delivers more gas than is inspired (i.e. >30 L/min). Consequently, F_iO_2 is less affected by the breathing pattern. The resulting masks are high flow, low concentration and fixed performance

Used in patients with COPD and respiratory failure to avoid CO_2 retention

(c) Risks associated with high dose oxygen therapy

1. **Carbon dioxide retention:**
   ~10% of breathless patients, mainly COPD, have type II respiratory failure (RF). ~40–50% of COPD patients are at risk of type II RF
2. **Rebound hypoxaemia:**
   occurs if oxygen is suddenly withdrawn in type II RF
3. **Absorption collapse**
   O_2 in poorly ventilated alveoli is rapidly absorbed causing collapse; whereas N_2 absorption is slow
4. **Pulmonary oxygen toxicity**
   F_iO_2>60% may damage alveolar membranes causing ARDS if inhaled for > 24–48hrs (chapter 26). Hyperoxia can cause coronary and cerebral vasospasm
5. **Fire**
   Deaths and burns occur in smokers during O_2 therapy
6. **Paul-Bert effect**
   Hyperbaric O_2 can cause cerebral vasoconstriction and epileptic fits

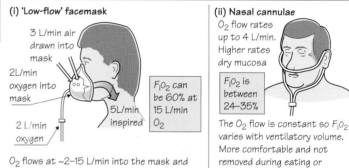

(i) 'Low-flow' facemask

3 L/min air drawn into mask
2L/min oxygen into mask
2 L/min oxygen
5L/min inspired
F_iO_2 can be 60% at 15 L/min O_2

O_2 flows at ~2–15 L/min into the mask and is supplemented by air drawn into the mask. Flow rate must be > 5 L/min to prevent CO_2 rebreathing

(ii) Nasal cannulae

O_2 flow rates up to 4 L/min. Higher rates dry mucosa

F_iO_2 is between 24–35%

The O_2 flow is constant so F_iO_2 varies with ventilatory volume. More comfortable and not removed during eating or coughing. O_2 inhaled even when mouth breathing

(iii) Non-rebreathing and anaesthetic masks

One way valve stops exhaled air entering reservoir bag
Reservoir bag
O_2 flow 10–15 L/min
F_iO_2 is 60–100% at O_2 flow rates of 10–15 L/min

High (10–15 L/min) flow rates of O_2 provide high F_iO_2 > 60% and up to 100%

Non-rebreathing masks have a reservoir bag which should be filled before use. They increase F_iO_2 by preventing O_2 loss during expiration

(iv) 'High-flow' (Venturi), low concentration facemask

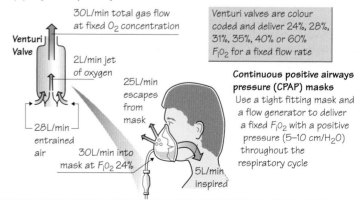

30L/min total gas flow at fixed O_2 concentration
Venturi Valve
2L/min jet of oxygen
25L/min escapes from mask
28L/min entrained air
30L/min into mask at F_iO_2 24%
5L/min inspired

Venturi valves are colour coded and deliver 24%, 28%, 31%, 35%, 40% or 60% F_iO_2 for a fixed flow rate

Continuous positive airways pressure (CPAP) masks
Use a tight fitting mask and a flow generator to deliver a fixed F_iO_2 with a positive pressure (5–10 cm/H_2O) throughout the respiratory cycle

Management of arterial hypoxaemia requires: (a) treatment of the cause (e.g. pneumonia); (b) supplemental oxygen to increase inspired oxygen concentration (F_iO_2); and (c) reduction of V/Q mismatch (Chapter 11) by ensuring optimal ventilation, sputum clearance, bronchodilation and alveolar recruitment.

Oxygen therapy

Oxygen is widely available and commonly prescribed. When given correctly it is a life-saving drug, but it is often used without appropriate evaluation of potential benefits and side effects. Figure (a) lists indications for initiating oxygen therapy. It should be prescribed on the drug chart (i.e. dose, delivery method, duration, target saturation), signed for by the doctor and documented by the nursing staff at each drug round (Fig. b). Initial oxygen saturation (S_aO_2) and associated F_iO_2 should be recorded. In emergency situations oxygen is often started without prescription but therapy should be documented retrospectively. Immediate 'ABCDE' assessment (i.e. airway, breathing, circulation) is essential and confirms airway patency and good circulation.

Figure (d) illustrates the important features of oxygen delivery systems. The therapeutic aims of oxygen therapy depend on the risk of developing hypercapnic respiratory failure (HCRF):

• **In normal patients** (i.e. low risk of HCRF) aim to achieve a S_aO_2 of 94–98% if aged <70 years and 92–98% if aged >70 years (i.e. wider normal range in the elderly). These ranges are on the plateau of the oxygen–haemoglobin dissociation curve where haemoglobin is fully saturated. Consequently, increasing P_aO_2 further has no impact on oxygen delivery as little oxygen is dissolved in plasma.

• **In patients at risk of hypercapnic respiratory failure** (e.g. neuromuscular disease, COPD) the target saturation should be 88–92% pending arterial blood gas (ABG) analysis. A higher S_aO_2 has few advantages but results in hypoventilation, hypercapnia and respiratory acidosis in patients dependent on hypoxaemic respiratory drive.

Initial oxygen dose and delivery method depends on cause:

• **High dose supplemental oxygen (>60%)** is delivered through a non-rebreathing, reservoir mask at 10–15 L/min. It is given during cardiac or respiratory arrests, shock, major trauma, sepsis, carbon monoxide (CO) poisoning and other critical illness. Once clinical stability has been restored, the oxygen dose is reduced, whilst maintaining a S_aO_2 of 92–98%. Seriously ill patients at risk of HCRF are initially treated with high dose oxygen pending ABG analysis.

• **Moderate dose supplemental oxygen (40–60%)** is given in serious illnesses (e.g. pneumonia), through nasal cannulae (2–6 L/min) or simple facemasks (5–10 L/min), aiming for a S_aO_2 of 92–98% (see above). A reservoir mask is substituted if target saturations are not achieved. Those at risk of HCRF (e.g. COPD) are managed as below.

• **Low-dose (controlled) supplemental oxygen (24–28%)** is delivered through a fixed performance Venturi mask. It is indicated in patients at risk of HCRF including COPD, neuromuscular disease, chest wall disorders, morbid obesity and cystic fibrosis. Long-term smokers, >50 years old, with exertional dyspnoea and without another cause for breathlessness are treated as COPD. The target saturation is 88–92% whilst awaiting ABG results. If P_aCO_2 is normal, S_aO_2 is adjusted to 92–98% (except in patients with previous HCRF) and ABG

rechecked at 1 hour. If an air compressor is not available, nebulizers are driven with oxygen but only for 6 minutes to limit the risk of HCRF. A raised P_aCO_2 and bicarbonate with normal pH suggests long-standing hypercapnia and the target S_aO_2 should be 88–92% with repeat ABG at 1 hour. If the patient is hypercapnic (P_aCO_2 > 6 kPa) and acidotic (pH < 7.35) consider non-invasive ventilation (NIV), especially if the acidosis has persisted for >30 minutes despite appropriate medical treatment. Venturi masks are replaced with nasal cannulae (1–2 L/min) when the patient is stable. An oxygen alert card and Venturi mask are issued to patients with previous HCRF to warn future emergency staff of the potential risk.

Oxygen therapy is of little benefit in 'normoxic' patients because haemoglobin is fully saturated and oxygen solubility is low even at high P_aO_2. Early restoration of tissue blood flow is often more important in these cases. In myocardial infarction, drug overdoses, metabolic disorders, hyperventilation or during labour in non-hypoxic pregnant women oxygen therapy is of little value. It may be harmful in normoxic patients with strokes, paraquat poisoning, bleomycin lung injury or acid inhalation and to the foetus in normoxic obstetric emergencies. However, in **CO poisoning** high dose oxygen is essential, despite a normal P_aO_2, to reduce carboxyhaemoglobin half-life (Chapter 57). Figure (c) reports the dangers of oxygen therapy.

Monitoring S_aO_2 should be measured regularly in all breathless patients and recorded on the observation chart with the oxygen dosage. In unstable patients, S_aO_2 is monitored continuously in high dependency areas. S_aO_2 is observed for 5 minutes after starting or changing oxygen dose and adjusted to achieve the target saturation. If possible, an ABG is measured before and within 1 hour of starting oxygen therapy, especially in those at risk of HCRF, and then at intervals to assess therapeutic response.

Stop oxygen therapy when the patient is clinically stable on low dose oxygen (e.g. 1–2 L/min) and S_aO_2 is within the desired range on two consecutive occasions. Monitor S_aO_2 for 5 minutes after stopping oxygen and recheck at 1 hour. If S_aO_2 remains within the desired range, oxygen has been safely discontinued.

Other techniques to improve oxygenation

1 Anaemia: Failure of tissue oxygen delivery is best corrected by blood transfusion (Chapter 4).

2 Secretion retention requires physiotherapy, mucolytic agents (e.g. N-acetylcysteine) and occasionally bronchoscopy to remove impacted sputum plugs and improve alveolar ventilation.

3 Fluid restriction reduces alveolar oedema in settings of increased alveolar permeability (e.g. ARDS).

4 Alveolar recruitment improves oxygenation by reducing V/Q mismatch and shunt (Chapter 11). Simple postural changes may improve oxygenation. Sitting upright optimizes V/Q matching in the alert patient. Regular turning and prone positioning improve secretion drainage and oxygenation in supine patients. Techniques that increase mean alveolar pressures (e.g. PEEP, CPAP, increased I:E ratio) also improve alveolar recruitment and oxygenation (Chapters 16, 35).

5 Ventilatory support (e.g. NIV) improves oxygenation by correcting hypoventilation and associated hypercapnia (Chapter 14).

13 Airways obstruction and management

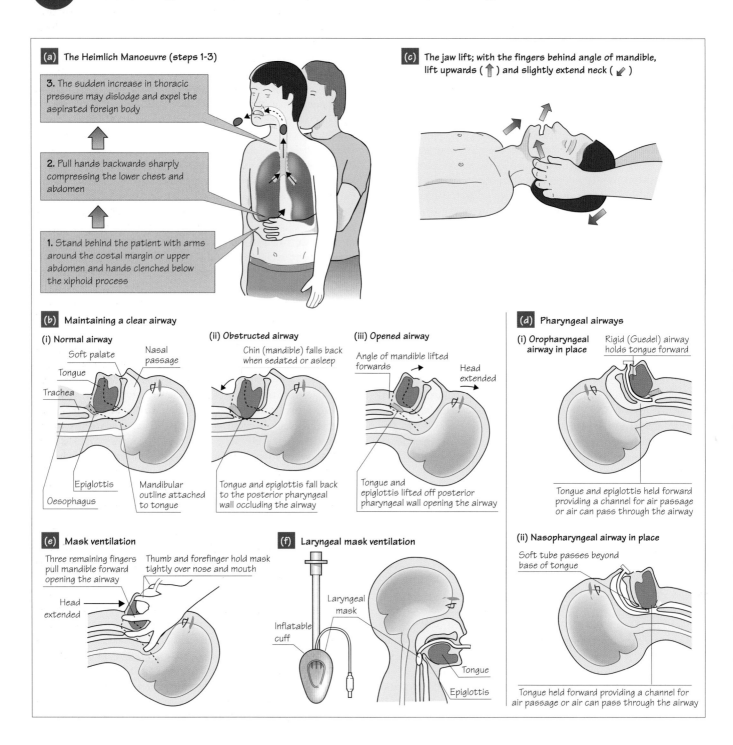

(a) The Heimlich Manoeuvre (steps 1-3)

3. The sudden increase in thoracic pressure may dislodge and expel the aspirated foreign body

2. Pull hands backwards sharply compressing the lower chest and abdomen

1. Stand behind the patient with arms around the costal margin or upper abdomen and hands clenched below the xiphoid process

(c) The jaw lift; with the fingers behind angle of mandible, lift upwards (↑) and slightly extend neck (↙)

(b) Maintaining a clear airway

(i) Normal airway
Soft palate
Nasal passage
Tongue
Trachea
Epiglottis
Oesophagus
Mandibular outline attached to tongue

(ii) Obstructed airway
Chin (mandible) falls back when sedated or asleep
Tongue and epiglottis fall back to the posterior pharyngeal wall occluding the airway

(iii) Opened airway
Angle of mandible lifted forwards
Head extended
Tongue and epiglottis lifted off posterior pharyngeal wall opening the airway

(d) Pharyngeal airways

(i) Oropharyngeal airway in place
Rigid (Guedel) airway holds tongue forward
Tongue and epiglottis held forward providing a channel for air passage or air can pass through the airway

(ii) Nasopharyngeal airway in place
Soft tube passes beyond base of tongue
Tongue held forward providing a channel for air passage or air can pass through the airway

(e) Mask ventilation
Three remaining fingers pull mandible forward opening the airway
Thumb and forefinger hold mask tightly over nose and mouth
Head extended

(f) Laryngeal mask ventilation
Laryngeal mask
Inflatable cuff
Tongue
Epiglottis

Airways obstruction is a life-threatening emergency and is particularly perilous when cardiorespiratory function is compromised. Within minutes it causes arterial hypoxaemia, hypoxic brain injury, coma and death. Consequently, all emergency personnel must be able to establish and maintain a patent airway and ventilation.

Upper airways obstruction (UAO)

Complete or partial UAO may occur at any level in the respiratory tract from the mouth to the trachea.

• **Complete obstruction** is characterized by absent air flow and breath sounds, chest wall intercostal recession, accessory muscle use and

34 *Acute and Critical Care Medicine at a Glance, 2e.* By R. Leach. Published 2009 by Blackwell Publishing. ISBN 978-1-4051-6139-8.

paradoxical abdominal movement (i.e. as the chest inflates the abdomen is pulled in, rather than the normal abdominal movement outwards as the diaphragm descends).
• **Partial obstruction** reduces air flow despite increased respiratory effort and is usually noisy. Inspiratory stridor suggests laryngeal obstruction, snoring follows partial nasopharyngeal occlusion by the tongue (± palate), a distressing 'crowing' occurs during laryngeal spasm and expiratory wheeze indicates airways obstruction.

Recognition of airways obstruction utilizes the 'look, listen and feel' approach:
• **Look** for respiratory effort, paradoxical chest and abdominal wall movement, accessory muscle use (e.g. neck, shoulder) and tracheal tug. Examine the mouth for the cause of the obstruction (e.g. foreign bodies, secretions). Central cyanosis is a late sign.
• **Listen and feel** for airflow and reduced, absent, noisy or characteristic (e.g. stridor) breath sounds. Movement of air at the patient's mouth is detected by placing your cheek or hand immediately in front of the patient's mouth.
Oropharyngeal obstruction is often caused by the tongue, which falls backwards when normal muscle tone is reduced in drowsy, sedated or unconscious patients, obstructing normal airflow. Solid particulate matter (e.g. food, coins, teeth or vomit), laryngeal oedema (e.g. allergy, burns, inflammation), tumours and laryngeal spasm (e.g. due to foreign bodies, blood, secretions, inhaled toxic gas) also cause oropharyngeal obstruction.
   Tracheobronchial obstruction is caused by aspiration of particulate matter, bronchospasm, tumours or pulmonary oedema.

Airways management

In many cases of UAO, simple measures open the airway and aid ventilation. These include:
• **The Heimlich Manoeuvre** (Fig. a): following aspiration of an object (e.g. food, marble) that completely occludes the larynx or trachea, the subject is unable to speak or breathe and becomes rapidly cyanosed; a scenario that is characteristically termed the 'café coronary' when partially masticated food is aspirated during swallowing. If a sharp blow to the back of the chest fails to dislodge the object, the Heimlich manoeuvre is attempted. The attendant stands behind the patient with his arms around the upper abdomen, just adjacent to the costal margin, and the hands clenched below the xiphoid process. The hands are pulled backwards sharply, compressing the upper abdomen and lower costal margin. The sudden increase in thoracic pressure may dislodge the object, which is then exhaled.
• **Airway clearance:** foreign bodies (e.g. dentures) and secretions are detected and removed by sweeping the index finger around the oral cavity. Head tilt, chin lift and jaw thrust (Fig. b), slightly extend the neck and lift the mandible forward, relieving nasopharyngeal obstruction due to the tongue and upper airway structures. This restores the airway and airflow. Jaw thrust is the technique of choice in patients with potential cervical spine injury (Fig. c).

• **Mechanical oropharyngeal airways** are firm plastic tubes, inserted through the nose and mouth, to bypass the relaxed tongue and establish an airway when manipulation of the mandible and neck is unsuccessful. They are useful during mask ventilation (see below), especially in edentulous patients.
   • **Rigid oropharyngeal (Guedel) airway:** lifts the tongue and epiglottis away from the posterior pharyngeal wall (Fig. d(i)) and serves as a 'bite-block' to reduce damage during jaw clenching. The airway is inserted upside down and rotated 180° into the functional position. Care is required to avoid damaging the teeth or increasing obstruction by pushing the tongue backwards. Guedel airways should only be used in obtunded patients as they provoke gag reflexes, vomiting and laryngospasm and are removed when consciousness returns.
   • **Soft nasopharyngeal airways (SNPA):** firm (but compressible) tubes available in different sizes and diameters. After insertion they extend beyond the base of the tongue creating an airway and facilitating nasopharyngeal secretion removal (Fig. d(ii)). As they provoke less gag reflex SNPA are useful in alert patients. Topical nasal anaesthesia and lubrication (e.g. lidocaine (lignocaine) gel) reduce insertion discomfort although traumatic epistaxis is not uncommon. Continuous use risks infective (e.g. sinusitis) and erosive complications. Contraindications to SNPA include coagulopathy, nasal obstruction and basilar skull fractures.
• **Mask ventilation:** enables ventilatory support and supplemental oxygen delivery in non-intubated patients. In conjunction with jaw lift, the increased oropharyngeal pressure delivered during ventilation alleviates UAO. **Anaesthetic facemasks** are available in many shapes and sizes to ensure a tight fit. An oropharyngeal airway alleviates difficulty associated with edentulous patients. Firm downward pressure on the mask with the thumb and forefinger maintains a seal whilst the mandible is simultaneously lifted with the three remaining fingers and the head extended to optimize the airway during ventilation (Fig. e). A two-handed technique with an assistant to squeeze the bag may be required. Unfortunately, mask ventilation may occasionally be impossible.
• **Laryngeal mask airways:** useful when intubation fails or is difficult. They sit over the laryngeal inlet allowing temporary positive pressure ventilation in sedated or obtunded patients (Fig. f). Potential problems (e.g. aspiration, laryngospasm, gastric inflation, poor ventilation) limit ICU use.
• **Combitube:** an oesophageal-tracheal double lumen airway for use in pre-hospital emergencies by those without specialist airways skills. It is blindly inserted into the oropharynx up to the indicated markings and following inflation of the appropriate cuffs may aid ventilation.
If a patent airway and adequate ventilation cannot be achieved, **endotracheal intubation** performed by an appropriately trained clinician is indicated (Chapter 15). Occasionally an **emergency cricothyroidotomy** or **surgical tracheostomy** is required to establish an airway (Chapter 17).

14 Non-invasive ventilation

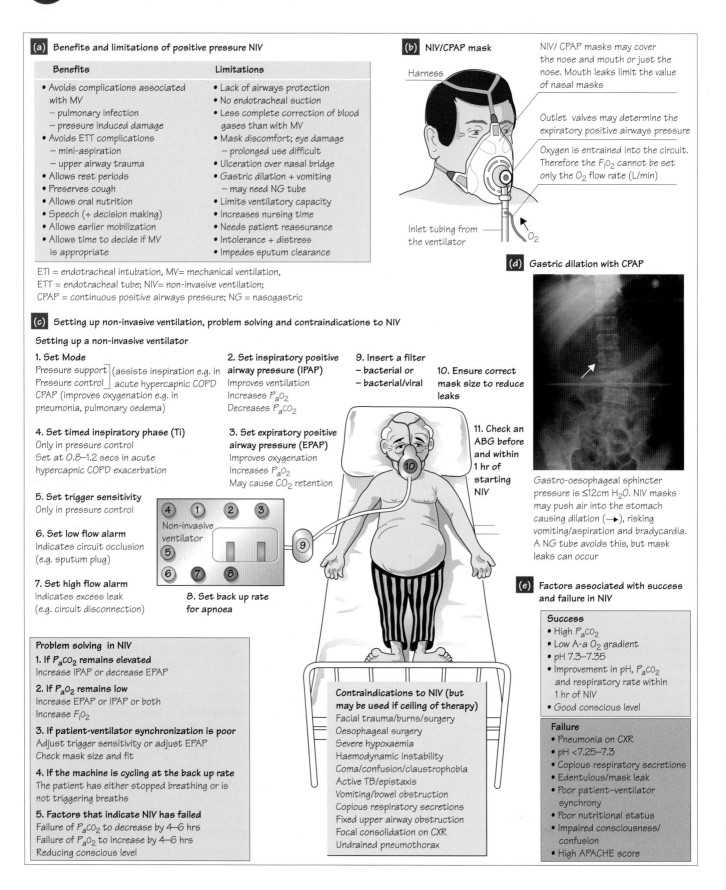

(a) Benefits and limitations of positive pressure NIV

Benefits	Limitations

• Avoids complications associated with MV
  – pulmonary infection
  – pressure induced damage
• Avoids ETT complications
  – mini-aspiration
  – upper airway trauma
• Allows rest periods
• Preserves cough
• Allows oral nutrition
• Speech (+ decision making)
• Allows earlier mobilization
• Allows time to decide if MV is appropriate
	• Lack of airways protection
	• No endotracheal suction
	• Less complete correction of blood gases than with MV
	• Mask discomfort; eye damage
	  – prolonged use difficult
	• Ulceration over nasal bridge
	• Gastric dilation + vomiting
	  – may need NG tube
	• Limits ventilatory capacity
	• Increases nursing time
	• Needs patient reassurance
	• Intolerance + distress
	• Impedes sputum clearance

ETI = endotracheal intubation, MV= mechanical ventilation,
ETT = endotracheal tube; NIV= non-invasive ventilation;
CPAP = continuous positive airways pressure; NG = nasogastric

(b) NIV/CPAP mask

Harness

NIV/ CPAP masks may cover the nose and mouth or just the nose. Mouth leaks limit the value of nasal masks

Outlet valves may determine the expiratory positive airways pressure

Oxygen is entrained into the circuit. Therefore the F_iO_2 cannot be set only the O_2 flow rate (L/min)

Inlet tubing from the ventilator

O_2

(c) Setting up non-invasive ventilation, problem solving and contraindications to NIV

Setting up a non-invasive ventilator

1. Set Mode
Pressure support ⎤ (assists inspiration e.g. in
Pressure control ⎦ acute hypercapnic COPD
CPAP (improves oxygenation e.g. in pneumonia, pulmonary oedema)

2. Set inspiratory positive airway pressure (IPAP)
Improves ventilation
Increases P_aO_2
Decreases P_aCO_2

9. Insert a filter
– bacterial or
– bacterial/viral

10. Ensure correct mask size to reduce leaks

4. Set timed inspiratory phase (Ti)
Only in pressure control
Set at 0.8–1.2 secs in acute hypercapnic COPD exacerbation

3. Set expiratory positive airway pressure (EPAP)
Improves oxygenation
Increases P_aO_2
May cause CO_2 retention

11. Check an ABG before and within 1 hr of starting NIV

5. Set trigger sensitivity
Only in pressure control

6. Set low flow alarm
Indicates circuit occlusion (e.g. sputum plug)

Non-invasive ventilator

7. Set high flow alarm
Indicates excess leak (e.g. circuit disconnection)

8. Set back up rate for apnoea

Problem solving in NIV

1. If P_aCO_2 remains elevated
Increase IPAP or decrease EPAP

2. If P_aO_2 remains low
Increase EPAP or IPAP or both
Increase F_iO_2

3. If patient-ventilator synchronization is poor
Adjust trigger sensitivity or adjust EPAP
Check mask size and fit

4. If the machine is cycling at the back up rate
The patient has either stopped breathing or is not triggering breaths

5. Factors that indicate NIV has failed
Failure of P_aCO_2 to decrease by 4–6 hrs
Failure of P_aO_2 to increase by 4–6 hrs
Reducing conscious level

Contraindications to NIV (but may be used if ceiling of therapy)
Facial trauma/burns/surgery
Oesophageal surgery
Severe hypoxaemia
Haemodynamic instability
Coma/confusion/claustrophobia
Active TB/epistaxis
Vomiting/bowel obstruction
Copious respiratory secretions
Fixed upper airway obstruction
Focal consolidation on CXR
Undrained pneumothorax

(d) Gastric dilation with CPAP

Gastro-oesophageal sphincter pressure is ≤12cm H_2O. NIV masks may push air into the stomach causing dilation (→), risking vomiting/aspiration and bradycardia. A NG tube avoids this, but mask leaks can occur

(e) Factors associated with success and failure in NIV

Success
• High P_aCO_2
• Low A-a O_2 gradient
• pH 7.3–7.35
• Improvement in pH, P_aCO_2 and respiratory rate within 1 hr of NIV
• Good conscious level

Failure
• Pneumonia on CXR
• pH <7.25–7.3
• Copious respiratory secretions
• Edentulous/mask leak
• Poor patient–ventilator synchrony
• Poor nutritional status
• Impaired consciousness/ confusion
• High APACHE score

 Acute and Critical Care Medicine at a Glance, 2e. By R. Leach. Published 2009 by Blackwell Publishing. ISBN 978-1-4051-6139-8.

Non-invasive ventilation provides respiratory support, aids alveolar recruitment and reduces work of breathing (WoB) without the need for endotracheal intubation (ETI), laryngeal mask or tracheostomy. Negative and positive pressure techniques are available.

Negative pressure ventilation

Negative pressure ventilation (NPV) developed to support victims of poliomyelitis-induced respiratory paralysis. Affected patients were placed in **tank ventilators** ('iron lungs') sealed at the neck. Lowering tank pressures expanded the chest causing inspiration; expiration was passive. However, inadequate nursing access, poor CO_2 clearance and secretion retention with airways obstruction (± pneumonia) limited use. Current techniques include **jacket (cuirass) ventilators** which localize external negative pressure to the chest region and **rocking beds** that utilize gravity to enhance diaphragmatic movement. NPV has been superseded by positive pressure ventilation (PPV) and use is usually limited to specialist centres for rehabilitation (e.g. spinal injury) or chronic hypoventilation (e.g. kyphoscoliosis).

Positive pressure ventilation

Positive pressure ventilation is particularly effective in acute respiratory failure. It is delivered through the upper airway using full facemasks or helmets (Fig. b). Nasal masks are more comfortable in stable patients. Figure (a) lists the benefits and disadvantages. PPV is most successful in alert, co-operative, haemodynamically stable patients who can protect and clear their airways (Fig. e):

1 **Non-invasive ventilation (NIV)** refers to PPV which assists inspiration. Pressure controlled (PC) modes of ventilation compensate for mask leaks and have largely replaced volume controlled modes (Chapter 16). Tidal volume is determined by lung (± chest wall) compliance and circuit resistance.

• **Pressure support (PS):** the patient determines breath timing and frequency as respiratory effort 'triggers' the ventilator on and off (i.e. assisted spontaneous breathing). Only pressure (~10–30 cmH$_2$O) is adjusted to support inspiration. Most PS ventilators incorporate a back up breath rate of 6–8/min to ensure ventilation in patients who make no respiratory effort.

• **Bi-level pressure support** combines inspiratory positive airways pressure (IPAP; ~30 cmH$_2$O) to aid inspiration and expiratory positive airways pressure (EPAP; ~5 cmH$_2$O) to recruit underventilated lung and stent open upper airways. EPAP also offsets intrinsic positive end expiratory pressure (PEEP) which aids ventilator triggering (Chapter 34). These ventilators are simple to use, cheap and have been used in most major studies.

• **Pressure controlled ventilation:** the decelerating flow of a PC breath improves distribution of ventilation. Inflation pressure, frequency and inspiratory time (T_i) are selected according to patient requirements (e.g. T_i is usually set at ~0.8–1.2 seconds in acute hypercapnic COPD). A preset number of mandatory breaths are delivered in the absence of patient effort. Although patient triggering can occur, delivered breaths are identical to mandatory breaths. Triggered breaths delay the next machine-determined breath (i.e. synchronization), the spontaneous/timed (S/T) mode on NIV machines.

2 **Continuous positive airways pressure (CPAP)** is maintained throughout inspiration and expiration (e.g. 5–10 cm/H$_2$O) by a flow generator; it does not assist inspiration. Resulting alveolar recruitment (i.e. inflation of collapsed lung) reduces V/Q mismatch and improves oxygenation. Consequently CPAP is most successful in cardiogenic pulmonary oedema or acute lung injury (ALI). In obstructive sleep apnoea (OSA) it prevents upper airways collapse during sleep. Although CPAP is not usually considered respiratory support, the increase in functional residual capacity reduces WoB by making the lungs easier to inflate (i.e. the steep upstroke of the lung pressure–volume relationship). In patients with hyperinflation due to airways obstruction further increases in lung volume may be detrimental, but by offsetting intrinsic PEEP (e.g. in COPD), CPAP can reduce WoB, increase ventilation and reduce $P_a CO_2$ (Chapters 33, 34).

Indication for NIV and CPAP

NIV is most beneficial in patients with respiratory acidosis (pH < 7.35; H$^+$ > 45 nmol/L). Arterial blood gas (ABG) measurement is usually required in patients with acute breathlessness, neuromuscular disease, chest wall deformity, obesity or acute confusional states. Before starting, decide whether NIV will be the ceiling of treatment (e.g. end-stage COPD) or a therapeutic trial leading to ETI in the event of failure. Figure (c) illustrates how to optimize NIV and lists contraindications to NIV. A trial of NIV/CPAP is required if ABG do not rapidly improve with oxygen and medical therapy in patients with:

1 **Acute hypercapnic respiratory failure:**
• **COPD exacerbations** – mortality, ETI rates and complications (e.g. pneumonia) are substantially reduced with early NIV. In addition, pH, $P_a CO_2$ and respiratory rate usually improve within 1 hour.
• **Neuromuscular disease and chest wall deformity (e.g. kyphoscoliosis)** – NIV is the treatment of choice in acute decompensation. In chronic respiratory failure, home NIV achieves 80% 5-year survival depending on bulbar involvement and severity.

2 **Cardiogenic pulmonary oedema:** CPAP reduces mortality and ETI rates in patients who are hypoxaemic despite maximal medical treatment. NIV is less effective and used when CPAP is unsuccessful.

3 **Obstructive sleep apnoea:** CPAP and NIV are equally effective in decompensated OSA. Bi-level pressure support is required in patients with respiratory acidosis.

4 **Weaning:** NIV may aid weaning of COPD patients from mechanical ventilation.

5 **Other conditions:** NIV is used with varying success in chest wall trauma, ALI, post-operative respiratory failure and pneumonia. It should only be used in critical care units in patients for ETI if NIV fails.

6 **When ETI is considered inappropriate** (e.g. end-stage respiratory disease).

Monitoring includes clinical evaluation (e.g. comfort, conscious level, respiratory rate, chest wall motion), continuous $S_a O_2$ monitoring (i.e. $S_a O_2$ 88–92% with oxygen therapy) and ABG measurements 1 hour after starting NIV and at 4–6 hours if the earlier sample showed little improvement.

Treatment success and failure (Fig. c and e) Patients who benefit from NIV are ventilated as much as possible during the first 24 hours, with breaks for meals, drugs and physiotherapy. A nasogastric tube prevents gastric distension and reduces aspiration risk (Fig. d). Benefit is usually evident at 1 hour and certainly after 4–6 hours of NIV. The point at which treatment is considered to have failed and should be withdrawn, or ETI considered, depends on severity of respiratory failure, patient wishes and whether other factors (e.g. secretions) could be better managed following ETI. **Follow-up:** spirometry and ABG are measured before discharge in those who benefit. Patients with chronic hypercapnic hypoventilation (e.g. obesity) should be referred for home NIV assessment.

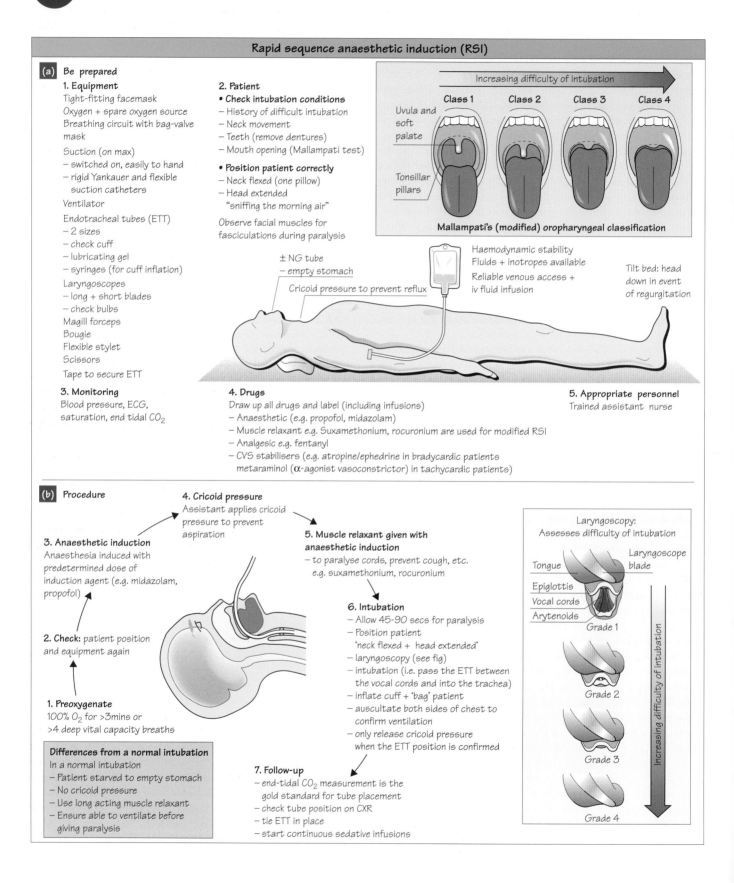

Rapid sequence anaesthetic induction (RSI)

(a) **Be prepared**

1. Equipment
Tight-fitting facemask
Oxygen + spare oxygen source
Breathing circuit with bag-valve mask
Suction (on max)
– switched on, easily to hand
– rigid Yankauer and flexible suction catheters
Ventilator
Endotracheal tubes (ETT)
– 2 sizes
– check cuff
– lubricating gel
– syringes (for cuff inflation)
Laryngoscopes
– long + short blades
– check bulbs
Magill forceps
Bougie
Flexible stylet
Scissors
Tape to secure ETT

2. Patient
• **Check intubation conditions**
– History of difficult intubation
– Neck movement
– Teeth (remove dentures)
– Mouth opening (Mallampati test)

• **Position patient correctly**
– Neck flexed (one pillow)
– Head extended "sniffing the morning air"

Observe facial muscles for fasciculations during paralysis

± NG tube
– empty stomach

Cricoid pressure to prevent reflux

Haemodynamic stability
Fluids + inotropes available
Reliable venous access + iv fluid infusion

Tilt bed: head down in event of regurgitation

Increasing difficulty of intubation

Class 1   Class 2   Class 3   Class 4

Uvula and soft palate

Tonsillar pillars

Mallampati's (modified) oropharyngeal classification

3. Monitoring
Blood pressure, ECG, saturation, end tidal CO_2

4. Drugs
Draw up all drugs and label (including infusions)
– Anaesthetic (e.g. propofol, midazolam)
– Muscle relaxant e.g. Suxamethonium, rocuronium are used for modified RSI
– Analgesic e.g. fentanyl
– CVS stabilisers (e.g. atropine/ephedrine in bradycardic patients
  metaraminol (α-agonist vasoconstrictor) in tachycardic patients)

5. Appropriate personnel
Trained assistant nurse

(b) **Procedure**

3. Anaesthetic induction
Anaesthesia induced with predetermined dose of induction agent (e.g. midazolam, propofol)

2. Check: patient position and equipment again

1. Preoxygenate
100% O_2 for >3mins or >4 deep vital capacity breaths

4. Cricoid pressure
Assistant applies cricoid pressure to prevent aspiration

5. Muscle relaxant given with anaesthetic induction
– to paralyse cords, prevent cough, etc.
  e.g. suxamethonium, rocuronium

6. Intubation
– Allow 45–90 secs for paralysis
– Position patient 'neck flexed + head extended'
– laryngoscopy (see fig)
– intubation (i.e. pass the ETT between the vocal cords and into the trachea)
– inflate cuff + 'bag' patient
– auscultate both sides of chest to confirm ventilation
– only release cricoid pressure when the ETT position is confirmed

7. Follow-up
– end-tidal CO_2 measurement is the gold standard for tube placement
– check tube position on CXR
– tie ETT in place
– start continuous sedative infusions

Laryngoscopy:
Assesses difficulty of intubation

Tongue   Laryngoscope blade
Epiglottis
Vocal cords
Arytenoids
Grade 1
Grade 2
Grade 3
Grade 4

Increasing difficulty of intubation

Differences from a normal intubation
In a normal intubation
– Patient starved to empty stomach
– No cricoid pressure
– Use long acting muscle relaxant
– Ensure able to ventilate before giving paralysis

Most intubations in critically ill patients are emergency procedures rendered particularly hazardous by haemodynamic instability, hypovolaemia, hypoxaemia, co-existing disease and potential aspiration of stomach contents. Whenever possible, appropriately trained clinicians, skilled in airways management, should perform endotracheal intubation (ETI). However, in order to assist during emergencies, all critical care team members should be familiar with basic airways management (Chapter 13), ETI techniques and failed intubation drills.

Indications for ETI

- **Clinical indications** include respiratory failure (Chapter 11), airways protection from aspiration of oral secretions or gastric contents, decreased conscious level (Glasgow Coma Score ≤8), sputum clearance, upper airways obstruction and surgical procedures.
- **Objective measures** suggesting the need for ventilatory support and ETI (if non-invasive ventilation is not possible), include a respiratory rate >35/min; vital capacity <15 ml/kg; $P_aO_2 < 8\,kPa$ on >50% O_2 and $P_aCO_2 > 7.5\,kPa$ (except in chronic retainers).

Preparation for ETI (Fig. a)

- **Airways assessment** only predicts ~50% of difficult ETI (incidence ≤1:65). **History:** when feasible, review anaesthetic notes and ask about previous difficult ETI. **General examination:** assesses cardio-respiratory status including oxygen therapy requirements. Patients with obesity, short necks, distorted neck anatomy (e.g. goitres), beards or pregnancy often present problems. **Airway examination:** evaluates features associated with difficult ETI including: (a) absence of key anatomical landmarks during oropharyngeal inspection with tongue protrusion (e.g. faucial pillars, soft palate, uvula) as described in Mallampati's modified classification (Fig. a); (b) short thyromental distance (i.e. <3 fingerbreadths or 6 cm from thyroid cartilage to chin); (c) restricted mouth opening (i.e. <4 cm); (d) reduced neck extension; (e) oral factors (e.g. large tongue, buck teeth).
- **Routes of intubation:** oral endotracheal tubes are preferred in most circumstances. They are relatively wide which reduces airways resistance and improves secretion clearance. Nasotracheal tubes are rarely used (e.g. oral trauma).
- **Preparation for ETI:** all equipment and drugs must be immediately available (Fig. a). Intravenous access is established and fluid (± electrolyte correction) commenced but clinical circumstances rarely permit full resuscitation in emergencies. **Preoxygenation** increases the time available before desaturation fivefold and is achieved using tight fitting facemasks to deliver 100% O_2 (Chapters 12, 13). **Suction apparatus:** is required to clear oropharyngeal secretions. **Laryngoscopes:** enable laryngeal visualization (Fig. b). In adults curved Macintosh blades are most popular. **Endotracheal tubes (ETT):** should be available in a number of sizes. The usual tube size in adult males is 8–9 mm (internal diameter in mm) and 7–8 mm in adult females. Most ETT have low-pressure, high-volume cuffs to limit tracheal mucosal damage. **Drugs:** include anaesthetic, analgesic, muscle relaxant and vasoactive agents (e.g. atropine, ephedrine, metaraminol) because most anaesthetic agents are vasodilators. **Monitoring equipment:** should include capnography for end-tidal CO_2 measurement.

Intubation

All critically ill patients are assumed to be at high risk of aspiration (i.e. full stomach) because fasting status is either unknown or <6 hours and/or gastric emptying may be impaired (e.g. obstruction, diabetic or opiate-induced gastric paresis). These patients require rapid sequence rather than normal induction.

- **Rapid sequence induction (RSI;** Fig. b) rapidly secures the airway after loss of consciousness reducing the risk of aspiration. Following preoxygenation, an induction agent (e.g. propofol) is administered, quickly followed by a rapidly acting muscle relaxant (e.g. suxamethonium). Simultaneously, an assistant applies anterior pressure to the cricoid cartilage, which closes the oesophagus preventing gastric regurgitation (Sellick manoeuvre). The patient is positioned with the **neck flexed** (i.e. one pillow beneath the occiput) and **head extended** ('sniffing the morning air') to align the glottis, pharynx and oral cavity and achieve the best view on laryngoscopy. Intubation rapidly follows *without mask ventilation*. Cricoid pressure is released only after confirmation of correct tube placement and cuff inflation. A **modified RSI** using a non-depolarizing muscle relaxant (e.g. rocuronium) is recommended in situations where suxamethonium is contraindicated (i.e. hyperkalaemia in renal failure, neuromuscular disorders, trauma).
- **Normal intubation** differs from RSI in that the patient is usually stable (i.e. haemodynamically, metabolically), fasted for >6 hours to ensure an empty stomach, does not require cricoid pressure and mask ventilation is established before giving the muscle relaxant, then continued for 2–3 minutes to ensure complete paralysis before intubation.

Difficult intubation

- **Difficult intubation aids** include **gum elastic bougies/flexible stylets** which aid ETI when the tracheal opening is anterior to the visual axis. **Fibreoptic endoscopy, video laryngoscopes:** allow direct visualization of intubation. **Specialist laryngoscope blades** (e.g. McCoy blade) lift the epiglottis improving the laryngoscopic view.
- **Failed intubation drill (FID):** initial intubation attempts fail in ≤1:300 intubations. The FID is as follows:
  1. Summon experienced help. Consider waking the patient, but this may not be an option in emergencies.
  2. Mask-ventilate the patient, or if this is not possible consider laryngeal mask ventilation (Chapter 13), until senior help arrives.
  3. If ventilation is inadequate with these methods consider an emergency cricothyroidotomy (Chapter 17).

Experienced personnel may consider alternative approaches to intubation (e.g. fibreoptic endoscopy).

Complications

ETI complications include failure, oesophageal intubation, hypoxaemia, gastric aspiration, bronchospasm and trauma (e.g. lips, teeth, mucosa, vocal cords, cervical spine).

Endotracheal tube (ETT) care

ETT position is checked on CXR and the tip should be level with the lower border of the clavicles. The right main bronchus is intubated if the ETT is inserted too far, impairing ventilation of the opposite lung. The distance from the lips to the tube tip should be ~22–24 cm and the tip will move ~4 cm from full neck flexion to extension. High cuff inflation pressures (>20 cmH₂O), head movement and prolonged intubation (>7–14 days) are avoided as these cause pressure-induced ischaemic ulcers, granulation tissue and eventually tracheal stenosis. Avoid long ETT tubes which increase airways resistance and impair ventilation.

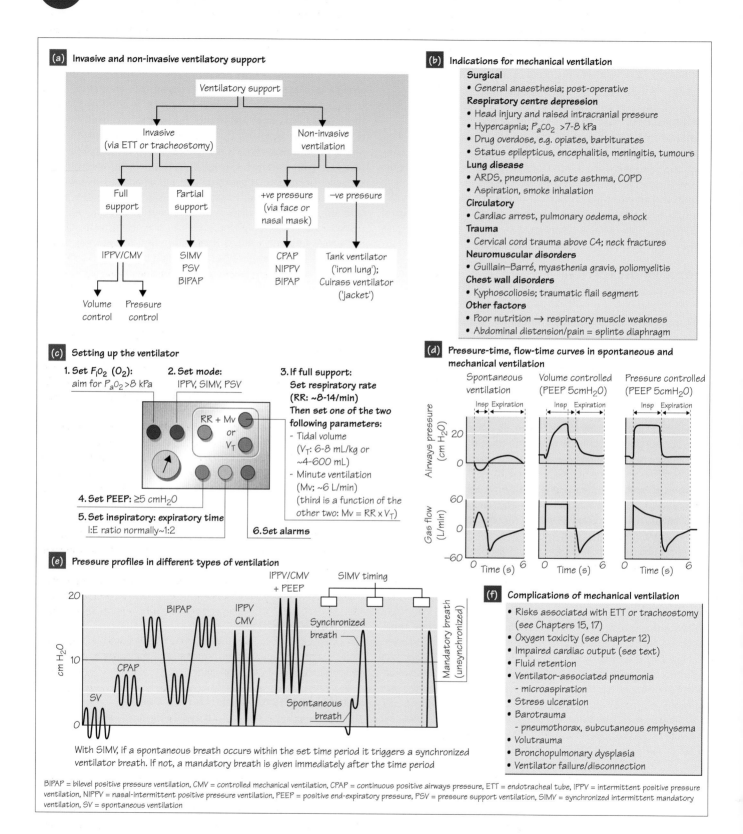

(a) Invasive and non-invasive ventilatory support

Ventilatory support

Invasive (via ETT or tracheostomy)
- Full support → IPPV/CMV → Volume control / Pressure control
- Partial support → SIMV, PSV, BIPAP

Non-invasive ventilation
- +ve pressure (via face or nasal mask) → CPAP, NIPPV, BIPAP
- −ve pressure → Tank ventilator ('iron lung'); Cuirass ventilator ('jacket')

(b) Indications for mechanical ventilation

Surgical
- General anaesthesia; post-operative

Respiratory centre depression
- Head injury and raised intracranial pressure
- Hypercapnia; P_aCO_2 >7-8 kPa
- Drug overdose, e.g. opiates, barbiturates
- Status epilepticus, encephalitis, meningitis, tumours

Lung disease
- ARDS, pneumonia, acute asthma, COPD
- Aspiration, smoke inhalation

Circulatory
- Cardiac arrest, pulmonary oedema, shock

Trauma
- Cervical cord trauma above C4; neck fractures

Neuromuscular disorders
- Guillain–Barré, myasthenia gravis, poliomyelitis

Chest wall disorders
- Kyphoscoliosis; traumatic flail segment

Other factors
- Poor nutrition → respiratory muscle weakness
- Abdominal distension/pain = splints diaphragm

(c) Setting up the ventilator

1. Set F_iO_2 (O_2): aim for P_aO_2 >8 kPa
2. Set mode: IPPV, SIMV, PSV
3. If full support:
   Set respiratory rate (RR: ~8-14/min)
   Then set one of the two following parameters:
   - Tidal volume (V_T: 6-8 mL/kg or ~4-600 mL)
   - Minute ventilation (Mv; ~6 L/min)
   (third is a function of the other two: Mv = RR x V_T)
   RR + Mv or V_T
4. Set PEEP: ≥5 cmH$_2$O
5. Set inspiratory: expiratory time I:E ratio normally ~1:2
6. Set alarms

(d) Pressure-time, flow-time curves in spontaneous and mechanical ventilation

Spontaneous ventilation | Volume controlled (PEEP 5cmH$_2$O) | Pressure controlled (PEEP 5cmH$_2$O)

Airways pressure (cm H$_2$O): 20, 0
Gas flow (L/min): 60, 0, −60
Time (s): 0 ... 6
Insp / Expiration

(e) Pressure profiles in different types of ventilation

cmH$_2$O: 0, 10, 20

SV, CPAP, BIPAP, IPPV CMV, IPPV/CMV + PEEP, SIMV timing
Synchronized breath, Spontaneous breath
Mandatory breath (unsynchronized)

With SIMV, if a spontaneous breath occurs within the set time period it triggers a synchronized ventilator breath. If not, a mandatory breath is given immediately after the time period

(f) Complications of mechanical ventilation

- Risks associated with ETT or tracheostomy (see Chapters 15, 17)
- Oxygen toxicity (see Chapter 12)
- Impaired cardiac output (see text)
- Fluid retention
- Ventilator-associated pneumonia
  - microaspiration
- Stress ulceration
- Barotrauma
  - pneumothorax, subcutaneous emphysema
- Volutrauma
- Bronchopulmonary dysplasia
- Ventilator failure/disconnection

BIPAP = bilevel positive pressure ventilation, CMV = controlled mechanical ventilation, CPAP = continuous positive airways pressure, ETT = endotracheal tube, IPPV = intermittent positive pressure ventilation, NIPPV = nasal-intermittent positive pressure ventilation, PEEP = positive end-expiratory pressure, PSV = pressure support ventilation, SIMV = synchronized intermittent mandatory ventilation, SV = spontaneous ventilation

During critical illness, ventilatory support (Fig. a) may be required to maintain gas exchange and reduce WoB. Mechanical ventilation (MV) is usually delivered through an endotracheal tube or tracheostomy and provides complete or partial respiratory support. Non-invasive ventilation (NIV) aids spontaneous ventilation (SV) and avoids the need for endotracheal intubation (Chapter 14).

Indications for mechanical ventilation (Fig. b)

The main indication for MV, excluding surgical procedures, is respiratory failure. However, its value in the support of other organs, especially during shock or cardiac failure, is increasingly being recognized. Apart from in emergencies (e.g. cardiac arrest), the difficult decision is when and whether to ventilate a deteriorating patient. There are no simple guidelines but hypoxaemia ($P_aO_2 < 8\,kPa$ on $F_iO_2 > 0.5$), hypercapnia ($P_aCO_2 > 7.5\,kPa$), respiratory/metabolic acidosis (pH < 7.2) and physical factors (e.g. confusion, exhaustion, poor cough) may indicate the need for MV. Trends in these variables are often more helpful than absolute values. In general, MV is only appropriate when there is a reasonable chance of survival. In terminal illness, support is often limited to NIV, after discussion with the patient and/or relatives (Chapter 14).

Ventilator set-up (Fig. c)

Typical initial adult intermittent positive pressure ventilation (IPPV) settings are: tidal volume (V_T) ~6–8 ml/kg; respiratory frequency (f) ~8–14 breaths/min and minute ventilation ($M_V = V_T \times f$) ~6 L/min. F_iO_2 and M_V are adjusted to maintain $P_aO_2 > 8\,kPa$ and $P_aCO_2 < 7\,kPa$ respectively, but acceptable values depend on individual diseases. Initially PEEP is set at $\geq 5\,cmH_2O$ and the inspiratory:expiratory time (I:E) ratio at ~1:2. Disease-specific ventilatory strategies are discussed in individual chapters.

Ventilatory mode (Fig. e)

Mode of ventilation describes whether a breath is: (a) fully or partially supported; (b) volume or pressure controlled; (c) mandatory (delivered by the ventilator regardless of patient respiratory effort) or spontaneously triggered (Figs a, e). Duration of a breath may be fixed (i.e. timed) or variable (i.e. dependent on T_v delivery). Modern ventilators with microprocessor controls provide considerable flexibility allowing a change from mandatory, full-support modes to partial support modes that minimize sedation requirements and allow patients to be conscious but comfortable.

• **Full (mandatory) support modes** (e.g. IPPV, controlled mechanical ventilation (CMV)) are uncomfortable and may require sedation as no allowance is made for spontaneous respiration. They are used in severe respiratory disease, in circulatory instability or when respiratory drive is absent. Volume or pressure-controlled (VC, PC) modes are available but the pattern of gas flow in PC ventilation achieves better gas exchange.
  • **Volume-controlled IPPV/CMV** (Fig. d) is often used postoperatively. Each breath is delivered at a preset volume over a fixed time. Airway pressure varies with lung compliance.
  • **Pressure-controlled IPPV/CMV** (Fig. d) delivers preset pressures and there is no direct control of T_v, which depends on inspiratory time, lung compliance and airways resistance. PC ventilation protects lungs by limiting peak inspiratory pressures (PIP) and encourages alveolar recruitment.
• **Partial support modes** 'support' spontaneous ventilation and are preferable as they reduce sedation requirements. Breaths are patient initiated and detected by sensitive flow/pressure triggers in the ventilator, which then provides inspiratory support.
  • **Assist control** – the ventilator delivers a breath when triggered by inspiratory effort or independently if the patient does not breathe within a certain time.
  • **Synchronized intermittent mandatory ventilation (SIMV)** – delivers a set number of mechanically imposed breaths to achieve a minimum M_V but also allows pressure-supported spontaneous breathing. Imposed breaths are reduced as the patient becomes ventilator independent during weaning.
  • **Pressure support** – a preset pressure supports each spontaneous breath. The patient determines breath rate. Gradual pressure reductions make it a comfortable and effective mode of weaning (Chapter 17).
• **Positive end-expiratory pressure (PEEP)** describes a positive pressure, maintained throughout expiration that increases functional residual capacity (i.e. alveolar recruitment), prevents alveolar collapse at end expiration, reduces V/Q mismatch and decreases alveolar oedema by increasing lymphatic drainage. PEEP improves oxygenation for any given mode of ventilation, provided that CO is not significantly reduced by the associated increase in intrathoracic pressure.

Physiological responses to mechanical ventilation

1 Cardiovascular responses are due to alveolar overdistention and two effects of increased intrathoracic pressure (IP):
  • **Right ventricular (RV) preload reduction** is due to increased right atrial pressure which reduces venous return and RV cardiac output. However, fluid infusion rapidly restores venous return and CO.
  • **Left ventricular (LV) afterload reduction** is due to reduced LV transmural pressure, which decreases LV work. In the normal heart any beneficial effect of LV afterload reduction is offset by reduced venous return. However, in the failing heart, CO is relatively insensitive to preload changes but very sensitive to afterload reduction (Chapter 28). Consequently, MV may increase CO in heart failure, a useful therapeutic effect.

The overall response to raised IP depends on the state of the heart, vasomotor tone and fluid status (e.g. hypovolaemia). MV also increases lung volumes but overinflated alveoli compress alveolar blood vessels increasing pulmonary vascular resistance and causing pulmonary hypertension. Subsequent RV distension displaces the septum into the LV cavity, reducing LV filling and CO, an effect known as interventricular dependence.

2 Respiratory effects: MV reduces WoB, which increases the proportion of CO going to other potentially ischaemic organs. Re-expansion of collapsed alveoli also improves oxygenation. Unfortunately supine position, reduced surfactant and ventilation of poorly perfused lung increases V/Q mismatch.

3 Fluid retention is due to antidiuretic hormone secretion.

Complications of mechanical ventilation (Fig. f)

'Barotrauma' refers to pressure-induced lung damage (e.g. pneumothorax). High PIP ($>35\,cmH_2O$) due to reduced lung compliance (e.g. ARDS) may cause airways disruption and interstitial gas formation. 'Volutrauma' describes damage to healthy alveoli due to overdistention. 'Protective' ventilation strategies use low T_v (~6 ml/kg) to avoid volutrauma, PIP < 35 cmH$_2$O and maintain alveolar recruitment with PEEP > 5 cmH$_2$O (Chapter 35). Disease-specific complications are discussed in relevant chapters.

17 Respiratory management, weaning and tracheostomy

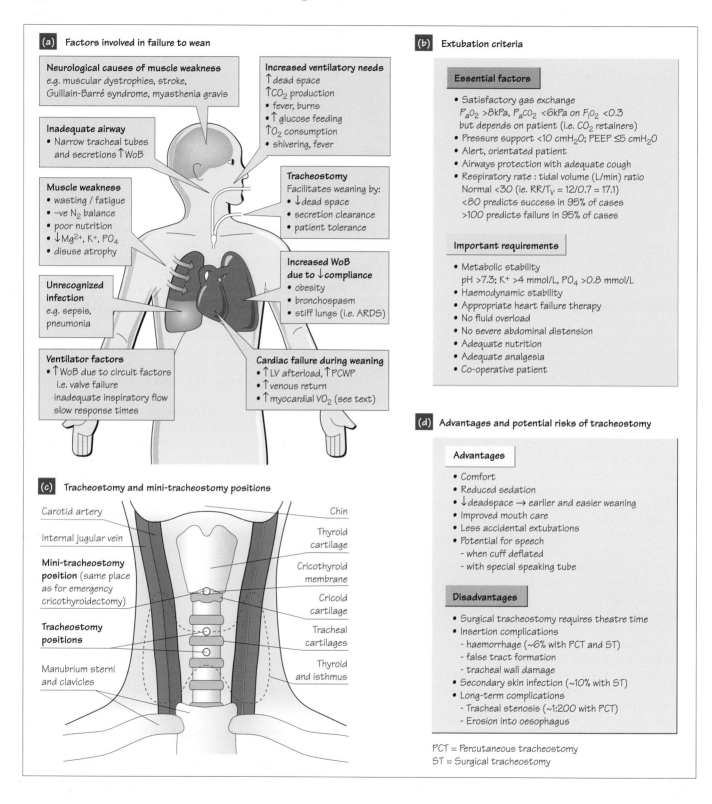

(a) Factors involved in failure to wean

Neurological causes of muscle weakness
e.g. muscular dystrophies, stroke, Guillain-Barré syndrome, myasthenia gravis

Increased ventilatory needs
- ↑dead space
- ↑CO_2 production
  - fever, burns
  - ↑glucose feeding
- ↑O_2 consumption
  - shivering, fever

Inadequate airway
- Narrow tracheal tubes and secretions ↑WoB

Muscle weakness
- wasting / fatigue
- –ve N_2 balance
- poor nutrition
- ↓Mg^{2+}, K^+, PO_4
- disuse atrophy

Tracheostomy
Facilitates weaning by:
- ↓dead space
- secretion clearance
- patient tolerance

Unrecognized infection
e.g. sepsis, pneumonia

Increased WoB due to ↓compliance
- obesity
- bronchospasm
- stiff lungs (i.e. ARDS)

Ventilator factors
- ↑WoB due to circuit factors i.e. valve failure inadequate inspiratory flow slow response times

Cardiac failure during weaning
- ↑LV afterload, ↑PCWP
- ↑venous return
- ↑myocardial VO_2 (see text)

(b) Extubation criteria

Essential factors
- Satisfactory gas exchange
  P_aO_2 >8kPa, P_aCO_2 <6kPa on F_iO_2 <0.3 but depends on patient (i.e. CO_2 retainers)
- Pressure support <10 cmH$_2$O; PEEP ≤5 cmH$_2$O
- Alert, orientated patient
- Airways protection with adequate cough
- Respiratory rate : tidal volume (L/min) ratio
  Normal <30 (ie. RR/T$_V$ = 12/0.7 = 17.1)
  <80 predicts success in 95% of cases
  >100 predicts failure in 95% of cases

Important requirements
- Metabolic stability
  pH >7.3; K^+ >4 mmol/L, PO_4 >0.8 mmol/L
- Haemodynamic stability
- Appropriate heart failure therapy
- No fluid overload
- No severe abdominal distension
- Adequate nutrition
- Adequate analgesia
- Co-operative patient

(c) Tracheostomy and mini-tracheostomy positions

Carotid artery

Internal jugular vein

Mini-tracheostomy position (same place as for emergency cricothyroidectomy)

Tracheostomy positions

Manubrium sterni and clavicles

Chin

Thyroid cartilage

Cricothyroid membrane

Cricoid cartilage

Tracheal cartilages

Thyroid and isthmus

(d) Advantages and potential risks of tracheostomy

Advantages
- Comfort
- Reduced sedation
- ↓deadspace → earlier and easier weaning
- Improved mouth care
- Less accidental extubations
- Potential for speech
  - when cuff deflated
  - with special speaking tube

Disadvantages
- Surgical tracheostomy requires theatre time
- Insertion complications
  - haemorrhage (~6% with PCT and ST)
  - false tract formation
  - tracheal wall damage
- Secondary skin infection (~10% with ST)
- Long-term complications
  - Tracheal stenosis (~1:200 with PCT)
  - Erosion into oesophagus

PCT = Percutaneous tracheostomy
ST = Surgical tracheostomy

General respiratory management includes: (i) oxygen therapy (Chapter 12); (ii) secretion clearance; (iii) treatment of infection; (iv) decreasing work of breathing (WoB) by reducing airways resistance (e.g. bronchodilator therapy) and improving compliance (e.g. oedema treatment); (v) optimizing functional residual capacity (FRC) by recruiting alveoli (e.g. CPAP) when FRC is low (e.g. pneumonia) and preventing hyperinflation and raised intrathoracic pressure (Chapters 33, 34) when FRC is high (e.g. asthma).

 Acute and Critical Care Medicine at a Glance, 2e. By R. Leach. Published 2009 by Blackwell Publishing. ISBN 978-1-4051-6139-8.

Management of ventilated patients

Important considerations are:

- **Sedation (± paralysis):** during uncomfortable ventilatory strategies to improve synchronization and prevent patients 'fighting the ventilator'. In agitated or restless subjects other problems (e.g. pneumothorax, pulmonary oedema, pain) should be excluded before administering sedation.
- **Ventilator dependence:** control of breathing is abolished in sedated (± paralysed) patients. Ventilator alarms must be set for:
  - *Minimum acceptable ventilation:* to identify ventilator disconnection/failure.
  - *Maximum acceptable airways pressures:* to avoid barotrauma.

Ventilated patients cannot compensate for metabolic derangements (e.g. hyperventilation in acidosis). Therefore, ventilator settings must be adjusted and treatment instituted (e.g. bicarbonate infusion) to correct for monitored blood gas abnormalities.

- **Airways management:** regular suctioning, physiotherapy and 'positioning' facilitate secretion clearance and prevent airways obstruction or distal alveolar collapse. Inspired gas is humidified and warmed to minimize viscid secretions. Endotracheal tube (ETT) care is essential (Chapter 15). CXR confirms ETT position and monitors ongoing respiratory disease. Bronchoscopy facilitates removal of airways obstructions (e.g. secretions), sampling (e.g. microbiology) and investigation.
- **Ventilator management (Chapters 16, 31–37)** includes:
- **'Protective' strategies** – which aim to reduce ventilator-induced damage (e.g. barotrauma) when high distending pressures are required to achieve normal tidal volumes (T_V) in diseased lungs (e.g. fibrosis, consolidation, atelectasis, ARDS). Low T_V (~6 ml/kg) ventilation and low peak inspiratory pressures (i.e. <30 cmH$_2$O) decrease both volutrauma and barotrauma respectively. Increased mean airways pressures (e.g. PEEP, CPAP) and reversed I : E ratios (i.e. >1 : 1) promote alveolar recruitment and improve oxygenation.
- **'Asthma' strategies** – which increase alveolar ventilation and CO_2 clearance by reducing gas trapping when airways resistance or FRC are high (e.g. asthma, COPD). Reduced breathing frequency and low I : E ratios (<1 : 2) increase expiratory time and hence expiratory volume. Likewise, modest PEEP levels may hold open potentially collapsible airways during expiration increasing expiratory volume. The resulting fall in FRC allows greater inspiratory volume and improves minute ventilation.
- **'Oxygenation' strategies** – which aim to reduce shunt fraction (Chapters 11, 12). Rarely, **nitric oxide,** an inhaled vasodilator, is used to increase blood flow through ventilated alveolar capillaries, briefly reducing hypoxaemia (~24 hours). Likewise, **prone positioning,** (i.e. face down) improves oxygenation in >50% of severely hypoxaemic patients with dependent consolidation by improving V/Q matching and recruiting poorly ventilated basal lung segments. Neither therapy improves survival.

Extubation and weaning

Weaning is the process of reducing and then removing respiratory support. It is usually required in patients who have undergone prolonged ventilation with associated muscle weakness. It is rarely necessary following short periods of ventilation (i.e. post-operative). A simple trial of breathing through the ETT and comparing the ratio of respiratory rate (RR) to T_V (L/min) often determines the likelihood of successful extubation. The normal RR/T_V ratio is <30 (i.e. 12/0.7 = 17.1); <80 or >100 strongly predicts success or failure, respectively. **Extubation criteria:** Fig. (b) lists essential requirements prior to extubation.

Weaning techniques improve respiratory muscle strength by slowly reducing respiratory support.

1 **Partial support modes** (Chapters 14, 16) include:
- **Synchronized intermittent mandatory ventilation (SIMV)** which allows supported spontaneous breaths between gradually decreasing mandatory (i.e. imposed) breaths.
- **Pressure support (PS) ventilation** – PS for patient triggered breaths is slowly decreased until the patient is doing all the work. A small amount of PS compensates for the work imposed by the ETT and breathing circuit.
- **Bilevel positive pressure ventilation (BIPAP)** which delivers two levels of pressure in phase with respiration. The higher pressure provides inspiratory support and augments T_V; the lower pressure is applied during expiration and increases FRC. It can be delivered via an ETT or facemask.

2 **Continuous positive airways pressure (CPAP)** increases FRC, in the same way as PEEP, in a spontaneously breathing patient (Chapter 14). It can be delivered through an ETT or facemask.

3 **Non-invasive ventilation (NIV)** allows weaning to continue after ETT removal (Chapter 14).

Potential weaning difficulties are illustrated in Fig. (a). After extubation, cardiac dysfunction and pulmonary oedema may occur due to: (i) increases in LV afterload, pulmonary capillary 'wedge' pressure and venous return (Chapter 7); or (ii) inability to sustain the increased cardiac output, myocardial oxygen consumption and work required for spontaneous breathing. Cardiac support with diuretics, after-load reduction (e.g. ACE inhibitors) and inotropes may be necessary.

Tracheostomy (Fig. c)

Despite the low pressure, high volume cuffs used in modern ETT's, prolonged intubation risks damage to the vocal cords and/or tracheal stenosis. Tracheostomy is usually advisable after 7–14 days, or earlier, if it is evident that a patient will require prolonged intubation.

- **Advantages and potential risks** are reported in Fig. (d). Bedside **percutaneous tracheostomy** has the advantages of simplicity, reduced cost, saved theatre time and fewer complications (e.g. infection, tracheal stenosis) compared to surgical tracheostomy.
- **Tracheostomy tubes (± cuffs)** are available in a variety of sizes and types. Some have inner tubes that facilitate cleaning, prevent obstruction and reduce the frequency of tube changes (i.e. ~30 days). Others have long flanges for obese necks.
- **Removal** follows a period of cuff deflation and tube capping to ensure respiratory independence. The remaining stoma is covered with an airtight dressing and heals with a few days.
- **Mini-tracheostomy:** a small tube (~5 mm) is inserted through the cricothyroid membrane (Fig. c), through which a suction catheter can be passed. They are useful for short-term secretion clearance when cough or conscious level is temporarily impaired in high dependency areas.

(a) Calculating arterial oxygen partial pressure (PaO₂) from the alveolar gas equation

The simplified alveolar gas equation

$$P_AO_2 = F_iO_2 (P_b - P_{H_2O}) - (1.25 \times P_aCO_2)$$

Breathing air at sea-level where P_b ~101 kPa

$$P_AO_2 = 0.21 (101 - 6.2) - (1.25 \times 5.3)$$
$$= 19.9 - 6.63 = \text{~13-14 kPa}$$

P_aO_2 slightly lower than P_AO_2 because of normal shunt fraction (~3%) ~12.5-13 kPa

Thus, P_AO_2 (and P_bO_2) breathing air at 4500 m altitude where Pb ~53 kPa will be ~7-8 kPa

P_AO_2 = alveolar oxygen tension,
F_iO_2 = fractional concentration of oxygen in inspired air,
P_b = barometric pressure,
P_{H_2O} = water vapour pressure (6.2 kPa),
P_aO_2 = arterial oxygen tension,
P_aCO_2 = arterial CO₂ tension

(b) The bicarbonate buffer system and the Henderson-Hasselbach equation

The bicarbonate buffer system

Carbonic anhydrase
$$CO_2 + H_2O \leftrightarrow H_2CO_3 \leftrightarrow HCO_3^- + H^+$$

The Henderson-Hasselbach equation

→ $K = [HCO_3^-] \times [H^+] / [H_2CO_3]$
  From the law of mass action
  K = dissociation constant

→ $K_A = [HCO_3^-] \times [H^+] / [H_2CO_3]$
  At equilibrium $[CO_2] \alpha [H_2CO_3]$
  K_A = corrected dissociation constant

→ $\log K_A = \log [H^+] + \log ([HCO_3^-] / [CO_2])$

→ $-\log [H^+] = -\log K_A + \log ([HCO_3^-] / [CO_2])$

→ $pH = pK_A + \log ([HCO_3^-] / [CO_2])$
  (Henderson-Hasselbach equation)

(c) The relationship between pH, HCO₃⁻ and PCO₂

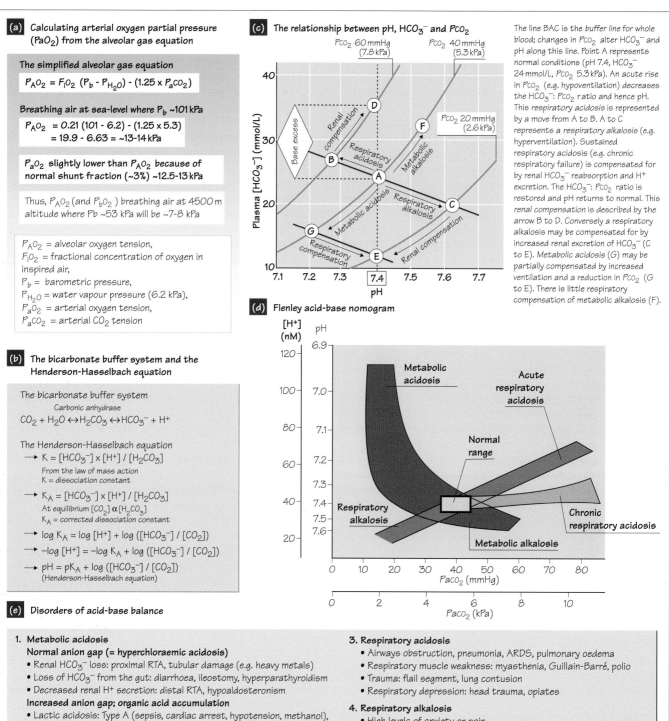

The line BAC is the buffer line for whole blood; changes in PCO₂ alter HCO₃⁻ and pH along this line. Point A represents normal conditions (pH 7.4, HCO₃⁻ 24 mmol/L, PCO₂ 5.3 kPa). An acute rise in PCO₂ (e.g. hypoventilation) decreases the HCO₃⁻: PCO₂ ratio and hence pH. This respiratory acidosis is represented by a move from A to B. A to C represents a respiratory alkalosis (e.g. hyperventilation). Sustained respiratory acidosis (e.g. chronic respiratory failure) is compensated for by renal HCO₃⁻ reabsorption and H⁺ excretion. The HCO₃⁻: PCO₂ ratio is restored and pH returns to normal. This renal compensation is described by the arrow B to D. Conversely a respiratory alkalosis may be compensated for by increased renal excretion of HCO₃⁻ (C to E). Metabolic acidosis (G) may be partially compensated by increased ventilation and a reduction in PCO₂ (G to E). There is little respiratory compensation of metabolic alkalosis (F).

(d) Flenley acid-base nomogram

(e) Disorders of acid-base balance

1. Metabolic acidosis
Normal anion gap (= hyperchloraemic acidosis)
- Renal HCO₃⁻ loss: proximal RTA, tubular damage (e.g. heavy metals)
- Loss of HCO₃⁻ from the gut: diarrhoea, ileostomy, hyperparathyroidism
- Decreased renal H⁺ secretion: distal RTA, hypoaldosteronism

Increased anion gap; organic acid accumulation
- Lactic acidosis: Type A (sepsis, cardiac arrest, hypotension, methanol), Type B (insulin deficiency, metformin, decreased hepatic metabolism)
- Ketoacidosis: insulin deficiency (e.g. diabetic ketoacidosis), starvation
- Exogenous acids: salicylates

2. Metabolic alkalosis
- H⁺ loss: vomiting, renal loss (with hypokalaemia, hyperaldosteronism), diuretics, low Cl⁻ states
- HCO₃⁻ gain: sodium HCO₃⁻ (excess antacid), lactate, citrate administration

3. Respiratory acidosis
- Airways obstruction, pneumonia, ARDS, pulmonary oedema
- Respiratory muscle weakness: myasthenia, Guillain-Barré, polio
- Trauma: flail segment, lung contusion
- Respiratory depression: head trauma, opiates

4. Respiratory alkalosis
- High levels of anxiety or pain
- Altitude
- Excessive mechanical ventilation
- Respiratory stimulants: salicylate overdose
- Pulmonary embolism, asthma, oedema

HCO₃⁻ = bicarbonate, H⁺ = hydrogen ion, RTA = renal tubular acidosis, Cl⁻ = chloride ion, ARDS = acute respiratory distress syndrome

Arterial blood gases (ABG)

Understanding ABG is essential to the management of acutely ill patients. Full interpretation requires knowledge of the clinical context, serum electrolyte concentrations and occasionally serum albumin and lactate levels. The blood gas analyser typically displays the following

1 Arterial partial pressure of oxygen (P_aO_2), which is measured directly. Its relationship with the fractional inspired oxygen concentration (F_iO_2) is described by the alveolar gas equation (Fig. a). When breathing air at sea level (i.e. barometric pressure ~101 kPa) the partial pressure of inspired oxygen (P_iO_2) is ~21 kPa. This falls to ~19.9 kPa when fully saturated with water in the upper airways. In the alveolus, oxygen is taken up and replaced with CO_2, which reduces the alveolar oxygen partial pressure (P_AO_2) to ~13–14 kPa. The P_aO_2 is slightly lower than the P_AO_2 due to the normal pulmonary shunt fraction (~3%). Normal P_aO_2 is ~13 kPa (~100 mmHg) at the age of 20 years and ~11 kPa at 65 years.

2 Arterial partial pressure of carbon dioxide (P_aCO_2), which is measured directly and is normally ~5.3 kPa (40 mmHg).

3 pH, the negative logarithm$_{10}$ of the hydrogen ion concentration ([H$^+$] = 40 nM = pH 7.4).

4 Standard bicarbonate, which is calculated from the CO_2 and pH using the Henderson–Hasselbach equation (Fig. b). It is the concentration of bicarbonate [HCO$_3^-$] in a sample equilibrated to 37 °C and P_aCO_2 5.3 kPa. It allows assessment of the metabolic component of acid–base balance. Normal values are ~21–27 mmol/L.

5 Actual bicarbonate, which reflects the contribution of both respiratory and metabolic components. In venous blood the normal value is 21–28 mmol/l.

6 Base excess (BE), which is a measure of the amount of acid or alkali (in mmol/L) that must be added to a sample, under standard conditions (37 °C, P_aCO_2 5.3 kPa), to return the pH to 7.4. It quantifies metabolic acid–base status by comparing the 'corrected' HCO$_3^-$ with the 'normal' HCO$_3^-$ (i.e. ~24 mmol/L at pH 7.4). It is calculated automatically from pH and P_aCO_2 and adjusted for haemoglobin. The normal range is +2 mmol/L to −2 mmol/L.

A simple method to analyse arterial blood gases

1 Note the P_aO_2 and F_iO_2.

2 Assess pH: a pH outside the normal range defines acidaemia (<7.35) or alkalaemia (>7.45).

3 Assess the respiratory component: P_aCO_2 > 6 kPa (45 mmHg) defines respiratory acidosis, P_aCO_2 < 4.5 kPa (35 mmHg) defines respiratory alkalosis.

4 Assess the metabolic component: HCO$_3^-$ > 33 mmol/L defines metabolic alkalosis, HCO$_3^-$ < 23 mmol/L defines metabolic acidosis.

5 Determine if there is metabolic or respiratory compensation: see section 'Acid–base balance' below.

6 Consider the anion gap (AG): this is the difference between the sum of serum sodium and potassium ion concentrations (cations) and sum of serum chloride and bicarbonate ions concentration (anions): [(Na$^+$) + (K$^+$)] − [(Cl$^-$) + (HCO$_3^-$)]. The normal AG (~12 ± 2 mmol/L) is a reflection of the kidney excreted mineral acids (e.g. phosphates). An increased AG indicates an accumulation of anions including keto-, lactic and exogenous (i.e. salicylates) acids. A normal or reduced AG (i.e. hyperchloraemic acidosis) suggests HCO$_3^-$ loss or renal tubular acidosis.

Acid–base balance

Maintenance of a stable hydrogen ion concentration (45–35 nM) or pH between 7.35 and 7.45 is essential for intracellular enzyme function. Normally acids are generated by the hydration of CO_2 ('respiratory acids') or metabolic processes ('metabolic' acids; typically phosphoric, sulphuric and lactic). In disease states [H$^+$] can rise due to lactate production (e.g. ischaemia), ketoacid generation (e.g. diabetes), alcohol ingestion (e.g. methanol) or failure of normal excretion (e.g. renal, respiratory or liver failure). Loss of H$^+$ (e.g. vomiting) or HCO$_3^-$ (e.g. diarrhoea) also effects acid–base balance. **Causes** are listed in Fig. (e).

Control of acid–base balance

The body prevents pH changes by regulating two pathways for eliminating acid; respiratory and renal. However, ~100 times more acid equivalents are expired each day in the form of CO_2/carbonic acid than are excreted as fixed acids by the kidneys. **Buffers** bind or release H$^+$ according to the pH; this limits the change in pH that occurs when acid is added. The relationship between the amount of acid added to a buffer-containing solution and the change in pH is known as the **buffer line** (Fig. c). Buffers are most effective when pH is close to their pK_A (log of the dissociation constant K_A; Fig. b). The most important blood buffers systems are:

1 Bicarbonate (HCO$_3^-$; Fig. b): CO_2 combines with water to form carbonic acid (H$_2$CO$_3$) which dissociates to HCO$_3^-$ and H$^+$. The relationship between pH, PCO$_2$ and [HCO$_3^-$] is described by the Henderson–Hasselbach equation. In normal blood, [HCO$_3^-$] is 24 mmol/L, PCO$_2$ 5.3 kPa and pH calculates to 7.4. If the ratio [HCO$_3^-$]:PCO$_2$ remains at 20, pH will remain at 7.4. Although the pK_A of the bicarbonate system (6.1) is further away from the blood pH (7.4) than would seem ideal for a buffer, the fact that PCO$_2$ and HCO$_3^-$ can be independently controlled by ventilation and the kidneys respectively means that in practice it makes an effective buffer system.

2 Haemoglobin (Hb): particularly when deoxygenated. It significantly improves buffering capacity in whole blood compared with plasma. All other blood proteins have <20% of the buffering capacity of Hb.

The relationship between pH, HCO$_3^-$ and PCO$_2$ (Fig. c)

This is illustrated using Davenport diagrams (Fig. c). Acute CO_2 changes cause **respiratory acidosis or alkalosis**. When CO_2 changes persist (e.g. type 2 respiratory failure) pH is slowly corrected by renal compensation (i.e. increase/decrease [HCO$_3^-$]). The terms **metabolic acidosis and alkalosis** are used to describe alterations in acid–base status due to changes in HCO$_3^-$ rather than CO_2: – as a result, for example, of renal disease or increased H$^+$ production (e.g. diabetic ketoacidosis). A metabolic acidosis may be partially compensated by increased ventilation. However, there is little respiratory compensation for a metabolic alkalosis which may require unsustainable falls in ventilation. **Mixed metabolic and respiratory** acid–base disorders may occur. For example respiratory acidosis due to respiratory failure (i.e. increased PCO$_2$) may be combined with a metabolic acidosis due to the associated hypoxia. The **Flenley nomogram** is a useful diagnostic aid as only one type of disturbance is likely if pH and PCO$_2$ fall within a band (Fig. d).

19 Analgesia, sedation and paralysis

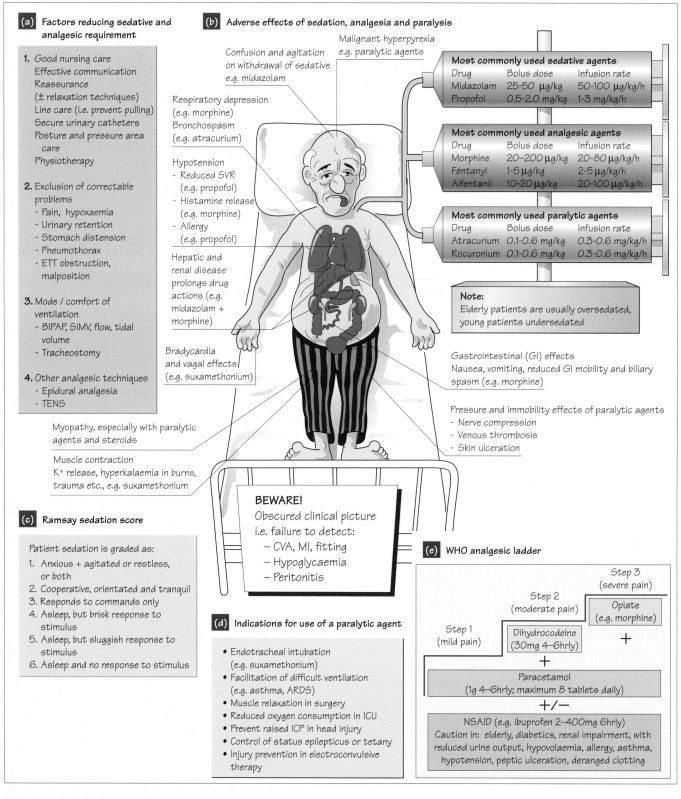

(a) Factors reducing sedative and analgesic requirement

1. Good nursing care
   Effective communication
   Reassurance
   (± relaxation techniques)
   Line care (i.e. prevent pulling)
   Secure urinary catheters
   Posture and pressure area care
   Physiotherapy

2. Exclusion of correctable problems
   - Pain, hypoxaemia
   - Urinary retention
   - Stomach distension
   - Pneumothorax
   - ETT obstruction, malposition

3. Mode / comfort of ventilation
   - BIPAP, SIMV, flow, tidal volume
   - Tracheostomy

4. Other analgesic techniques
   - Epidural analgesia
   - TENS

(b) Adverse effects of sedation, analgesia and paralysis

Confusion and agitation on withdrawal of sedative e.g. midazolam

Malignant hyperpyrexia e.g. paralytic agents

Respiratory depression (e.g. morphine)
Bronchospasm (e.g. atracurium)

Hypotension
- Reduced SVR (e.g. propofol)
- Histamine release (e.g. morphine)
- Allergy (e.g. propofol)

Hepatic and renal disease prolongs drug actions (e.g. midazolam + morphine)

Bradycardia and vagal effects (e.g. suxamethonium)

Myopathy, especially with paralytic agents and steroids

Muscle contraction
K⁺ release, hyperkalaemia in burns, trauma etc., e.g. suxamethonium

Gastrointestinal (GI) effects
Nausea, vomiting, reduced GI mobility and biliary spasm (e.g. morphine)

Pressure and immobility effects of paralytic agents
- Nerve compression
- Venous thrombosis
- Skin ulceration

Most commonly used sedative agents		
Drug	Bolus dose	Infusion rate
Midazolam	25-50 µg/kg	50-100 µg/kg/h
Propofol	0.5-2.0 mg/kg	1-3 mg/kg/h

Most commonly used analgesic agents		
Drug	Bolus dose	Infusion rate
Morphine	20–200 µg/kg	20-80 µg/kg/h
Fentanyl	1-5 µg/kg	2-5 µg/kg/h
Alfentanil	10-20 µg/kg	20-100 µg/kg/h

Most commonly used paralytic agents		
Drug	Bolus dose	Infusion rate
Atracurium	0.1-0.6 mg/kg	0.3-0.6 mg/kg/h
Rocuronium	0.1-0.6 mg/kg	0.3-0.6 mg/kg/h

Note:
Elderly patients are usually oversedated, young patients undersedated

BEWARE!
Obscured clinical picture i.e. failure to detect:
– CVA, MI, fitting
– Hypoglycaemia
– Peritonitis

(c) Ramsay sedation score

Patient sedation is graded as:
1. Anxious + agitated or restless, or both
2. Cooperative, orientated and tranquil
3. Responds to commands only
4. Asleep, but brisk response to stimulus
5. Asleep, but sluggish response to stimulus
6. Asleep and no response to stimulus

(d) Indications for use of a paralytic agent

- Endotracheal intubation (e.g. suxamethonium)
- Facilitation of difficult ventilation (e.g. asthma, ARDS)
- Muscle relaxation in surgery
- Reduced oxygen consumption in ICU
- Prevent raised ICP in head injury
- Control of status epilepticus or tetany
- Injury prevention in electroconvulsive therapy

(e) WHO analgesic ladder

Step 1 (mild pain)

Step 2 (moderate pain)
Dihydrocodeine (30mg 4–6hrly)
+

Step 3 (severe pain)
Opiate (e.g. morphine)
+

Paracetamol (1g 4–6hrly; maximum 8 tablets daily)
+/–

NSAID (e.g. ibuprofen 2–400mg 6hrly)
Caution in: elderly, diabetics, renal impairment, with reduced urine output, hypovolaemia, allergy, asthma, hypotension, peptic ulceration, deranged clotting

Effective relief of pain and anxiety is essential. Analgesic and sedative requirements vary according to patient psychology, pathology, surgical procedure and need for mechanical ventilation. Good nursing care, comfortable modes of ventilation and epidural analgesia reduce drug doses and side-effects (Fig. a). The aims, type and route of therapy depend on the clinical scenario:

1 Self-ventilating patients usually communicate their needs, which aids selection of appropriate therapy (i.e. drug type, route of administration), guides dosage and permits early recognition of side-effect. Oral therapy and regional anaesthesia (e.g. epidural) may be feasible options.

2 Ventilated patients should be comfortable but able to communicate and co-operate. Heavy sedation is occasionally required for intracranial pressure reduction, uncomfortable ventilatory modes (i.e. inverse I : E ratio) or epilepsy. Sedation levels are assessed regularly and sedative infusions stopped briefly each day to allow a degree of 'awakening'. The Ramsay Scale (Fig. c) is the most frequently used sedation-scoring system. Levels 2–5 are appropriate for most patients. Adverse effects of over-sedation are illustrated in Fig. (b). Under-sedation with unrelieved pain and/or anxiety causes hypertension, tachycardia, atelectasis, immobility, thromboembolism and reduced immunity.

3 Paralysed, ventilated patients are sedated to unconsciousness. Distress in 'awake' patients is only recognized as hypertension, tachycardia, sweating and lacrimation. Limited electroencephalography helps confirm adequate sedation. A peripheral nerve stimulator is the best objective index of level of paralysis. Paralytic agents are used infrequently (Fig. d) and with caution as unrecognized extubation is fatal.

Analgesics

The WHO analgesic ladder recommends a stepwise approach to pain relief (Fig. e), using regularly prescribed, preferably oral, medication, tailored to the patient's needs.

• **Step 1. Non-opioid analgesia:** regular **paracetamol** (1 g 6 hourly) is an effective first-line antipyretic analgesic with few side-effects. **Non-steroidal anti-inflammatory drugs** (NSAID) inhibit cyclo-oxygenases (COX) and are added at any step of the analgesic ladder to enhance paracetamol and opioid analgesic efficacy and for their independent analgesic effect. Renal toxicity, peptic ulceration, drug interactions and deranged clotting limit use.

• **Step 2. Add mild opioid analgesic:** regular **dihydrocodeine or codeine** (30 mg 6 hourly) is added to regular paracetamol (± NSAID) if pain remains uncontrolled. Combined paracetamol and weak opioid tablets (e.g. coproxamol) may not allow adequate doses of paracetamol to be given.

• **Step 3. Use strong opioid analgesic:** a strong opioid, replaces the mild opioid, in combination with regular paracetamol (± NSAID) if pain is uncontrolled. Analgesic and sedative responses to opioid receptor (μ, κ, σ) stimulation are very variable and gradual titration is essential in elderly or debilitated patients. **Side-effects** include hypotension, respiratory depression, constipation, euphoria, biliary spasm, meiosis, histamine release, tolerance and withdrawal symptoms. Nausea, vomiting and gastroparesis hamper enteral nutrition.

(a) **Tramadol** is an intermediate strength opioid analgesic, useful in post-operative or protracted pain. It has fewer side-effects, notably constipation, respiratory depression and addiction.

(b) **Morphine** produces potent, rapid onset analgesia and anxiolysis with minimal cardiovascular instability. Renal or hepatic impairment impairs clearance and prolongs action. Ventilated patients require high doses, with benzodiazepines, to produce unconsciousness. Reduced respiratory drive may aid patient-ventilator synchronization but can cause apnoea.

(c) **Fentanyl**, a synthetic opioid, has a short duration of action after single doses. Protracted use allows accumulation in, and subsequent slow release from, fat stores which prolongs action.

(d) **Alfentanil and remifentanil** are short-acting, rapidly cleared agents.

Naloxone is an effective but short-acting opioid antagonist.

Sedative-anxiolytics

No drug fulfils the properties of an ideal sedative (i.e. anxiolysis, analgesia, amnesia, predictability, titratability, minimal side-effects and rapid elimination) in the ventilated patient. A multi-drug approach using analgesics, anxiolytic-sedatives and occasional paralysing agents is required. Choice depends on patient needs, drug properties and side-effects. Most are administered as bolus or continuous intravenous infusions and titrated to the required effect.

• **Benzodiazepines** provide excellent sedation, anxiolysis, amnesia, muscle relaxation and anticonvulsant effects with few cardiorespiratory consequences. They have no analgesic properties but decrease analgesic requirements by relieving anxiety. **Midazolam** is lipid soluble allowing rapid onset of action (i.e. blood–brain barrier penetration) but fat accumulation prolongs drug withdrawal. Hepatic metabolism and excretion prolong action in liver disease, whereas liver enzyme induction (e.g. alcoholics, epileptics) necessitates large doses to achieve therapeutic effects. **Lorazepam** is the exception, as it has no hepatic metabolism or active metabolites. **Flumazenil** is a short-acting benzodiazepine antagonist but may precipitate withdrawal.

• **Propofol** is an easily titrated sedative, with no analgesic properties, short duration of action and rapid reversibility. Hypotension occurs in 30% of patients limiting use in haemodynamic instability. The drug vehicle (i.e. egg and soyabean emulsion) can cause allergic reactions and supports bacterial growth with subsequent bacteraemia. Infusions must be prepared under sterile conditions and changed at short intervals. Metabolism is neither hepatic or renal.

• **Haloperidol:** gradually titrated combinations of haloperidol and benzodiazepine are usually better than either agent alone in agitated patients. Barbiturates and phenothiazines have few advantages over other sedatives and cause significant side-effects (e.g. dystonic reactions).

Neuromuscular paralytic agents

• **Depolarizing neuromuscular agents** resemble acetylcholine (ACH), depolarize neuromuscular junctions (NMJ) but are not metabolized by acetylcholinesterases. Depolarization persists until the drug diffuses out of the NMJ and is degraded by plasma cholinesterases. **Suxamethonium/succinylcholine:** has a rapid onset and short duration of action (<10 min) which is ideal for intubation. Depolarization causes muscle contraction and associated K^+ release limits use in renal failure, rhabdomyolysis, burns or trauma patients. Vagal stimulation prevents use of continuous infusions.

• **Non-depolarizing neuromuscular agents** passively occupy ACH-binding sites, prevent ACH action and block depolarization. Onset takes 2–3 minutes and duration of action is 20–60 minutes. Atracurium and rocuronium infusions are non-cumulative and often used in ICU. Prolonged paralysis, particularly with steroid therapy, results in severe myopathy. Side-effects include vagal blockade (e.g. pancuronium) and histamine release with bronchospasm (e.g. atracurium).

Many factors potentiate (e.g. acidosis, hyponatraemia, gentamicin) and inhibit (e.g. oedema, phenytoin) neuromuscular blockade. **Complications** (Fig. b) include malignant hyperthermia (Chapter 21). **Pseudocholinesterase deficiency** occurs in 1 in 2500 people and extends paralysis for 6–8 hours.

(a) Nutritional requirements

1. Energy (calorie) requirement

a. Determine basal metabolic rate (BMR) from Schofield equation

BMR in kcal/day by age and gender

Age (yrs)	Female	Male
15–18	13.3W + 690	17.6W + 656
18–30	14.8W + 485	15.0W + 690
30–60	8.1W + 842	11.4W + 870
>60	9.0W + 656	11.7W + 585

W = weight in kg, #=fractures
IBD = inflammatory bowel disease

b. Adjust BMR for stress, activity and thermogenesis

Starvation (>10% weight loss)	– 0–15%
Mild infection, IBD, post-operative	+ 0–13%
Moderate infection, long bone #	+ 10–30%
Severe sepsis, multiple trauma	+25–50%
Burns 10-90%	+10–70%
Bed-bound, immobile	+10%
Bed-bound, mobile/sitting	+20%
Mobile around the ward	+25%

Or determine energy expenditure from:
- (a) Direct bedside calorimetry: measures O_2 consumption + CO_2 production
- (b) The Fick principle in patients with pulmonary artery catheters

Or calculate from lean body weight:
Normally ~30 kcal/kg/day, increasing to >60 kcal/kg/day in severe stress (e.g. burns). Non-protein sources supply ~80% of calories (e.g. carbohydrate 30-70%, fat 15-30%)

2. Protein requirement:
Can be determined from 24 hour urinary nitrogen loss; but not necessary Nitrogen intake should be ~0.2g/kg/day, given as protein ~1.25g/kg/day.

3. Vitamin and trace elements
Especially Vitamin K, thiamine, folic acid and zinc. Other trace elements serve key physiological and metabolic roles

4. Basal water and electrolyte requirements/kg/day
Water 30ml, sodium ~1mmol, potassium 0.7–1mmol, magnesium 0.1mmol, calcium 0.1mmol, phosphorus 0.4mmol

(c) Starter feeding regime

Initially feed at 30mls/hr
Check gastric aspirates 4hrly

⬇

If GRV <200mls increase feed to 60mls/hr
Check gastric aspirates 4hrly

⬇

If GRV <200mls increase feed to 75mls/hr or target volume
Check gastric aspirates 4hrly

⬇

Feed with target volume for 20hrs
Daily rest period 4hrs
Check gastric aspirates 4hrly
until feeding established

GRV=gastric residual volume

(b) Disease specific nutritional requirements

Starvation
Electrolyte depletion (PO_4^-, K^+, Mg^{2+}) and glucose intolerance result in impaired cardiac contractility and respiratory muscle function. Electrolyte and glucose imbalance must be corrected. Refeeding syndrome occurs after prolonged starvation

Renal failure (RF)
High energy feed is used (i.e. 2 kcal/mL) to reduce volume. In TPN essential amino acids (AA) may stimulate protein synthesis and reduce urea by recycling nitrogen into non-essential AA. Low Na^+ and K^+ feeds with supplemental vitamins may be required

⟺ Nutritional requirements in disease states ⟺

COPD
Malnutrition is common. Ventilation in respiratory failure has a high energy expenditure. Overfeeding with carbohydrate causes high CO_2 production. Feeds should contain less carbohydrate and more fat. Fat oxidation produces 30% less CO_2

Hepatic failure
Impaired fat metabolism and carbohydrate intolerance are common. Use of branched chain (instead of aromatic) amino acids may improve mental status in hepatic encephalopathy. TPN must contain less sodium and volume due to aldosterone-induced water retention

(d) Complications of enteral and parenteral nutrition

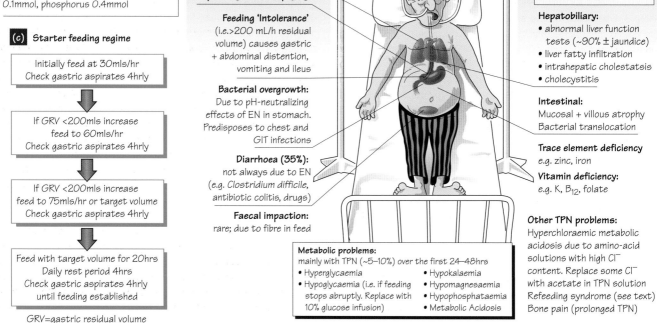

Enteral nutrition (EN)

NG tube problems:
sinusitis, tube obstruction, perforation + ulceration

Aspiration pneumonia:
Prevented by avoiding gastric distention + 30 elevation of the head of the bed

Impaired gastric emptying

Feeding 'Intolerance'
(i.e.>200 mL/h residual volume) causes gastric + abdominal distention, vomiting and ileus

Bacterial overgrowth:
Due to pH-neutralizing effects of EN in stomach. Predisposes to chest and GIT infections

Diarrhoea (35%):
not always due to EN (e.g. Clostridium difficile, antibiotic colitis, drugs)

Faecal impaction:
rare; due to fibre in feed

Parenteral nutrition (TPN)

Catheter-related:
- line infection, sepsis
- thrombosis, phlebitis
- air embolism, occlusion

Fluid overload

$\downarrow K^+$, $\downarrow Mg$, $\downarrow PO_4$ especially in the first 24hrs

Hepatobiliary:
- abnormal liver function tests (~90% ± jaundice)
- liver fatty infiltration
- intrahepatic cholestatsis
- cholecystitis

Intestinal:
Mucosal + villous atrophy
Bacterial translocation

Trace element deficiency
e.g. zinc, iron

Vitamin deficiency:
e.g. K, B_{12}, folate

Other TPN problems:
Hyperchloraemic metabolic acidosis due to amino-acid solutions with high Cl^- content. Replace some Cl^- with acetate in TPN solution Refeeding syndrome (see text) Bone pain (prolonged TPN)

Metabolic problems:
mainly with TPN (~5–10%) over the first 24–48hrs
- Hyperglycaemia
- Hypoglycaemia (i.e. if feeding stops abruptly. Replace with 10% glucose infusion)
- Hypokalaemia
- Hypomagnesaemia
- Hypophosphataemia
- Metabolic Acidosis

Nutritional assessment is essential in the acute or critically ill patient. Clinical evaluation (e.g. weight loss, subcutaneous fat loss, muscle wasting, oedema, ascites, gastro-intestinal symptoms) is more effective than either objective measurements (e.g. skin-fold thickness) which may be obscured by oedema, or laboratory features (e.g. transferrin, albumin, lymphocyte count) which are independently reduced by acute illness. **Effects of malnutrition** include impaired immune function, reduced plasma protein and oncotic pressure, delayed wound healing and impaired respiratory muscle strength. **Refeeding syndrome** occurs when food intake is resumed after a period of starvation. As glucose is reintroduced, increased insulin promotes cellular ion uptake, resulting in hypophosphataemia, hypokalaemia, hypomagnesaemia and metabolic acidosis. Depletion of ATP and 2,3-DGP (± thiamine) causes tissue hypoxia and inhibits metabolism which manifests as cardiorespiratory failure, paraesthesia and seizures. **Timing the onset of nutritional support (NS)** is controversial although it reduces protein catabolism and improves markers of nutritional status (e.g. lymphocyte counts, plasma proteins), evidence that specific regimes improve outcome is limited and complications may outweigh benefits. Generally early NS is recommended for pre-existing malnutrition, hypermetabolic states and protracted illness but is unnecessary in well-nourished, short-stay patients. Current guidelines recommend that nutritional support be started in any patient unlikely to regain oral intake within 5–10 days. **Nutritional route:** enteral nutrition (EN) is always preferred as it is cheaper and reduces infective complications (e.g. in abdominal trauma patients). Likewise in pancreatitis, transpyloric feeding reduces sepsis and mortality. However, complications occur with both EN (e.g. tube misplacement, aspiration) and total parenteral nutrition (TPN).

Assessment of nutritional requirements

• **Energy expenditure (calories):** usually calculated from predictive equations which determine basal metabolic rate (BMR) from weight, age and sex and correct for stress, activity and fever. The Schofield equation, an update of the Harris–Benedict equation, is currently used (Fig. a). Indirect calorimetry (i.e. which measures O_2 consumption and CO_2 production) or calculation from the Fick principle (i.e. pulmonary artery catheter measurements) offer little additional benefit. Adjustments are required in COPD, renal and hepatic failure (Fig. b). Many clinicians have dispensed with energy expenditure measurements and simply aim to deliver ~30 kcal/kg/day.
• **Protein:** a daily nitrogen provision of 0.2 g/kg/day (equivalent to 1.25 g protein/kg/day) is usually adequate but 0.3 g/kg/day (2 g protein/kg/day) may be required in severely catabolic patients (e.g. severe burns). Urinary urea nitrogen measurements are generally unhelpful.
• **Vitamins and micronutrients:** requirements of vitamins A, K, thiamine (B_1), B_3, B_6, C and folic acid increase in severe illness. Vitamin K, folic acid and thiamine are prone to deficiency during TPN. Deficiencies of zinc, iron and selenium have been reported. Renal replacement therapy risks loss of water soluble vitamins.
• **Water and electrolytes:** requirements vary considerably. Basal intakes are shown in Fig. (a).

Enteral nutrition

Enteral nutrition (EN) increases splanchnic perfusion, prevents stress ulceration, ensures mucosal integrity which protects against bacterial translocation (± sepsis), increases gut-associated lymphoid tissue enhancing immunity, supplies complex nutrients (e.g. medium chain fatty acids), stimulates gallbladder emptying and promotes insulin (i.e. reduces hyperglycaemia), gastrin (± other gut hormones) and pancreatic secretions. **Feeding formulas:** standard commercial feeds provide 1–1.5 kcal/ml (~45% carbohydrate, ~25% lipid) and most electrolytes and micronutrients. They are isotonic, polymeric (i.e. complex protein, fat and carbohydrate molecules) and gluten/lactose free, which reduces the potential for diarrhoea. Elemental diets (i.e. amino acids, oligosaccharides) require minimal digestion (e.g. chronic pancreatitis). **Administration** is by continuous infusion. Initially, a wide bore (12–14F) nasogastric tube allows gastric residual volumes to be aspirated at 4-hourly intervals but is replaced with a more comfortable fine bore when feeding is established. A daily 4-hour feeding rest period prevents stomach bacterial overgrowth by allowing restoration of normal gastric pH (<7.1) and reduces the risk of aspiration-related pneumonia. EN can be achieved in most patients despite abdominal distension, absence of bowel sounds or diarrhoea. Figure (c) illustrates a typical starter feeding regime. **Complications** are illustrated in Fig. (d). **Contraindications** include intestinal obstruction, ischaemia and anatomical disruption. **Failure to establish EN:** gastric aspirates are measured every 4 hours at the onset of EN. Gastric residual volumes (GRV) >400 ml risk pulmonary aspiration and feeding should be stopped and re-introduced at a lower infusion rate. GRV consistently >200 ml are treated with prokinetic agents, initially metoclopramide (10 mg 8 hourly), a dopamine antagonist and then erythromycin (250 mg 12 hourly), a motilin-receptor agonist to stimulate gastric emptying. Endoscopically placed nasojejunal or surgical jejunostomy tubes bypass the stomach and feed directly into the bowel.

'Total' parenteral nutrition

'Total' parenteral nutrition (TPN) is required if EN is contraindicated or cannot be established (e.g. ileus) but benefit has not been convincingly established. The main energy source is fat emulsion (i.e. ~35% non-protein energy source) because excess glucose causes metabolic derangement (i.e. hyperglycaemia, CO_2 production, lipogenesis). Unfortunately lipid infusions impair neutrophil function and TPN may be immunosuppressive. Insulin is often added to ensure normoglycaemia. Nitrogen is supplied as amino acids but glutamine and tyrosine are unstable and absent. Consequently TPN is nutritionally incomplete, irritant and often hyperosmolar. **Administration:** most solutions are prepared aseptically in hospital pharmacies as a single bag which is infused continuously over 24 hours through the dedicated lumen of a central venous catheter. When TPN is given into a peripheral vein, large volumes with low glucose concentrations are used to reduce osmolality-induced phlebitis. Nevertheless, new line sites may still be required at 2- to 3-day intervals. **Complications** are illustrated in Fig. (d). Catheter-related sepsis is reduced by using antimicrobial-coated lines, a dedicated lumen and strict aseptic handling (Chapter 23). Subcutaneous tunnelling is not of benefit. Liver dysfunction is reduced by decreasing TPN glucose content.

Immunonutrition uses compounds that, although unproven, may improve metabolic and immune responses in critical illness. Glutamine, an amino acid and primary energy source for enterocytes, preserves intestinal integrity. Arginine stimulates immune (e.g. T-cell) function and nitrogen balance. Omega-3-polyunsaturated fatty acids, from fish oils, are anti-inflammatory agents and immune modulators.

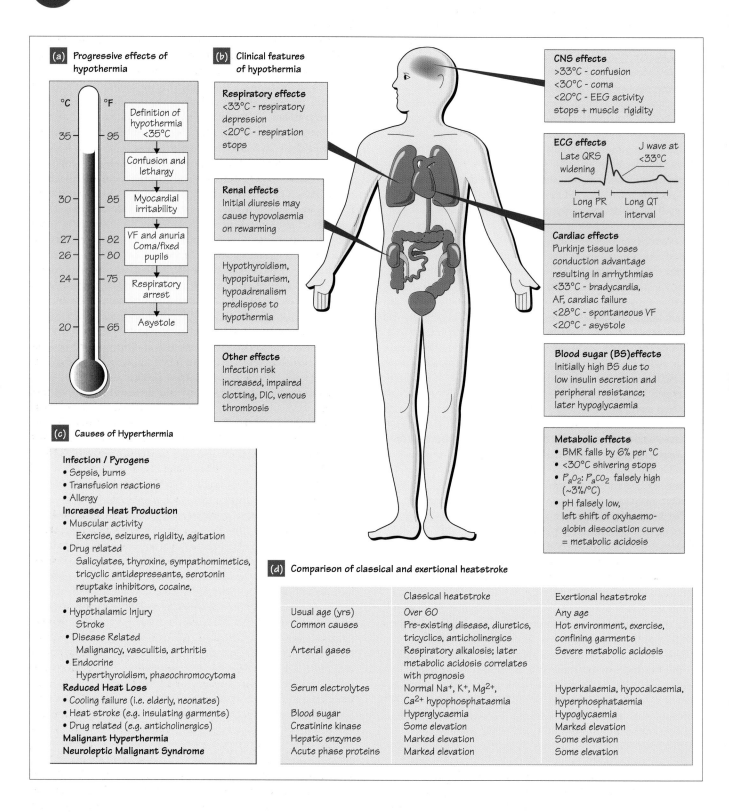

(a) Progressive effects of hypothermia

Definition of hypothermia <35°C → Confusion and lethargy → Myocardial irritability → VF and anuria Coma/fixed pupils → Respiratory arrest → Asystole

°C / °F scale: 35/95, 30/85, 27/82, 26/80, 24/75, 20/65

(b) Clinical features of hypothermia

Respiratory effects
<33°C - respiratory depression
<20°C - respiration stops

Renal effects
Initial diuresis may cause hypovolaemia on rewarming

Hypothyroidism, hypopituitarism, hypoadrenalism predispose to hypothermia

Other effects
Infection risk increased, impaired clotting, DIC, venous thrombosis

CNS effects
>33°C - confusion
<30°C - coma
<20°C - EEG activity stops + muscle rigidity

ECG effects
Late QRS widening
J wave at <33°C
Long PR interval
Long QT interval

Cardiac effects
Purkinje tissue loses conduction advantage resulting in arrhythmias
<33°C - bradycardia, AF, cardiac failure
<28°C - spontaneous VF
<20°C - asystole

Blood sugar (BS) effects
Initially high BS due to low insulin secretion and peripheral resistance; later hypoglycaemia

Metabolic effects
- BMR falls by 6% per °C
- <30°C shivering stops
- P_aO_2: P_aCO_2 falsely high (~3%/°C)
- pH falsely low, left shift of oxyhaemoglobin dissociation curve = metabolic acidosis

(c) Causes of Hyperthermia

Infection / Pyrogens
- Sepsis, burns
- Transfusion reactions
- Allergy

Increased Heat Production
- Muscular activity
  Exercise, seizures, rigidity, agitation
- Drug related
  Salicylates, thyroxine, sympathomimetics, tricyclic antidepressants, serotonin reuptake inhibitors, cocaine, amphetamines
- Hypothalamic Injury
  Stroke
- Disease Related
  Malignancy, vasculitis, arthritis
- Endocrine
  Hyperthyroidism, phaeochromocytoma

Reduced Heat Loss
- Cooling failure (i.e. elderly, neonates)
- Heat stroke (e.g. insulating garments)
- Drug related (e.g. anticholinergics)

Malignant Hyperthermia
Neuroleptic Malignant Syndrome

(d) Comparison of classical and exertional heatstroke

	Classical heatstroke	Exertional heatstroke
Usual age (yrs)	Over 60	Any age
Common causes	Pre-existing disease, diuretics, tricyclics, anticholinergics	Hot environment, exercise, confining garments
Arterial gases	Respiratory alkalosis; later metabolic acidosis correlates with prognosis	Severe metabolic acidosis
Serum electrolytes	Normal Na^+, K^+, Mg^{2+}, Ca^{2+} hypophosphataemia	Hyperkalaemia, hypocalcaemia, hyperphosphataemia
Blood sugar	Hyperglycaemia	Hypoglycaemia
Creatinine kinase	Some elevation	Marked elevation
Hepatic enzymes	Marked elevation	Some elevation
Acute phase proteins	Marked elevation	Some elevation

Hypothermia

Hypothermia is defined as a core temperature <35 °C. Mild hypothermia is defined as 32–35 °C, moderate 28–32 °C and severe <28 °C. **Mortality** varies according to severity and cause (e.g. hypothermia (28–32 °C) alone ~20%; with an underlying cause >60%). **Causes:** accidental hypothermia is usually multifactorial, involving exposure to low environmental or water immersion temperatures (e.g. drowning), alcohol intoxication, a primary neurological insult (e.g. CVA), thermoregulatory compromise (e.g. spinal cord injury), predisposing factors (e.g. hypopituitarism), surgery (i.e. exposure, anaesthetic drugs, impaired shivering) and drugs that alter cold perception, cause vasodilation or inhibit heat generation (e.g. barbiturates). Hypothyroidism, which depresses heat production, impairs temperature perception and blunts shivering, is involved in ~10% of cases. Hypothermia is induced during cardiac or neurosurgery to provide cerebral protection.

Clinical features

Hypothermia initially stimulates protective peripheral vasoconstriction, shivering and increased metabolism. However, as core body temperature falls, progressive physiological and organ dysfunction follow (Fig. a) including cardiorespiratory and neurological depression, renal diuresis, tissue hypoperfusion and metabolic derangement (Fig. b). Cardiac conduction and pacemaker activity are progressively impaired and myocardial irritability increases, with atrial fibrillation and heart block common below 33 °C. Ventricular fibrillation, resistant to cardioversion, is precipitated by rough handling or cardiopulmonary resuscitation (CPR) below 28 °C. Cardiac output falls by 50% at 28 °C due to reduced heart rate and contractility. Initial neurological responses include reduced respiratory drive, lethargy and confusion; coma and fixed pupils occur below 30 °C. Cerebral oxygen consumption halves during a 10 °C temperature fall, which partially protects against the associated decrease in cerebral perfusion.

Management

1 General management: includes oxygen therapy, gentle handling, close monitoring and treatment of underlying causes. Fluid resuscitation often requires central access due to intense peripheral vasoconstriction. Arrhythmias and heart block usually respond to rewarming alone. Prolonged CPR is often successful in hypothermic patients but cardioversion is often ineffective below 30 °C. Consequently rewarming to >35 °C is essential before death is declared.

2 Rewarming: determined by the severity of the hypothermia:
- **Passive, external rewarming:** (i.e. warm environment (>30 °C), insulating covers) usually adequate in mild (i.e. >33 °C) hypothermia without circulatory compromise.
- **Active, external rewarming:** (i.e. warming blankets, immersion) recommended in moderate to severe hypothermia with no evidence of circulatory collapse. However, caution is required as rapid peripheral vasodilation may increase organ hypoperfusion (± mortality). Convective (forced air) warming (e.g. Bair Hugger) at 43 °C has been shown to increase body temperature by 2–3 °C/h.
- **Internal, core rewarming:** indicated in severe hypothermia with poor physiological tolerance, circulatory failure or cardiac arrest when rapid rewarming is necessary. Techniques include warm intravenous fluids or inhaled gas (1 °C/h), bladder, pleural or peritoneal lavage (2–3 °C/h) and haemodialysis (5 °C/h). Cardiopulmonary bypass (10 °C/h) is only necessary during cardiac arrest.

Hyperthermia

Hyperthermia is defined as a core temperature >37.5 °C (99 °F). Fever increases metabolic rate and CO_2 production. Sweating and vasodilation cause hypovolaemia. Metabolic acidosis, epilepsy, neurological impairment, renal failure, rhabdomyolysis and myocardial ischaemia

may follow. Severe hyperthermia (>42 °C) is potentially lethal and even short periods may cause permanent cerebral damage.

Causes

Figure (c) lists the causes of hyperthermia; ~50% are due to infection. In addition to thyroid storm (Chapter 41), five non-infectious causes of hyperthermia require immediate recognition and treatment:
- **Exertional heatstroke:** follows prolonged exercise in warm, humid environments. It often affects athletes, firefighters and military recruits or those wearing garments that restrict heat loss. It presents with hyperthermia, confusion, hypotension and tachypnoea followed by shock, rhabdomyolysis and renal failure. Figure (d) presents the metabolic consequences. Mortality is ~10% even with rapid cooling.
- **Classical (non-exertional) heatstroke:** usually affects sedentary, elderly, inner-city dwellers with co-existent illness during heat-waves. Patients with thermoregulatory disorders (e.g. hypothalamic stroke), inability to dissipate heat (e.g. heart failure, skin disease) and those using drugs that impair heat loss (e.g. anticholinergics, diuretics) or generate heat (e.g. tricyclics) are at greater risk. It presents with hyperthermia, hot (dry) skin and altered mental status followed by shock and organ failure. Figure (d) reports metabolic effects. Volume depletion and rhabdomyolysis occasionally cause renal failure. About 80% of deaths occur in those >50 years old.
- **Drug-induced hyperthermia:** may be due to serotonin receptor stimulation by amphetamine derivatives (e.g. methylene dioxymethamphetamine (MDMA; 'ecstasy')), serotonin reuptake inhibitors (e.g. fluoxetine, imipramine) or serotonin agonists (e.g. lithium).
- **Malignant hyperthermia (MH):** a rare autosomal dominant trait causing excessive muscle heat production due to altered calcium kinetics, during or shortly after anaesthetic drug exposure. Muscle rigidity, sudden hyperpyrexia (41–45 °C), tachycardia, metabolic acidosis and hypercarbia occur. Halothane and succinylcholine precipitate 80% of cases. Early recognition has reduced mortality to <10%.
- **Neuroleptic malignant syndrome (NMS):** an idiosyncratic reaction to neuroleptic drugs (e.g. haloperidol, phenothiazines, metoclopramide). It may be due to hypothalamic dopamine-receptor blockade. Muscle rigidity, encephalopathy, catatonia, extrapyramidal symptoms and autonomic effects (e.g. sweating, labile hypertension, tachycardia) are common. Organ failure (e.g. renal) and death (10–15%) may occur.

Management

Early recognition can be lifesaving. **General management** includes stopping causative drugs, replacing fluid and correcting electrolyte imbalance. Renal replacement therapy and seizure prophylaxis may be indicated. **Cooling** is best achieved by spraying unclothed skin with tepid water and using a fan to encourage evaporation. Ice packs (e.g. axilla, groin) are often useful. Cold water immersion causes cutaneous vasoconstriction and may prevent heat loss. Additional measures include cold intravenous fluids, iced gastric or peritoneal lavage and haemofiltration. **Drug therapy:** paracetamol (±NSAID) is usually ineffective. Intravenous dantrolene, a muscle relaxant that uncouples excitation-contraction mechanisms by inhibiting calcium release from sarcoplasmic reticulum is the only specific therapy for MH, NMS and MDMA toxicity. Bromocriptine in NMS, anticholinergics and muscle relaxants may be helpful. Alkaline diuresis and mannitol may reduce myoglobin-induced renal damage.

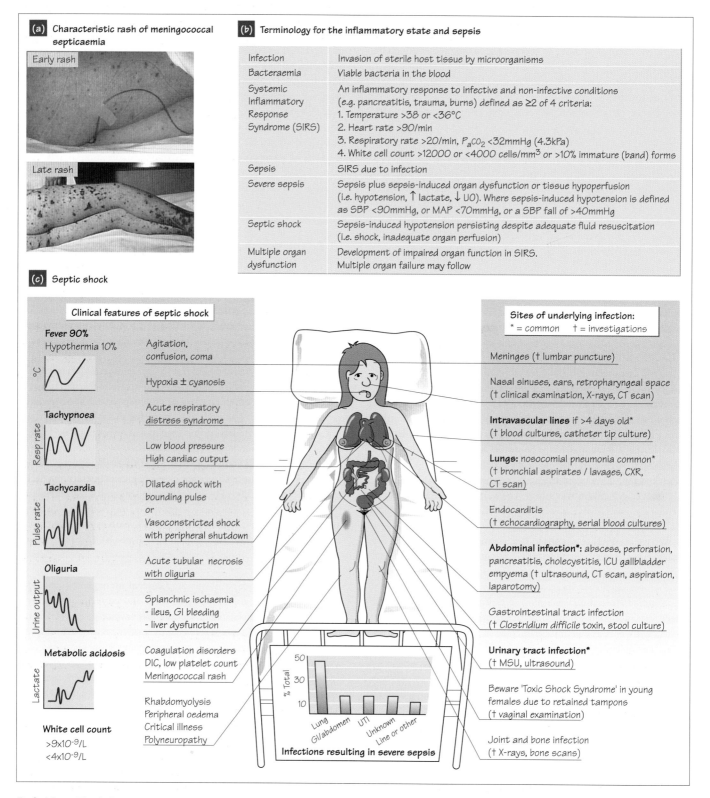

(a) Characteristic rash of meningococcal septicaemia

Early rash

Late rash

(b) Terminology for the inflammatory state and sepsis

Infection	Invasion of sterile host tissue by microorganisms
Bacteraemia	Viable bacteria in the blood
Systemic Inflammatory Response Syndrome (SIRS)	An inflammatory response to infective and non-infective conditions (e.g. pancreatitis, trauma, burns) defined as ≥2 of 4 criteria: 1. Temperature >38 or <36°C 2. Heart rate >90/min 3. Respiratory rate >20/min, P_aCO_2 <32mmHg (4.3kPa) 4. White cell count >12000 or <4000 cells/mm³ or >10% immature (band) forms
Sepsis	SIRS due to infection
Severe sepsis	Sepsis plus sepsis-induced organ dysfunction or tissue hypoperfusion (i.e. hypotension, ↑ lactate, ↓ UO). Where sepsis-induced hypotension is defined as SBP <90mmHg, or MAP <70mmHg, or a SBP fall of >40mmHg
Septic shock	Sepsis-induced hypotension persisting despite adequate fluid resuscitation (i.e. shock, inadequate organ perfusion)
Multiple organ dysfunction	Development of impaired organ function in SIRS. Multiple organ failure may follow

(c) Septic shock

Clinical features of septic shock

Fever 90%
Hypothermia 10%
°C

Tachypnoea
Resp rate

Tachycardia
Pulse rate

Oliguria
Urine output

Metabolic acidosis
Lactate

White cell count
>9x10⁻⁹/L
<4x10⁻⁹/L

Agitation, confusion, coma

Hypoxia ± cyanosis

Acute respiratory distress syndrome

Low blood pressure
High cardiac output

Dilated shock with bounding pulse
or
Vasoconstricted shock with peripheral shutdown

Acute tubular necrosis with oliguria

Splanchnic ischaemia
- ileus, GI bleeding
- liver dysfunction

Coagulation disorders
DIC, low platelet count
Meningococcal rash

Rhabdomyolysis
Peripheral oedema
Critical illness
Polyneuropathy

Sites of underlying infection:
* = common   † = investigations

Meninges († lumbar puncture)

Nasal sinuses, ears, retropharyngeal space († clinical examination, X-rays, CT scan)

Intravascular lines if >4 days old*
(† blood cultures, catheter tip culture)

Lungs: nosocomial pneumonia common*
(† bronchial aspirates / lavages, CXR, CT scan)

Endocarditis
(† echocardiography, serial blood cultures)

Abdominal infection*: abscess, perforation, pancreatitis, cholecystitis, ICU gallbladder empyema († ultrasound, CT scan, aspiration, laparotomy)

Gastrointestinal tract infection
(† *Clostridium difficile* toxin, stool culture)

Urinary tract infection*
(† MSU, ultrasound)

Beware 'Toxic Shock Syndrome' in young females due to retained tampons
(† vaginal examination)

Joint and bone infection
(† X-rays, bone scans)

% Total
50
30
10
Lung
GI/abdomen
UTI
Unknown
Line or other
Infections resulting in severe sepsis

Definitions The inflammatory response that characterizes 'sepsis' is not always due to infection. A potential infective cause is detected in ~65% of severe sepsis but blood cultures are positive in <25%. Figure (b) presents the current terminology used to describe the systemic inflammatory response syndrome (SIRS) and sepsis. **Severe sepsis** implies sepsis with sepsis-induced organ dysfunction or tissue hypoperfusion. **Septic shock** specifies persistent sepsis-induced hypotension despite adequate fluid resuscitation.

Epidemiology Sepsis causes significant morbidity and mortality on critical care units; at any one time ~50% of patients are on antibiotics, and infection was acquired after admission in about half. In the USA, ~500,000 patients, with an average age of 55 years, develop sepsis each year. It is the leading cause of multiple organ failure, ARDS, acute renal failure and late death following trauma. **Prognosis** deteriorates with age, lactic acidosis, low white cell count, cytokine elevation, reduced SVR and number of organ failures. **Mortality** is >40% in septic shock.

Pathophysiology

The host's immune response is stimulated by invasive microorganisms or bacterial endotoxins. Initial cytokine release (e.g. TNF-α) activates polymorphs, endothelium, platelets, complement and coagulation pathways. Activated white cells adhere to and damage vascular endothelium allowing fluid and cells to leak into the interstitial space and microcirculatory thrombosis impairs tissue oxygen delivery. Vasodilation follows release of inflammatory mediators (e.g. nitric oxide (NO)) from vascular endothelium. Myocardial dysfunction is due to reduced coronary perfusion and the negative inotropic effects of NO and inflammatory mediators. Tissue oxygen utilization is also impaired by sepsis-mediated cellular enzyme inhibition.

Clinical presentation

The clinical features of severe sepsis and potential sources of infection are illustrated in Figs (a) and (c). Haemodynamic changes are variable (Chapter 6) and circulatory assessment may reveal either a hyperdynamic (i.e. 'warm, dilated') patient with bounding pulses, or a hypotensive, vasoconstricted (i.e. 'cold, clammy') patient (i.e. mimics myocardial infarction (MI) or pulmonary embolism). **Examination** may detect a focus of infection or provide diagnostic clues (e.g. meningococcal rash, splinter haemorrhages in endocarditis). Chest infection is the commonest source of sepsis.

Management of severe sepsis

'The Surviving Sepsis Campaign' published updated guidelines for sepsis management in 2008. These apply to all acute wards. As in MI the speed and appropriateness of initial therapy influences outcome.

Diagnosis

• **Identify the cause of sepsis:** this informs subsequent therapy (e.g. antibiotic choice, abscess drainage, infected line removal).
• **Essential investigations:** include routine blood tests, C-reactive protein, plasma lactate, coagulation profile, arterial blood gases (ABG), central venous S_vO_2 ($S_{cv}O_2$), urinalysis, CXR and ECG. **Monitor:** vital signs, biochemistry, ABG, CVP (±CO) and urine output. **Cultures** of blood, sputum, urine, CSF and wound pus *must* be taken before starting antibiotics providing this does not delay therapy. At least two blood cultures (≥1 drawn percutaneously and one through each vascular access device >48 hours old) are required.
• **Specific investigations** (Fig. c): depend on the suspected cause (e.g. abdominal ultrasonography in abdominal sepsis) and patient mobility (e.g. CT scans).

Initial resuscitation (first 6 hours) and therapy

• **Protocolized fluid resuscitation:** should start *immediately* in patients with hypoperfusion (i.e. lactate > 4 mmol/L, raised $S_{cv}O_2$) or

hypotension. Crystalloid (1 L) or colloid (0.5 L) fluid challenges (Chapter 8) should aim to achieve: (a) CVP ≥ 8 mmHg (≥12 if ventilated); (b) MAP ≥ 65 mmHg; (c) urine output ≥ 0.5 ml/kg/h; (d) $S_{cv}O_2$ ≥ 70%. If the $S_{cv}O_2$ target is not achieved, consider packed red cell transfusion to a haemocrit ≥ 30% or a dobutamine infusion (max. 20 μg/kg/min) to increase oxygen delivery and hence $S_{cv}O_2$. Reduce fluid administration if CVP increases without haemodynamic improvement.
• **Antibiotic therapy:** started as early as possible and always within the first hour. It is initially *empiric* using broad spectrum agents active against the most likely causative pathogens and with good penetration into infected tissues. Antibiotic selection depends on the clinical features, whether community- or hospital-acquired, the site of primary infection and local antibiotic resistance patterns. Combination therapy is recommended in neutropenic patients and those infected with *Pseudomonas*. Microbiology results guide therapy and unnecessary antibiotics should be stopped (i.e. monotherapy after 3–5 days). Review antibiotics daily and limit treatment to 5–10 days.

Haemodynamic support and adjunctive therapy

• **Vasopressor and inotropic therapy** (Chapter 10): aims to maintain MAP ≥ 65 mmHg if initial fluid administration is unsuccessful. These drugs should be given through a central line and require an arterial line for blood pressure monitoring.
  • **In early sepsis** widespread vasodilation (i.e. low SVR) causes hypotension and relative hypovolaemia. Reduced left ventricular afterload increases cardiac output (CO) but inappropriate distribution can cause regional (i.e. splanchnic) ischaemia. At this stage a **vasopressor agent** (e.g. norepinephrine (noradrenaline)) with α-receptor agonist properties (Chapters 6, 10) increases SVR, MAP and organ perfusion pressure. Norepinephrine is supplemented with vasopressin if the initial pressor response is inadequate.
  • **In late sepsis** toxic myocarditis impairs myocardial contractility and reduces CO. At this stage fluid administration produces only small increases in CO and may precipitate pulmonary oedema (Chapters 8, 28), whilst increasing SVR with vasopressor therapy decreases CO. In this situation an **inotropic agent** is required to increase cardiac contractility and maintain CO. Dobutamine, often used in combination with norepinephrine, or dopamine are the agents of choice (Chapters 6, 10). Epinephrine (adrenaline) is second line therapy.
• **Additional therapies:** relative adrenocortical insufficiency may occur in severe sepsis. In these patients **low dose steroid therapy** (i.e. hydrocortisone 8 mg/h) can be beneficial if hypotension is refractory to fluid and vasopressor support. **Activated protein C** improves outcome in patients with septic shock (APACHE II ≥ 25), if there are no contraindications to use, by modifying microcirculatory thrombosis and preventing organ ischaemia.

Supportive therapy

General measures include oxygen therapy, respiratory support, glycaemic control (i.e. maintaining blood sugars < 7 mmol/L), renal support, nutrition and prophylaxis against stress ulceration and thromboembolism. **Sepsis prevention** includes infection control (e.g. hand washing), microbiological monitoring, appropriate prophylactic antibiotics and prompt management of suspected infection.

(a) Organisms responsible for most nosocomial infections

Methicillin-resistant *Staphylococcus aureus* (MRSA)	Increasing prevalence. Colonizes and infects. Easily treated but glycopepide resistance increasing
Coagulase negative staphylococcus (CNS)	Frequent skin colonization. Low virulence organisms. Increasing cause of nosocomial infections
Enterococcus faecalis (e.g. vancomycin resistant enterococcus (VRE))	Emerge with 3rd generation cephalosporin use. Often sensitive to ampicillin but resistance to aminoglycosides, ampicillin and vancomycin increasing (e.g. VRE)
Pseudomonas aeruginosa	Very broad spectrum of antibiotic resistance. Common in ICU and chronic lung disease
Stenotrophomonas maltophilia	Environmental organism. Increasingly common. Very broad spectrum of antibiotic resistance
Acinetobacter baumanii	Increasingly common. Multi-resistant to antibiotics but may be sensitive to carbapenems
Klebsiella spp.	Extended β-lactam resistance ± multi-resistant to antibiotics
Enterobacter sp	Occur in normal intestinal flora and develop extended β-lactam resistance
E.coli	Variable resistance seems to correspond with use of quinolones
Others: *Proteus spp, Serratia marcescens*	Broad spectrums of antibiotic resistance
Clostridium difficile	Spore forming, multi-antibiotic resistant bacillus that colonizes intestine in hospital patients
Candida species	Overgrowth due to antibiotic pressures. Diagnosis suggested by growth in more than 2 sites

(b) Risk factors for nosocomial infection

Patient factors
- Nutritional status, immunosuppression (e.g. steroids)
- Underlying disease (e.g. diabetes, SLE)
- Integrity of natural defences (e.g. burns, lines, open wounds)
- Multiple or prolonged antibiotic usage (i.e. resistant clone selection)

Environmental factors
- Inadequate infection control (e.g. hand washing, isolation)
- Inadequate staffing or inexperienced, new staff
- Transmission (e.g. overcrowding, frequent relocation, prolonged stay)
- Iatrogenic infection (e.g. during endotracheal tube or line insertion)

Organism factors
- Prevalence, resilience (e.g. spore formation, adherence), colonization
- Antibiotic resistance and selection
- Pathogenicity

(c) Control of endemic nosocomial infection

Reduce antibiotic use – Education – Restriction – Guidelines	**Identify carriers** – High risk patients – Early screening – Isolation
Stop transmission – Hand Hygiene – Infection control	**Eliminate reservoirs** – Decontamination – Cleaning/disinfection

(d) Prevention of central venous catheter or intra-arterial line infection

Strict aseptic insertion technique
- Mask
- Sterile gown
- Sterile gloves
- Sterile drapes

Skin antisepsis
Use 2% aqueous chlorhexidine to clean skin and allow to dry

Insertion site
- Firmly secure cannulae as movement risks infection
- Transparent dressings to allow regular inspection
- Change line if signs of local infection / cellulitis

Type of cannulae
Antimicrobial or antiseptic impregnated CVC (e.g. silver) may reduce catheter associated bacteraemia

Environment
Cleaning and disinfection

Line Management
- Use closed systems
- Avoid 3-way tap contamination
- Clean access ports with 70% alcohol before use
- Give TPN through a dedicated lumen
- Replace administration sets at ≥72hrs unless used to administer lipid, blood or blood products when they should be changed at 24hrs

Assistance during line insertion
Always ensure an assistant is available when inserting lines. This helps with maintaining sterility

HAND WASHING! HAND WASHING! HAND WASHING!

HAND WASHING
prevents transmission of organisms between patients

(e) Risk factors for line infection

- Non-sterile CVC insertion technique (e.g. emergency, skin preparation)
- Poor hand hygiene (i.e. peripheral catheters)
- >5 days since line insertion
- Iatrogenic (e.g. operator inexperience)
- Inadequate line-care
- Infection from distant sites (e.g. endocarditis)
- Contamination from infusions (e.g. propofol, TPN)
- Host risk factors (e.g. steroids, immunosuppression, diabetes)
- Catheter type (e.g. silver or antibiotic impregnation reduces risk, multilumen increases risk)
- Line material (e.g. silicone better than PVC or polythene lines)
- Line insertion site (e.g. subclavian at lower risk than femoral lines)

CVC=central venous catheter, TPN=total parenteral nutrition, PVC=polyvinyl chloride

Hospital-acquired infections are an increasingly important cause of morbidity and mortality in hospitals, nursing homes and critical care units. **Causative organisms** (Fig. a) are often virulent, antibiotic resistant and spore forming which impedes environmental eradication and encourages recurrent infection. Important examples include methicillin-resistant *Staphylococcus aureus* (MRSA), *Clostridium difficile* and multidrug-resistant (MDR) gram-negative bacilli (e.g. pseudomonas). **Commonest infection sites** are the urinary tract (~40%; but less common in ICU), surgical wounds (~15%), respiratory tract (~15%; Chapter 32), line-related bacteraemia (~10%) and colitis (<10%). **Risk factors** include host, environmental and pathogen-related factors (Fig. b). **Prevention** includes identification and isolation of carriers of causative organisms, elimination of reservoirs, prevention of transmission and appropriate antibiotic usage (Fig. c).

Line-related sepsis

Five days after insertion, ~10–20% of central venous catheters (CVC) are colonized and 2–5% develop bacteraemia. The average rate of CVC-associated bacteraemia is ~5/1000 CVC days but varies between critical care units, patient type (e.g. burns, surgical), severity of illness and CVC types (e.g. urgent, tunnelled, insertion site, antibiotic/silver-impregnation). Peripheral intra-arterial lines (e.g. radial) are less frequently colonized (~4–5% at day 5) and bacteraemia occurs on 2.9/1000 catheter days. Long, antecubital, peripheral venous catheters (PVC; >12 cm) are associated with bacteraemia on 0.8/1000 catheter days and short PVC (i.e. <12 cm) even less, although local phlebitis is common. **Microbiology:** *Staphylococcus epidermidis* (~35%), *S. aureus* (~15%) and gram-negative bacilli (e.g. *E. coli*; ~15%) are the commonest organisms. **Risk factors** for line infection are listed in Fig. (e). Figure (d) illustrates factors preventing infection. **Timing of line replacements:** PVC should be changed at 72–96 hours. Scheduled CVC and arterial line replacement does not reduce line-related bacteraemias and is not required for normally functioning catheters with no evidence of local or systemic complications. Lines must be inspected daily, replaced if infection is suspected and removed promptly when not needed. Always assess the risks of line replacement (e.g. pneumothorax). **Management:** if infection is suspected (i.e. sepsis ± positive blood cultures) remove the line and send the tip for culture. If needed, new lines should be inserted at different sites. Empiric antibiotic therapy is started whilst awaiting microbiology results, although fever and symptoms often resolve spontaneously after line removal.

Methicillin-resistant *Staphylococcus aureus* (MRSA)

MRSA infection has increased over the last 10 years. It is still largely associated with hospital and residential homes but is increasingly common in community settings, partly due to 'silent' healthcare acquisition during the previous year. Once established within healthcare environments it is difficult to eradicate. **Prevention** depends on the strategies in Fig. (c). Unrecognized MRSA carriage is present in ~3% of hospital and ~30% of ICU admissions (e.g. asymptomatic skin colonization) and constitutes the main reservoir and source of hospital transmission. **Detection** requires active surveillance especially in high risk patients (e.g. >75 years old, antibiotic use within <6 months, hospitalization within <1 year, urinary catheter at admission, critical care units). **Decolonization** aims to reduce MRSA carriage. Although intranasal mupirocin and chlorhexidine-based skin cleaning are commonly used, evidence for benefit is limited. However, environmental

cleaning and disinfection may be effective. **Early diagnosis** (e.g. rapid molecular screening techniques) and prompt patient isolation reduced MRSA acquisitions. **Antibiotic restriction** with reduced usage and avoidance of some antibiotics (e.g. quinolones, cephalosporins) decreases MRSA infection rates. **Antibiotic sensitivity:** MRSA resistance to fluoroquinolones occurs in ~80%, macrolides ~70%, trimethoprim ~35%, gentamicin 12% and mupirocin 12%. Most isolates are susceptible to tetracycline, fusidic acid and rifampicin. **MRSA therapy:** vancomycin, teicoplanin and linezolid should be reserved for patients with severe line-related or neutropenic sepsis, burns, serious soft tissue infections and prosthetic valve infections. A minimum treatment period of 14 days is required for bacteraemia and longer in endocarditis. Monitoring of levels is required during vancomycin and teicoplanin therapy. Tetracyclines, trimethoprim and combinations of rifampicin and fusidic acid are effective in cellulitis, urinary and respiratory tract infections and as part of eradication therapy. Inadequate therapy may contribute to excess mortality in critically-ill patients.

Clostridium difficile

C. difficile is a ubiquitous, gram-positive, anaerobic, motile, spore-forming bacillus that colonizes the intestines of nursing home or long-stay hospital patients (i.e. 13% and 50% acquisition at 2 and >4 weeks respectively). It is resistant to most antibiotics and forms heat- and disinfectant-resistant spores. Consequently, *C. difficile* survives for long periods in hospital environments. Fortunately bleach-containing disinfectants destroy the organism. **Clinical features:** spores are transmitted by the faecal–oral route. Following ingestion they pass through the stomach because they are acid resistance, then change to their active form and multiply in the colon. In small numbers *C. difficile* does not cause significant disease but after disruption of normal intestinal flora by broad-spectrum antibiotic therapy (especially quinolones, cephalosporins), overgrowth may cause a spectrum of symptoms. These range from asymptomatic to severe, life-threatening diarrhoea and pseudomembranous colitis. Pathogenic *C. difficile* produces toxins responsible for the diarrhoea and inflammation. The best characterized are toxins A and B. **Diagnosis** is based on clinical features (e.g. odorous diarrhoea, antibiotic exposure), detection of toxins A + B and characteristic CT scan features (e.g. colonic wall thickening > 4 mm). Delayed diagnosis risks bowel perforation and increases mortality. **Treatment:** the initial drug of choice is oral metronidazole which eliminates *C. difficile* in symptomatic patients. Oral vancomycin, and occasionally linezolid, is used in severe or resistant cases. Asymptomatic patients may not require antibiotic therapy. Antidiarrhoeal drugs (e.g. loperamide) are contraindicated as they prolong toxin-induced colonic damage. Probiotics (i.e. 'good' intestinal flora) may be beneficial. **Prevention** includes avoiding inappropriate antibiotic therapy (especially in the elderly), the use of gloves and appropriate infection control measures to reduce transmission. The value of prophylactic probiotics has not been established. **Mortality:** hospital outbreaks, often with virulent strains (e.g. Quebec strain), have caused many deaths, especially in the elderly or immunocompromised.

Urinary tract infections (UTI)

UTI follow introduction of perineal organisms into the bladder during catheterization. Although mortality rates are low, aseptic catheterization, closed unobstructed drainage and a well secured catheter to prevent movement and patient discomfort, reduce infection risk.

(a) Brainstem death can only be diagnosed if all the following preconditions and exclusion criteria are met

Essential preconditions include:
1) Apnoeic coma requiring mechanical ventilation
2) An established cause for the irreversible brain damage

Factors that must be excluded:
a) Sedative drugs, neuromuscular blocking agents + poisons
  • Test blood and urine for drugs if doubt exists
b) Significant metabolic, acid-base or endocrine abnormalities:
  • metabolic (e.g.uraemia, hyponatraemia, liver encephalopathy)
  • acid-base (e.g. acidosis, CO_2 retention)
  • endocrine (e.g. diabetic, thyroid, Addisonian crisis)
c) Hypothermia (temperature <35 °C)
d) Severe hypotension

(b) Potential complications during the period before operative organ harvesting

Cardiovascular instability
  • hypotension; due to myocardial depression + vasodilation
  • autonomic instability; arrhythmias + bradycardia
Endocrine disorders
  • diabetes insipidus; diuresis, hypovolaemia, hypernatraemia
  • thyroid hormone deficiency
  • adrenal (cortisol) deficiency
  • pancreatic (insulin) deficiency; hyperglycaemia
Temperature control
  • hypothermia; due to ↓ metabolic rate + ↓ muscle activity
Pulmonary oedema + hypoxaemia
Coagulopathy
Acid-base disorders + electrolyte imbalance

(c) Brainstem Function Testing: Criteria required to establish brain stem death (BSD) in the UK

The following 6 reflexes/responses must be absent to establish BSD

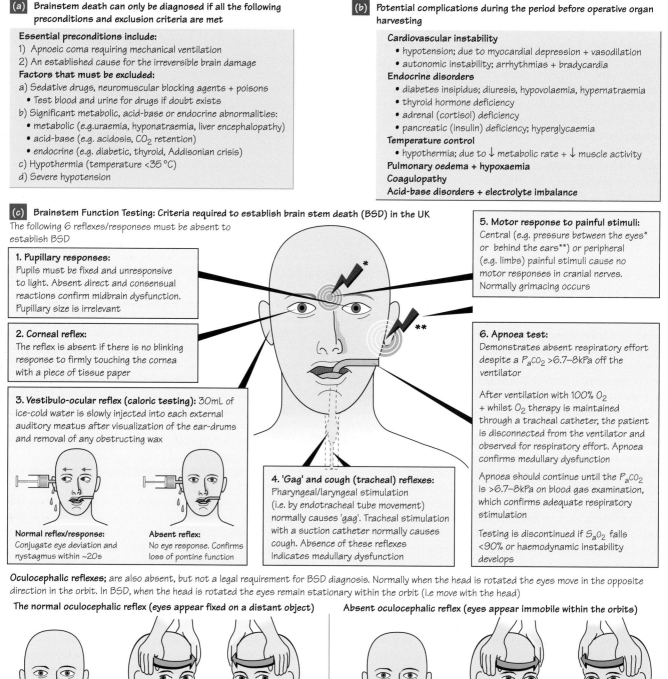

1. Pupillary responses:
Pupils must be fixed and unresponsive to light. Absent direct and consensual reactions confirm midbrain dysfunction. Pupillary size is irrelevant

2. Corneal reflex:
The reflex is absent if there is no blinking response to firmly touching the cornea with a piece of tissue paper

3. Vestibulo-ocular reflex (caloric testing): 30mL of ice-cold water is slowly injected into each external auditory meatus after visualization of the ear-drums and removal of any obstructing wax

Normal reflex/response:
Conjugate eye deviation and nystagmus within ~20s

Absent reflex:
No eye response. Confirms loss of pontine function

4. 'Gag' and cough (tracheal) reflexes:
Pharyngeal/laryngeal stimulation (i.e. by endotracheal tube movement) normally causes 'gag'. Tracheal stimulation with a suction catheter normally causes cough. Absence of these reflexes indicates medullary dysfunction

5. Motor response to painful stimuli:
Central (e.g. pressure between the eyes* or behind the ears**) or peripheral (e.g. limbs) painful stimuli cause no motor responses in cranial nerves. Normally grimacing occurs

6. Apnoea test:
Demonstrates absent respiratory effort despite a P_aCO_2 >6.7–8kPa off the ventilator

After ventilation with 100% O_2 + whilst O_2 therapy is maintained through a tracheal catheter, the patient is disconnected from the ventilator and observed for respiratory effort. Apnoea confirms medullary dysfunction

Apnoea should continue until the P_aCO_2 is >6.7–8kPa on blood gas examination, which confirms adequate respiratory stimulation

Testing is discontinued if S_aO_2 falls <90% or haemodynamic instability develops

Oculocephalic reflexes; are also absent, but not a legal requirement for BSD diagnosis. Normally when the head is rotated the eyes move in the opposite direction in the orbit. In BSD, when the head is rotated the eyes remain stationary within the orbit (i.e move with the head)

The normal oculocephalic reflex (eyes appear fixed on a distant object)

Neutral head position Eyes look forward at a fixed point

When head turned left Eyes move rightwards + continue to look at the same fixed point

When head turned right Eyes move leftwards + continue to look at the same fixed point

Absent oculocephalic reflex (eyes appear immobile within the orbits)

Neutral head position Eyeys look forward at a fixed point

If head is turned to the left or right, eyes do not move in the orbit (i.e. stare directly forward and away from the initial fixed point)

Acute and critical care medicine is often life-saving and many patients make a complete recovery or achieve a quality of life (QOL) which, although impaired, is tolerable for the patient. However, treatment that prolongs the dying process or results in an unacceptable QOL may cause unnecessary suffering, loss of dignity and undue emotional distress. Unfortunately, in emergency situations, it is often impossible to identify those individuals who will not benefit from therapy. In these patients, humane and cost-effective management requires a willingness to limit or withdraw treatment when it becomes clear that the prognosis is poor and that ongoing therapy is not in their best interests. These decisions are often difficult and based on accepted **ethical and moral principles**, including: (a) **beneficence:** the preservation of life, moderated by the need to relieve suffering; (b) **non-maleficence:** the duty to do no harm; (c) **respect for autonomy:** the right to make informed choices; (d) **justice:** fair allocation of medical resources; (e) **professional virtue:** including compassion and integrity. The **'duty of care'** expected from medical professionals has been documented by many statutory bodies including the American Medical Association and the General Medical Council (UK).

Brainstem death

Brainstem death (BSD) is defined as irreversible loss of brainstem function with associated unconsciousness and cessation of spontaneous respiration. In many countries (e.g. UK), BSD is considered to be a definition of death itself (i.e. despite a beating heart) as cardiac arrest (i.e. 'normal' death) always follows within ~1–21 days irrespective of ongoing mechanical ventilation. The purpose of establishing BSD is to demonstrate that continuing life support is futile and to meet the legal requirements for organ donation (see below). The following criteria are used in the UK although there are international variations.
• **Diagnosis:** requires that certain preconditions and exclusions are fulfilled (Fig. a).
• **Brainstem function tests (BSFT):** performed >6–24 hours after the precipitating event. Two doctors who are not part of the transplant team, one a consultant and both registered for >5 years, must complete two sets of BSFT either separately or together. The six legally required findings that establish BSD are illustrated in Fig. (c). These are absent **pupillary**, **corneal**, **vestibulo-ocular** and **gag/cough reflexes**, **no cranial nerve motor responses** in response to painful stimuli and **apnoea** following disconnection from the ventilator despite a $P_a\text{CO}_2 > 6.7$–8 kPa. Although not a legal requirement **oculocephalic reflexes** are also absent. Seizure activity and decerebrate or decorticate posturing are inconsistent with BSD but spinal reflexes may occur. Some countries require an **electroencephalogram**, **radioisotope scan** or **cerebral angiography** to confirm BSD. Although there is no evidence that these increase diagnostic accuracy, they are useful when cranial nerve injuries or severe hypoxia prevent normal BSFT.

Withdrawal of treatment (WOT)

The prognostic certainty of death associated with BSD relieves the anxiety associated with treatment discontinuation. However, prolonged self-ventilated survival without cognitive function is possible when the brainstem is intact but cortical function ceases due to ischaemic damage (e.g. prolonged cardiac arrest) or diffuse cerebral injury

(e.g. head trauma). This situation is termed **persistent vegetative state (PVS)**. In these patients WOT decisions are difficult because there is often prognostic uncertainty. Previous ethical and medicolegal deliberations recommend that decision-making should focus on 'the likelihood of return to cognitive function' and that life-sustaining therapy should be withdrawn when it is clear that the patient is 'unlikely to regain cognitive behaviour, the ability to communicate or purposeful environmental interaction'. In these circumstances, it is generally agreed that treatment other than basic medical and nursing care is inappropriate.

In '**severely disabled patients**' ethical dilemmas can be particularly complicated. It is important to appreciate that rational patients or legal surrogates have the right to refuse treatment even if this includes discontinuation of mechanical ventilation. Conversely, patients cannot demand life-saving therapy when clinicians consider it inappropriate. In practice, many patients cannot discuss treatment. Responsibility for WOT lies with the senior physician, who must review any such decisions made by other staff. These judgements are usually made in consultation with the family, taking into account prognosis, expected QOL, the opinions of the wider medical team (e.g. nursing staff) and the patient's previously expressed views (e.g. advance directives). It should be recognized that medical staff often underestimate a patient's willingness to undergo treatment independent of age or poor prognosis.

Once a WOT decision is made, **protocols** ensure patient comfort and dignity, reduce stress and reiterate the support required by relatives and junior staff. Physicians must decide which interventions to withdraw recognizing that this will influence the rapidity, comfort and dignity of the patient's death. The usual preference for the order of WOT is: renal replacement therapy, inotropic support, antibiotics, mechanical ventilation, feeding and finally intravenous fluids. Unfortunately, these biases can prolong dying causing unnecessary suffering. To prevent this WOT plans must be regularly updated. Liberal opiate therapy may be required to relieve discomfort particularly when ventilation is discontinued.

Organ donation

Organ donation is a successful treatment for end-stage organ failure, limited only by the shortfall of organs for transplantation. Organ retrieval from suitable BSD patients must be maximized but dying patients should not be ventilated simply to allow organ donation. The question of organ donation is usually raised with relatives at the time of BSFT. The decision should be autonomous and 'unpressured'. The process is easier if the patient is a Registered Organ Donor. Following consent, blood is sent for tissue typing, HIV, hepatitis and CMV testing. In the UK, each region has a transplant co-ordinator who, when contacted, will arrange retrieval and allocation of donated organs. Figure (b) lists **potential complications** prior to organ retrieval in the operating theatre. Graft survival is improved by maintaining pre-operative organ perfusion (e.g. fluids, inotropes, monitoring) and oxygenation (i.e. $P_a\text{O}_2 > 10$ kPa). Inotropes are selected to minimize organ dysfunction. Spinal reflexes and autonomic haemodynamic responses are controlled with neuromuscular blockers and opioids. Continuing emotional support for relatives and staff is essential.

25 Acute coronary syndromes I: clinical pathophysiology

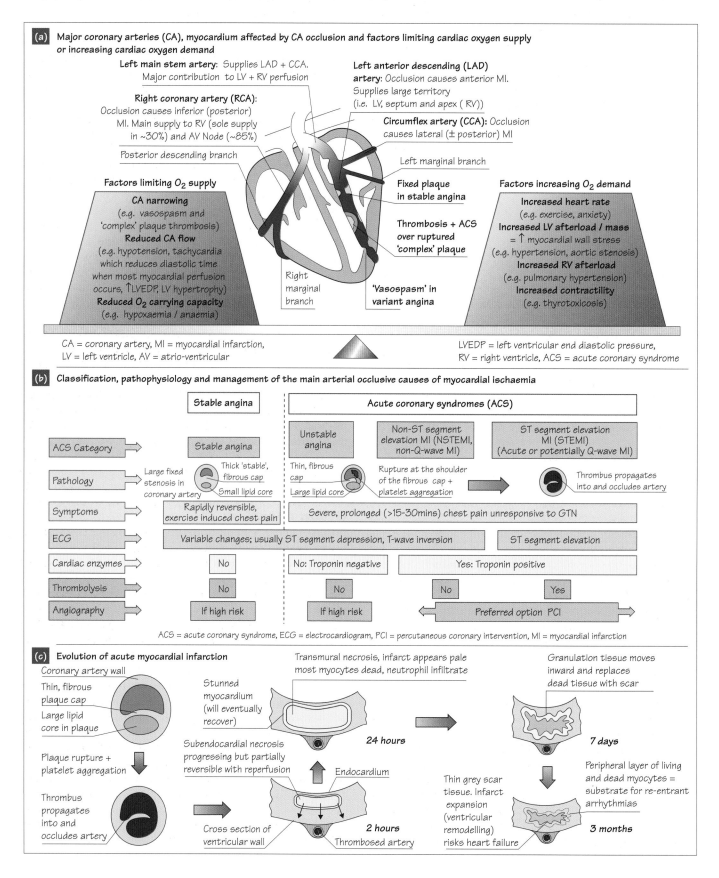

(a) Major coronary arteries (CA), myocardium affected by CA occlusion and factors limiting cardiac oxygen supply or increasing cardiac oxygen demand

Left main stem artery: Supplies LAD + CCA. Major contribution to LV + RV perfusion

Left anterior descending (LAD) artery: Occlusion causes anterior MI. Supplies large territory (i.e. LV, septum and apex (RV))

Right coronary artery (RCA): Occlusion causes inferior (posterior) MI. Main supply to RV (sole supply in ~30%) and AV Node (~85%)

Circumflex artery (CCA): Occlusion causes lateral (± posterior) MI

Posterior descending branch

Left marginal branch

Fixed plaque in stable angina

Thrombosis + ACS over ruptured 'complex' plaque

Right marginal branch

'Vasospasm' in variant angina

Factors limiting O₂ supply
- **CA narrowing** (e.g. vasospasm and 'complex' plaque thrombosis)
- **Reduced CA flow** (e.g. hypotension, tachycardia which reduces diastolic time when most myocardial perfusion occurs, ↑LVEDP, LV hypertrophy)
- **Reduced O₂ carrying capacity** (e.g. hypoxaemia / anaemia)

Factors increasing O₂ demand
- **Increased heart rate** (e.g. exercise, anxiety)
- **Increased LV afterload / mass** = ↑ myocardial wall stress (e.g. hypertension, aortic stenosis)
- **Increased RV afterload** (e.g. pulmonary hypertension)
- **Increased contractility** (e.g. thyrotoxicosis)

CA = coronary artery, MI = myocardial infarction, LV = left ventricle, AV = atrio-ventricular

LVEDP = left ventricular end diastolic pressure, RV = right ventricle, ACS = acute coronary syndrome

(b) Classification, pathophysiology and management of the main arterial occlusive causes of myocardial ischaemia

	Stable angina	Acute coronary syndromes (ACS)		
ACS Category	Stable angina	Unstable angina	Non-ST segment elevation MI (NSTEMI, non-Q-wave MI)	ST segment elevation MI (STEMI) (Acute or potentially Q-wave MI)
Pathology	Large fixed stenosis in coronary artery. Thick 'stable', fibrous cap. Small lipid core	Thin, fibrous cap. Large lipid core	Rupture at the shoulder of the fibrous cap + platelet aggregation	Thrombus propagates into and occludes artery
Symptoms	Rapidly reversible, exercise induced chest pain	Severe, prolonged (>15-30mins) chest pain unresponsive to GTN		
ECG	Variable changes; usually ST segment depression, T-wave inversion			ST segment elevation
Cardiac enzymes	No	No: Troponin negative	Yes: Troponin positive	
Thrombolysis	No	No	No	Yes
Angiography	If high risk	If high risk	Preferred option PCI	

ACS = acute coronary syndrome, ECG = electrocardiogram, PCI = percutaneous coronary intervention, MI = myocardial infarction

(c) Evolution of acute myocardial infarction

Coronary artery wall

Thin, fibrous plaque cap

Large lipid core in plaque

Plaque rupture + platelet aggregation

Thrombus propagates into and occludes artery

Stunned myocardium (will eventually recover)

Subendocardial necrosis progressing but partially reversible with reperfusion

Cross section of ventricular wall

Endocardium

Thrombosed artery

2 hours

Transmural necrosis, infarct appears pale most myocytes dead, neutrophil infiltrate

24 hours

Granulation tissue moves inward and replaces dead tissue with scar

7 days

Thin grey scar tissue. Infarct expansion (ventricular remodelling) risks heart failure

Peripheral layer of living and dead myocytes = substrate for re-entrant arrhythmias

3 months

Epidemiology of ischaemic heart disease (IHD)

Prevalence: IHD affects ~4–7% of the population in developed countries (~2.7 and ~18.5 million people in the UK and USA respectively). In the UK, >1.4 million people suffer with angina and 275,000 have a myocardial infarction (MI) annually. **Incidence** increases with age, male sex and following menopause in women. **Risk factors** include smoking, hypertension, diabetes, hypercholesterolaemia and family history. **Mortality:** IHD accounts for ~0.11, 0.53 and 0.75 million deaths annually in the UK, USA and European Union respectively (i.e. ~20% of all male and ~16% of all female deaths). Following MI, 33–66% of deaths occur before hospital admission, ~10% after admission and ~20% within 2 years due to heart failure or further MI.

Pathophysiology

Figure (a) illustrates the consequences of coronary artery occlusion and factors that result in myocardial ischaemia. Figure (b) illustrates the classification, characteristics and management of myocardial ischaemia.

1 Chronic stable (exertional) angina (SA) occurs when fixed, stable coronary artery occlusions (>70%) limit blood flow causing 'predictable', reversible cardiac ischaemia during exercise. These stenoses are caused by smooth, often circumferential atherosclerotic plaques with thick fibrous caps which are unlikely to rupture. Resulting ischaemia is usually subendocardial because systolic compression is greater in endocardial than epicardial arterioles. **Variant (Prinzmetal's) angina** is uncommon and caused by transient coronary artery vasospasm due to over-reactivity (e.g. to norepinephrine) or impaired flow-mediated vasodilation. It often occurs in the vicinity of atherosclerotic plaques but there may be no association with atherosclerosis.

2 Acute coronary syndrome (ACS) includes a spectrum of increasingly life-threatening conditions in which ischaemia (± myonecrosis) follows sudden coronary occlusion due to thrombosis (± vasoconstriction). ACS is initiated by stress-induced rupture (e.g. hypertension) of small, eccentric (i.e. non-circumferential), non-occlusive (i.e. <50%), 'complex' atherosclerotic plaques with lipid-rich cores and thin fibrous caps. Plaque rupture stimulates thrombus formation, vasospasm and arterial occlusion. The length of time and extent of the occlusion determine the severity of the ischaemia, which defines the clinical syndrome, associated symptoms, ECG changes and degree of myocardial necrosis as indicated by cardiac enzyme (CE) release (Fig. b):

- **Unstable angina (UA):** describes coronary artery occlusion of limited extent and/or duration (<20 min) which causes ischaemia but not necrosis. Symptoms occur but neither CE nor ST-segments are elevated.
- **Non-ST segment elevation MI (NSTEMI, non-Q wave MI):** describes occlusion which may be temporary, incomplete or alleviated by collateral vessels which limits ischaemia and necrosis to the subendocardium. This releases CE due to myocardial damage but does not cause ST elevation.
- **ST segment elevation MI (STEMI; Q-wave MI; acute MI):** describes coronary artery occlusion of sufficient severity to cause transmural cardiac ischaemia (i.e. immediate ST elevation on ECG and development of Q-waves in the absence of treatment). Figure (c) illustrates the evolution of an MI. Coronary angiography reveals complete occlusion in 87% of infarct-related arteries within 4 hours of onset of symptoms and the ECG ST-elevation. MI with normal coronary arteries is rare but may follow embolic occlusion (e.g. endocarditis), non-thrombotic vasospasm or cocaine abuse. Therapy aims to minimize infarct size and prevent transmural wall death (i.e. development of Q-waves on ECG).

Clinical features

Myocardial ischaemia causes 'crushing' or 'heavy' retrosternal chest pain radiating to the neck, medial aspect of the left arm and occasionally the right chest or shoulder blades. Pain may be atypical (i.e. burning), localized (i.e. jaw only) or absent in ~20% (e.g. diabetics, elderly). Pain severity, duration, relationship to exercise and the response to nitrates defines clinical subgroups but UA/NSTEMI and NSTEMI/STEMI show overlap:

- **Stable 'exercise-induced' angina (SA):** is 'predictably' precipitated by exercise or anxiety, is short-lived and relieved within 5 minutes by rest and sublingual nitrates.
- **Unstable angina and NSTEMI (UA/NSTEMI):** have clinical similarities and **do not** benefit from thrombolytic therapy. Symptoms occur 'unpredictably', are frequent, prolonged (>15 minutes) and less likely to respond to nitrates. 'New pain', 'altered SA pattern' (i.e. with less exercise), autonomic manifestations (e.g. nausea, sweating) and radiation to new sites (e.g. jaw) indicate UA/NSTEMI and increasing coronary artery occlusion. Typical presentations include crescendo angina (i.e. increasingly frequent episodes of prolonged, severe angina), angina at rest or on minimal exertion and post-MI angina. Both UA and NSTEMI may present with ST depression and/or T-wave inversion on ECG. The occurrence of UA/NSTEMI indicates a high risk of imminent coronary artery occlusion and death (i.e. within 4–6 weeks). In the USA ~4% of the 1.3 million people hospitalized with UA/NSTEMI die within 30 days and ~8% experience reinfarction.

Risk assessment: factors indicating increased risk of future cardiac events include ST depression, elevated troponin levels, recurrent angina, diabetes, previous STEMI, impaired LV function and heart failure. High risk patients require early cardiac angiography. Pain-free patients, without risk factors, should have an exercise ECG. Inducible ischaemia at a low workload indicates high risk and the need for early angiography.

- **Myocardial infarction (MI):** includes both NSTEMI and STEMI (i.e. 'troponin/CE positive' events). However, they are managed differently, in that thrombolytic therapy is only beneficial in STEMI. MI is characterized by abrupt onset of severe, prolonged pain unrelieved by nitrates, autonomic symptoms (e.g. 'cold, clammy appearance', sweating, nausea, vomiting), dyspnoea and anxiety. Most patients have previous IHD or risk factors but only 25% have preceding UA. Pain may not occur in elderly or diabetic patients who present with collapse, confusion, heart failure or metabolic dysfunction. Tachycardia often accompanies anterior MI whereas bradycardia (± heart block) is more frequent after inferior MI due to conducting tissue damage (Fig. a). Hypotension (systolic BP < 90 mmHg) suggests a large MI (>40% LV damage) and heralds cardiogenic shock (Chapters 6, 28). Auscultation may reveal a third or fourth heart sound (i.e. gallop rhythm) and a systolic murmur. **Early MI complications (<7 days)** include arrhythmias (Chapter 27), pericarditis, papillary muscle or free wall rupture (days 4–7) and ventricular septal defects. Heart failure may occur with >20% LV damage. **Late MI complications (>7 days)** include (a) mural thrombus over damaged myocardium (± thromboembolism) and (b) autoimmune pericarditis (Dressler's syndrome) which may require treatment with NSAIDs (± steroids).

Acute coronary syndromes II: investigations and management

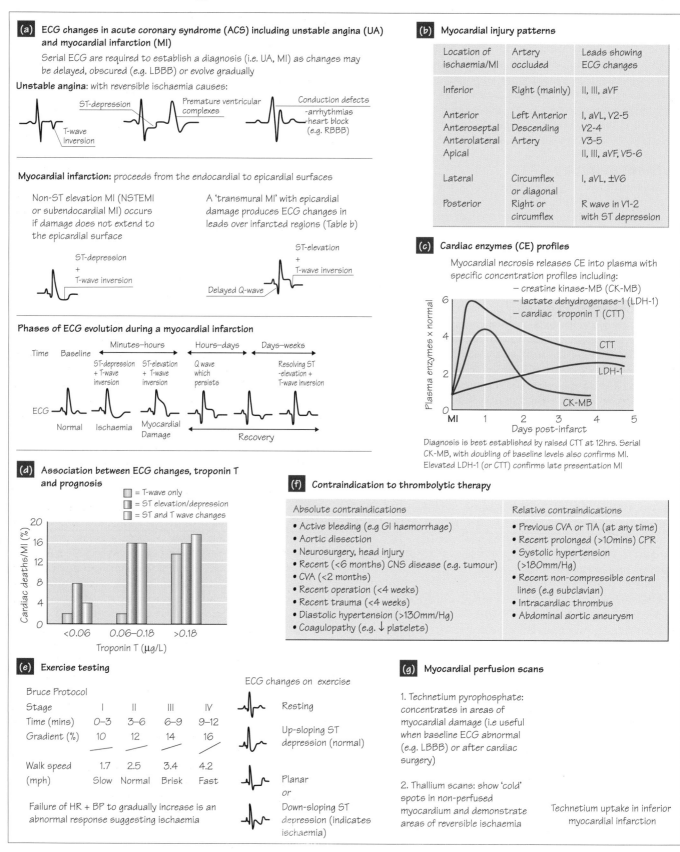

(a) ECG changes in acute coronary syndrome (ACS) including unstable angina (UA) and myocardial infarction (MI)

Serial ECG are required to establish a diagnosis (i.e. UA, MI) as changes may be delayed, obscured (e.g. LBBB) or evolve gradually

Unstable angina: with reversible ischaemia causes:

ST-depression
T-wave inversion
Premature ventricular complexes
Conduction defects -arrhythmias -heart block (e.g. RBBB)

Myocardial infarction: proceeds from the endocardial to epicardial surfaces

Non-ST elevation MI (NSTEMI or subendocardial MI) occurs if damage does not extend to the epicardial surface

A 'transmural MI' with epicardial damage produces ECG changes in leads over infarcted regions (Table b)

ST-depression + T-wave inversion

ST-elevation + T-wave inversion
Delayed Q-wave

Phases of ECG evolution during a myocardial infarction

Time	Baseline	Minutes–hours		Hours–days	Days–weeks
		ST-depression + T-wave inversion	ST-elevation + T-wave inversion	Q wave which persists	Resolving ST -elevation + T-wave inversion
ECG	Normal	Ischaemia	Myocardial Damage	Recovery	

(b) Myocardial injury patterns

Location of ischaemia/MI	Artery occluded	Leads showing ECG changes
Inferior	Right (mainly)	II, III, aVF
Anterior Anteroseptal Anterolateral Apical	Left Anterior Descending Artery	I, aVL, V2-5 V2-4 V3-5 II, III, aVF, V5-6
Lateral	Circumflex or diagonal	I, aVL, ±V6
Posterior	Right or circumflex	R wave in V1-2 with ST depression

(c) Cardiac enzymes (CE) profiles

Myocardial necrosis releases CE into plasma with specific concentration profiles including:
– creatine kinase-MB (CK-MB)
– lactate dehydrogenase-1 (LDH-1)
– cardiac troponin T (CTT)

Diagnosis is best established by raised CTT at 12hrs. Serial CK-MB, with doubling of baseline levels also confirms MI. Elevated LDH-1 (or CTT) confirms late presentation MI

(d) Association between ECG changes, troponin T and prognosis

= T-wave only
= ST elevation/depression
= ST and T wave changes

(f) Contraindication to thrombolytic therapy

Absolute contraindications	Relative contraindications
• Active bleeding (e.g GI haemorrhage) • Aortic dissection • Neurosurgery, head injury • Recent (<6 months) CNS disease (e.g. tumour) • CVA (<2 months) • Recent operation (<4 weeks) • Recent trauma (<4 weeks) • Diastolic hypertension (>130mm/Hg) • Coagulopathy (e.g. ↓ platelets)	• Previous CVA or TIA (at any time) • Recent prolonged (>10mins) CPR • Systolic hypertension (>180mm/Hg) • Recent non-compressible central lines (e.g subclavian) • Intracardiac thrombus • Abdominal aortic aneurysm

(e) Exercise testing

Bruce Protocol

Stage	I	II	III	IV
Time (mins)	0–3	3–6	6–9	9–12
Gradient (%)	10	12	14	16
Walk speed (mph)	1.7 Slow	2.5 Normal	3.4 Brisk	4.2 Fast

Failure of HR + BP to gradually increase is an abnormal response suggesting ischaemia

ECG changes on exercise

Resting
Up-sloping ST depression (normal)
Planar or
Down-sloping ST depression (indicates ischaemia)

(g) Myocardial perfusion scans

1. Technetium pyrophosphate: concentrates in areas of myocardial damage (i.e useful when baseline ECG abnormal (e.g. LBBB) or after cardiac surgery)

2. Thallium scans: show 'cold' spots in non-perfused myocardium and demonstrate areas of reversible ischaemia

Technetium uptake in inferior myocardial infarction

Acute chest pain accounts for ~15% of medical admissions. The initial diagnostic challenge is to differentiate ACS and other life-threatening conditions (e.g. aortic dissection) from benign causes of chest discomfort (e.g. gastro-oesophageal reflux, musculoskeletal).

Investigations

Serial electrocardiograms (ECG) and cardiac enzymes (CE) establish the diagnosis and have prognostic significance (Figs a, c, d).
- **ECG:** provides the earliest evidence of myocardial ischaemia, informs initial management and indicates the site and size of an infarct. Figures (a) and (b) illustrate typical ECG changes in ACS. ST-segment elevation (>0.1 mV in two chest leads or >0.2 mV in two limb leads) is the diagnostic hallmark of acute MI and indicates the need for immediate revascularization. However, ST-segment depression (ST↓) and T-wave inversion occur in ~20% of MI with raised CE. These non-ST-segment elevation (ST↑) MI (NSTEMI) do not benefit from thrombolysis. Although ACS patients with ST↓ have lower early mortality than those with ST↑, survival at >6 months is similar.
- **Cardiac enzymes:** a greater than twofold increase in plasma CE concentration indicates myocardial damage (Fig. c). Cardiac troponins (CT) measured at 12 hours are particularly sensitive and specific markers of myocardial necrosis and can detect MI after surgery or when the ECG is non-specific (e.g. left bundle branch block (LBBB)).
- **Chest radiography:** detects heart failure and aortic dissection.
- **Echocardiography:** assesses contractility and reveals dyskinesia, mural thrombus, septal defects and papillary muscle rupture.
- **Incremental exercise stress tests** (EST; e.g. Bruce protocol): reveal cardiac ischaemia as angina, ECG changes (i.e. >2 mm ↓, arrhythmias) or failure of appropriate heart rate or BP responses (Fig. e)
- **Myocardial perfusion scans (MPS):** detect reduced isotope uptake in poorly perfused myocardium using a gamma camera (Fig. g). It is a useful alternative to EST in immobile patients or those with LBBB.
- **Coronary angiography:** provides radiographic imaging and assessment of the severity of coronary artery disease.

Management

Treatment aims to reduce *myocardial oxygen consumption (MOC)* by decreasing heart rate (e.g. beta-blockers) and afterload (e.g. antihypertensives); whilst increasing *myocardial oxygen supply* with pharmacotherapy (± oxygen). Essential risk factor reduction includes smoking cessation, low fat diet, weight loss, exercise and control of diabetes or hypertension. Anti-platelet agents (e.g. aspirin) and lipid-lowering drugs (e.g. statins to reduce LDL to <2.6 mmol) are indicated in most patients. Angiotensin converting enzyme (ACE) inhibitors also reduce atherosclerosis and improve prognosis.

Stable angina (SA)

The following therapies improve symptoms:
- **Nitrovasodilators:** are very effective but tolerance develops without nitrate-free periods (~6 hours/day).
- **Beta-blockers:** improve prognosis and are first line therapy. They increase diastolic myocardial perfusion by slowing heart rate and lower left ventricular wall tension by reducing preload (± afterload). Sublingual, oral and intravenous routes are effective.
- **Calcium channel antagonists (CCA):** are useful when beta-blockers are contraindicated. They relieve coronary vasospasm but may cause tachycardia (e.g. nifedipine) and exacerbate heart failure (i.e. negatively inotropic). Only CCA that slow heart rate like diltiazem are given as monotherapy.

- **Revascularization:** is required if symptoms deteriorate, the EST is positive or angiography reveals >70% stenoses in all three main, left main or proximal LAD coronary arteries.

Unstable angina/NSTEMI

In UA/NSTEMI thrombolytic therapy (TT) is not beneficial. As in SA, therapy includes nitrates, beta-blockers (± CCA) and additional:
- **Antiplatelet therapy:** give all patients 300 mg **aspirin** immediately and continue at 75 mg/day indefinitely. Irreversible cyclo-oxygenase inhibition prevents platelet aggregation within 15 minutes of chewing an aspirin, reducing MI and sudden death by 50%. Clopidogrel inhibits ADP-stimulated platelet aggregation, reduces mortality by ~20%, and is combined with aspirin therapy for ≥30 days. **Glycoprotein IIb/IIIa antagonists** are the most effective platelet inhibitors and are used after percutaneous coronary interventions (PCI) to prevent stent-induced thrombosis.
- **Anticoagulant therapy:** intravenous **unfractionated heparin (UH)** or subcutaneous **low molecular weight heparin (LMWH)** prevent thromboembolic complications in immobile patients.
- **Consider PCI** after 48 hours if medical therapy fails.

Myocardial infarction/STEMI

Early reperfusion after MI limits infarct size and reduces hospital mortality from 13% to <10%.
- **Immediate management:** includes pain relief, monitoring and oxygen therapy (>60%). Patients without contraindications should be given aspirin, clopidogrel, beta-blockers (± heparin). Revascularization with PCI or TT should be commenced without delay.
- **Pharmacological therapies: Opiates** (e.g. morphine) relieve pain, reduce preload, lower MOC and lower anxiety-induced catecholamine release. **Aspirin** reduces 35-day mortality by 23% (42% when combined with TT). Immediate **beta-blockade** (e.g. metoprolol) reduces infarct size, arrhythmias and mortality, especially in hypertensive or tachycardic patients. Contraindications include asthma, heart failure and bradycardia. Early **nitrates** (<24 hours) reduce pain, infarct size and heart failure. **ACE inhibitors** after >24 hours improve LV remodelling and reduce heart failure in high risk patients. **Inotropic support** may be required in cardiogenic shock (Chapters 6, 28). Prophylactic antiarrhythmic therapy is not recommended.
- **Percutaneous coronary intervention:** within ≤90 minutes of presentation is the preferred method of revascularization after MI if facilities are available. Primary PCI (<6 hours) reopens >90% of occluded coronary arteries with few complications. Consider rescue PCI if TT fails but mortality is significant if unsuccessful.
- **Thrombolytic therapy:** dissipates thrombus, reverses ischaemia and limits myocardial injury and complications (e.g. heart failure). TT is most effective within <2 hours of symptom onset but benefit persists to 12 hours. It reduces mortality by ~25%. The main agents, **streptokinase** (SK) and **tissue plasminogen activator** (tPA), are given by infusion. SK is cheap but allergenic (i.e. single use). tPA has slight survival benefits and is given if SK has been used previously. Intravenous heparin is required for 48–72 hours after tPA because of its short half-life. Newer agents (e.g. reteplase, tenecteplase) have a longer half-life. The main risk of TT is haemorrhage (e.g. ~1% stroke). Contraindications (Fig. f) prevent use in half of cases.
- **Follow-up:** includes EST, risk factor reduction, anticoagulation after large MI and referral of high risk patients for angiography.

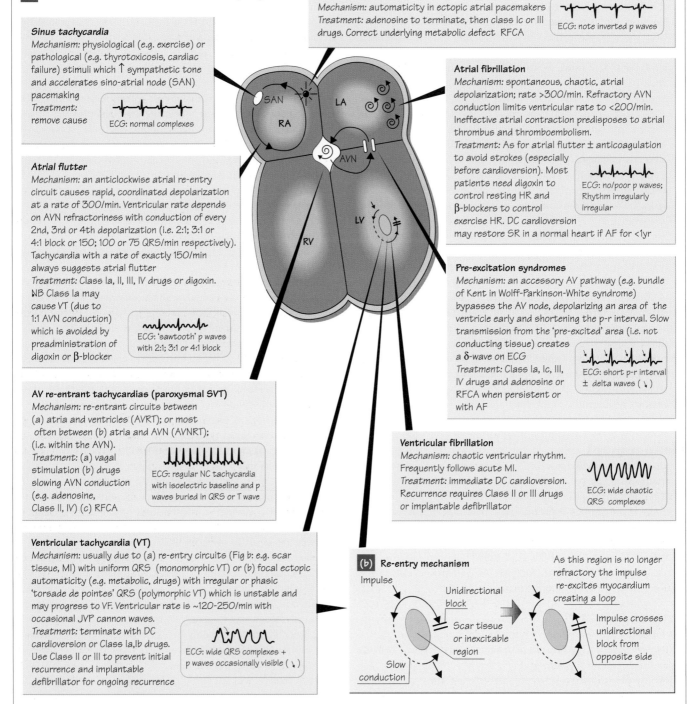

(a) Mechanisms and treatment of common tachyarrhythmias

Sinus tachycardia
Mechanism: physiological (e.g. exercise) or pathological (e.g. thyrotoxicosis, cardiac failure) stimuli which ↑ sympathetic tone and accelerates sino-atrial node (SAN) pacemaking
Treatment: remove cause

ECG: normal complexes

Atrial flutter
Mechanism: an anticlockwise atrial re-entry circuit causes rapid, coordinated depolarization at a rate of 300/min. Ventricular rate depends on AVN refractoriness with conduction of every 2nd, 3rd or 4th depolarization (i.e. 2:1; 3:1 or 4:1 block or 150; 100 or 75 QRS/min respectively). Tachycardia with a rate of exactly 150/min always suggests atrial flutter
Treatment: Class Ia, II, III, IV drugs or digoxin. NB Class Ia may cause VT (due to 1:1 AVN conduction) which is avoided by preadministration of digoxin or β-blocker

ECG: 'sawtooth' p waves with 2:1; 3:1 or 4:1 block

AV re-entrant tachycardias (paroxysmal SVT)
Mechanism: re-entrant circuits between (a) atria and ventricles (AVRT); or most often between (b) atria and AVN (AVNRT); (i.e. within the AVN).
Treatment: (a) vagal stimulation (b) drugs slowing AVN conduction (e.g. adenosine, Class II, IV) (c) RFCA

ECG: regular NC tachycardia with isoelectric baseline and p waves buried in QRS or T wave

Ventricular tachycardia (VT)
Mechanism: usually due to (a) re-entry circuits (Fig b: e.g. scar tissue, MI) with uniform QRS (monomorphic VT) or (b) focal ectopic automaticity (e.g. metabolic, drugs) with irregular and phasic 'torsade de pointes' QRS (polymorphic VT) which is unstable and may progress to VF. Ventricular rate is ~120-250/min with occasional JVP cannon waves.
Treatment: terminate with DC cardioversion or Class Ia,Ib drugs. Use Class II or III to prevent initial recurrence and implantable defibrillator for ongoing recurrence

ECG: wide QRS complexes + p waves occasionally visible (↓)

Atrial tachycardia
Mechanism: automaticity in ectopic atrial pacemakers
Treatment: adenosine to terminate, then class Ic or III drugs. Correct underlying metabolic defect RFCA

ECG: note inverted p waves

Atrial fibrillation
Mechanism: spontaneous, chaotic, atrial depolarization; rate >300/min. Refractory AVN conduction limits ventricular rate to <200/min. Ineffective atrial contraction predisposes to atrial thrombus and thromboembolism.
Treatment: As for atrial flutter ± anticoagulation to avoid strokes (especially before cardioversion). Most patients need digoxin to control resting HR and β-blockers to control exercise HR. DC cardioversion may restore SR in a normal heart if AF for <1yr

ECG: no/poor p waves; Rhythm irregularly irregular

Pre-excitation syndromes
Mechanism: an accessory AV pathway (e.g. bundle of Kent in Wolff-Parkinson-White syndrome) bypasses the AV node, depolarizing an area of the ventricle early and shortening the p-r interval. Slow transmission from the 'pre-excited' area (i.e. not conducting tissue) creates a δ-wave on ECG
Treatment: Class Ia, Ic, III, IV drugs and adenosine or RFCA when persistent or with AF

ECG: short p-r interval ± delta waves (↓)

Ventricular fibrillation
Mechanism: chaotic ventricular rhythm. Frequently follows acute MI.
Treatment: immediate DC cardioversion. Recurrence requires Class II or III drugs or implantable defibrillator

ECG: wide chaotic QRS complexes

(b) Re-entry mechanism

Impulse

Unidirectional block

Scar tissue or inexcitable region

Slow conduction

As this region is no longer refractory the impulse re-excites myocardium creating a loop

Impulse crosses unidirectional block from opposite side

RFCA=radiofrequency catheter ablation, AVN=atriventricular node, SAN=sinoatrial node, NC=narrow complex, RA=right atrium, LA=left atrium, RV=right ventricle, LV=left ventricle, SR=sinus rhythm, AV=atrioventricular, AF=atrial fibrillation. JVP=jugular venous pressure

Definition
Arrhythmias are abnormalities of the heart rate (HR) or rhythm due to aberrant impulse generation or conduction (e.g. re-entry circuits).

Tachycardia is a HR >100 beats/min and is supraventricular (SVT) or ventricular (VT) in origin. Tachycardias are caused by:

1 Increased pacemaker activity: faster spontaneous membrane depolarization, lower thresholds and oscillations during repolarization (e.g. digoxin toxicity) trigger early action potentials (AP).

2 Re-entry circuits: a depolarization wave travels around a circle of myocardial tissue; if the tissue is not refractory when the electrical impulse returns it will depolarize again producing a recurring circuit (Fig. b). This causes most paroxysmal tachycardias.

Bradycardia is a HR <60 beats/min and is due to delayed conduction.

Diagnosis

Diagnosis can be difficult. ECG interpretation is often complicated by electrical artifacts, shivering, seizures and tremor. Oesophageal or right-sided ECG leads occasionally aid diagnosis.

- **Narrow QRS complex (NC) tachycardias:** are usually SVTs and can be assessed (± terminated) with intravenous (i.v.) adenosine boluses.
- **Wide QRS complex (WC) tachycardias:** are usually due to VT but can be difficult to differentiate from SVT with abnormal conduction (SVT/AC). After excluding atrioventricular node (AVN) block, treat as VT if haemodynamic instability co-exists. Lack of response to DC cardioversion and/or i.v. lidocaine (lignocaine) suggests an SVT/AC, which is confirmed (± cardioverted) with i.v. adenosine. Ongoing treatment failure is managed with i.v. amiodarone (Appendix 1) and repeated cardioversion.

General management

Atrial fibrillation affects 10% of those aged > 75 years and arrhythmias, usually VT/VF, cause 15–40% of deaths in IHD. Rapid assessment and diagnosis are essential but not all arrhythmias require immediate intervention. Asymptomatic or stable rhythms can be observed whilst the cause (e.g. hypokalaemia) is corrected.

Prevention requires early correction of hypoxaemia, electrolyte disturbances (e.g. hypokalaemia), acid–base imbalance and cardiac ischaemia. Arrhythmogenic factors including vagal stimulation (e.g. pain), drugs (e.g. theophylline) and cardiac irritants (e.g. intracardiac catheters) must be addressed. **Tachyarrhythmias** are detrimental if they cause symptoms, hypotension, pulmonary oedema or reduce tissue perfusion and should be terminated immediately with cardioversion or drugs. **Bradyarrhythmias**, if symptomatic, are treated with atropine, β-agonists or pacing (see below).

- **Vagal stimulation** (e.g. carotid sinus massage): slows HR, allows diagnosis and may cardiovert some SVT.
- **Antiarrhythmic drugs** are classified by mechanism or site of action (Appendix 1). They are selected according to rhythm and underlying pathophysiology (Fig. a). Therapeutic windows are often narrow and side-effects common. Therapy is often ineffective (e.g. ~50% VT) and paradoxically causes new arrhythmias in ~20% of cases. These '**pro-arrhythmic**' effects are common with Class Ia and III drugs which increase AP duration (i.e. prolonged QT interval), trigger automaticity and precipitate VT (e.g. 'torsades de points'). **Prophylaxis:** beta-blockers reduce IHD mortality but anti-arrhythmics do not always improve outcome (e.g. after MI).
- **Non-pharmacological therapies:** can be more successful than protracted drug therapy and are often required in emergencies. In haemodynamically unstable VT or SVT, **direct current (DC) cardioversion** using 50–360J shocks delivered through sternal and cardiac apex electrodes, in anaesthetized patients, achieves rapid cardioversion (Chapter 5). In patients with recurrent VT **implantable defibrillators**

improve survival by >30% compared to drug therapy. **Radiofrequency catheter ablation** (RFCA) safely destroys >90% of treatable accessory pathways or ectopic pacemakers using radiofrequency energy delivered through a catheter tip. In refractory SVT **overdrive atrial pacing** may restore sinus rhythm.

Tachyarrhythmias

Mechanisms and treatments are summarized in Fig. (a).

1 Supraventricular tachyarrhythmias: originate above the AVN and present with dizziness, palpitations and breathlessness. They are rarely life-threatening, although sudden death can occur.
- **Sinus tachycardia** is a normal physiological response.
- **Atrial tachycardia** occurs in chronic cardiorespiratory disease due to ectopic atrial automaticity caused by metabolic, acid–base or drug (e.g. digoxin) toxicity.
- **Atrial flutter** and **fibrillation** may occur in isolation but are commonly associated with cardiac disease (e.g. atrial dilation, hypertension), thyrotoxicosis or thromboembolism.
- **AVN re-entrant tachycardias** are common and **pre-excitation syndromes** unusual causes of SVT.

2 Ventricular tachyarrhythmias: arise in the ventricles of patients with underlying IHD, cardiomyopathy or congenital heart disease. They are generally more serious than SVT.
- **Ventricular fibrillation (VF)** results in rapid loss of cardiac output (CO) and unconsciousness. Death follows without resuscitation and DC cardioversion (Chapter 5).
- **Ventricular tachycardia** may be well tolerated but often causes haemodynamic instability or degenerates into VF

Bradyarrhythmias

Bradycardia is often well tolerated but CO and BP fall if stroke volume cannot increase due to reduced compliance or contractility.

1 Sinus bradycardia: has normal ECG p-waves and 1:1 AVN conduction. It is treated by addressing potential causes including vagal reflexes (e.g. pain) or drug-toxicity (e.g. beta-blockers). Atropine, β-agonists (e.g. isoprenaline) or drug antidotes (e.g. digoxin antibodies) are occasionally required if symptoms persist.

2 Heart block (HB): is often due to AVN or conducting tissue ischaemia. It is common after inferior MI, because the right coronary artery supplies the AVN, but is usually transient and rarely requires treatment. By contrast, HB after an anterior MI suggests a large infarct and requires early pacemaker insertion.
- **First degree HB** slows AVN conduction causing p-r prolongation (>0.2 seconds) on ECG. It is unimportant except as an early warning of higher degrees of HB.
- **Second degree HB** occurs when some atrial beats are not conducted to the ventricles. *Mobitz 1 AVN block* (Wenkebach) causes progressive p-r interval lengthening, culminating in failure of transmission of an atrial impulse. This sequence is repetitive. Treatment is rarely required. *Mobitz II block* occurs below the AVN in the His-Purkinje system. Every second or third atrial impulse initiates ventricular contraction (2:1; 3:1 block). Pacemaker insertion is required (e.g. anterior MI) as complete HB often follows.
- **Complete (third degree) HB** – conduction between atria and ventricles ceases. Subsequent *AVN pacemaker activity* produces NC 'junctional' escape rhythms (HR ~40–60 beats/min), which are often transient and asymptomatic. *Infranodal WC pacemaker escape rhythms* are unstable, slower (HR ~30–45 beats/min) and symptomatic. Pacemaker insertion is essential.

28 Heart failure and pulmonary oedema

(a) Causes of heart failure and pulmonary oedema

Myocardial dysfunction	Ischaemic heart disease, cardiomyopathies, pregnancy and myocardial disease (e.g. amyloidosis). Isolated RVF follows ~33% of inferior MI as the RV blood supply is mainly from the right coronary artery
Pressure overload	*Left heart:* hypertension and aortic stenosis. Mitral stenosis does not often cause LVF *Right heart:* pulmonary hypertension due to chronic lung disease (cor pulmonale), pulmonary stenosis
Volume overload	Excessive fluid administration or retention (e.g. renal failure). Aortic or mitral valve regurgitation causes LVF. Tricuspid regurgitation causes RVF
Impaired filling	Constrictive pericarditis (e.g. TB; rheumatic heart disease) or cardiac tamponade (e.g. pericardial effusion)
Arrhythmias Tachycardia	Impair ventricular filling causing atrial hypertension. Cause myocardial ischaemia by reducing diastole (e.g. atrial fibrillation, supraventricular tachycardia)
High output	Thyrotoxicosis, arteriovenous shunts, anaemia, Paget's disease, beriberi (vitamin B deficiency), sepsis

(b) Cardiac output response of normal and failing hearts to loading conditions. Failing hearts respond well to afterload reduction but not preload increases

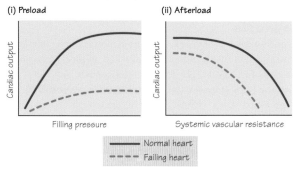

(i) Preload — Cardiac output vs Filling pressure
(ii) Afterload — Cardiac output vs Systemic vascular resistance

— Normal heart
-- Failing heart

(c) Cardiovascular compensatory mechanisms and the detrimental positive feedback effects they exert in heart failure. The location of action of key drugs is shown

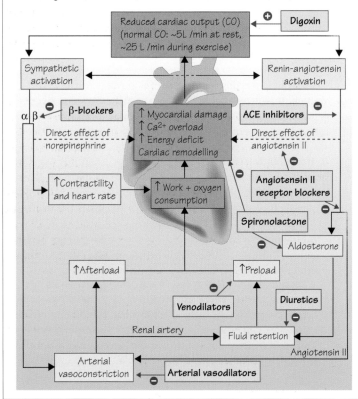

(d) New York Heart Association (NYHA) classification of heart failure

- **Class I (mild):** No limitation of physical activity. No symptoms (e.g. fatigue, dyspnoea, palpitations) from ordinary activity
- **Class II (mild):** Slight limitation of physical activity. Comfortable at rest but ordinary activity causes symptoms
- **Class III (moderate):** Marked limitation of physical activity. Only comfortable at rest; minimal activity causes symptoms
- **Class IV (severe):** Unable to carry out any physical activity without discomfort. Symptoms at rest

(e) The chest radiograph in heart failure shows an enlarged heart, pulmonary oedema with hilar 'bat's wing' shadowing, pleural effusions (usually right-sided) and upper lobe vein dilation due to increased venous pressure

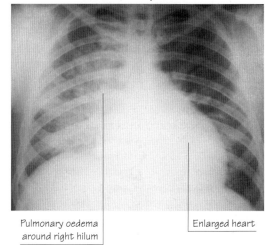

Pulmonary oedema around right hilum

Enlarged heart

Heart failure (HF) occurs when cardiac output (CO) is insufficient to meet the metabolic needs of the body, or can do so only with elevated filling pressures (**preload**; Chapter 7). Initially, compensatory mechanisms maintain CO at rest, but as HF (and CO) deteriorates, exercise tolerance falls and 'downstream' hydrostatic pressures increase. The left, right or both sides of the heart can fail.

- **Left ventricular failure** (LVF) is most common. If the resulting 'downstream' pulmonary capillary ('wedge') pressure (PCWP,

Chapters 3, 7) rises to >20–25 mmHg, fluid filters into alveolar and interstitial spaces causing **pulmonary oedema** and breathlessness. Low plasma oncotic pressure (e.g. hypoalbuminaemia) or increased membrane permeability (e.g. inflammation) can cause pulmonary oedema at lower PCWP.

- **Right ventricular failure** (RVF) causes systemic congestion (e.g. ankle oedema, hepatomegaly) and is usually associated with LVF. Resulting biventricular failure is termed **congestive cardiac failure**.
- 'Cor pulmonale' describes RVF due to chronic lung disease.

Epidemiology

HF affects 2–3% of the population and >10% of people >65 years old. It is commoner in men. **Causes** are listed in Fig. (a); the most common are IHD and hypertension. Volume overload can cause pulmonary oedema despite good contractile function. **Prognosis:** 5-year survival is <50%.

Pathophysiology

- **Systolic failure**, with reduced myocardial contractility and ejection fraction (EF; <50%), accounts for 70% of HF. It is often due to IHD, cardiomyopathy, metabolic toxicity, valve defects or arrhythmias. Initially CO is maintained by compensatory mechanisms including: (i) *increased sympathetic drive;* (ii) *raised circulating volume* (i.e. salt and water retention due to activation of the renin-angiotensin system by poor renal perfusion); (iii) *raised filling pressures* (Fig. b(i); Chapter 7). Unfortunately these mechanisms also have detrimental effects: failing hearts respond poorly to preload (Fig. b(i)) with subsequent pulmonary and peripheral congestion, whilst large ventricular volumes increase cardiac work and impair function (Fig. c). In pressure overload (e.g. aortic stenosis) compensatory hypertrophy initially improves ventricular EF but reduced compliance and capillary density eventually decreases blood supply and contractility.
- **Diastolic dysfunction** (DD) occurs when LV relaxation/filling, an energy-dependent process, is impaired due to myocardial ischaemia, fibrosis, LV hypertrophy (e.g. hypertension) and associated poor diastolic LV perfusion. Reduced LV compliance increases PCWP and can precipitate pulmonary oedema despite normal contractility and an EF >50%. DD affects ~30% of HF patients and may be precipitated by tachycardia (shorter diastolic perfusion time) or atrial fibrillation (impaired LV filling).

Clinical features

Presentation depends on speed of onset, underlying cause and ventricular involvement. HF can be precipitated or aggravated by stress, acute illness, arrhythmias, pregnancy or drugs. Severity is often classified as in Fig. (d). Whatever the cause, reduced CO causes fatigue, anorexia and exercise limitation.

- **LVF** is characterized by breathlessness, hypoxaemia, orthopnoea, paroxysmal nocturnal dyspnoea and cough productive of frothy 'pink' sputum. Auscultation may reveal a gallop rhythm (S_3/S_4 added sounds) and coarse crepitations at the lung bases.
- **RVF** causes systemic congestion with raised jugular venous pressure, hepatomegaly, ascites and ankle oedema.

Onset may be **acute** (e.g. MI) with cardiogenic shock (Chapter 6) or acute pulmonary oedema or **chronic** with fatigue and gradual fluid retention.

Diagnostic investigations

Investigations include cardiac enzymes, ECG and CXR (Fig. e).

Serum b-type natriuretic peptide (BNP) is increased by myocardial wall stress and is sensitive and specific for HF. Echocardiography may demonstrate wall hypokinesia and ventricular enlargement. Ejection fraction is usually reduced in HF although CO and BP may be normal (see above). Cardiac catheterization is often required.

Management

The cause (e.g. IHD, valve disease), underlying pathophysiology (e.g. DD), precipitating events (e.g. arrhythmias) must be treated. In general, **afterload reduction** rapidly improves LV function and CO in the failing heart (Fig. b(ii)) but may cause hypotension. By contrast, **preload reduction** relieves symptoms (e.g. pulmonary oedema) but CO is not increased (Fig. b(i)), except when afterload is indirectly reduced (e.g. decreased chamber size). **Non-invasive monitoring** and less frequently **pulmonary artery catheterization** may be required to measure filling pressures, CO and vascular resistances to optimize HF treatment (Chapters 3, 7).

Acute left ventricular failure

Immediate relief of breathlessness due to pulmonary oedema is a priority. The **sitting position** is most comfortable and **supplemental oxygen** (>60%) corrects hypoxaemia. **Loop diuretics** (e.g. furosemide i.v.) initially reduce LV preload and relieve dyspnoea by pulmonary venodilation. Subsequent diuresis lowers fluid load and cardiac filling pressures. **Nitrates** (i.v., sublingual) also increase venous capacitance whilst simultaneously dilating coronary arteries in IHD. **Diamorphine** decreases preload due to potent venodilator effects and reduces $\dot{V}o_2$ by relieving anxiety. **Bronchodilators** (e.g. salbutamol) reverse bronchospasm but aminophylline may precipitate arrhythmias. **CPAP** reduces hypoxaemia and work of breathing and is used with increasing frequency in HF (Chapter 14). **Arrhythmia** control is essential (Chapter 27).

Low-output left ventricular failure

When pulmonary oedema has been controlled, treatment aims to improve LV function, DD and prognosis. **ACE inhibitors** reduce afterload, increase CO, reduce symptoms (e.g. fatigue) and lengthen survival. They benefit most HF patients except when contra-indicated (e.g. renal artery stenosis) or if side-effects occur (e.g. cough). Selective **beta-blockers** (e.g. bisoprolol, carvedilol) improve prognosis by reducing myocardial ischaemia and arrhythmias but may precipitate pulmonary oedema, heart block or bronchospasm. **Calcium channel blockers (CCBs)** alleviate DD by reducing hypertension and coronary vasospasm. However, tachycardia and impaired contractility limit use. **Digoxin** has inotropic effects and is useful in HF with AF. **Prophylactic anticoagulants** reduce associated thromboembolic events.

Right ventricular failure

Diuresis reduces peripheral oedema but is detrimental if high RV filling pressures are required to maintain CO. Afterload reduction with pulmonary vasodilators (e.g. CCB) is usually limited by hypotension. **Oxygen therapy** relieves cor pulmonale (Chapter 34).

Cardiogenic shock

This may require **inotropic agents** or **intra-aortic balloon pumps** to maintain CO and perfusion pressures (Chapter 6). **Phosphodiesterase inhibitors** (milrinone) increase cAMP stimulating cardiac contractility and peripheral vasodilation. Similarly, new **calcium sensitizers** (e.g. levosimendan) enhance contractility. Early **ventilatory support** improves survival (Chapters 14, 16).

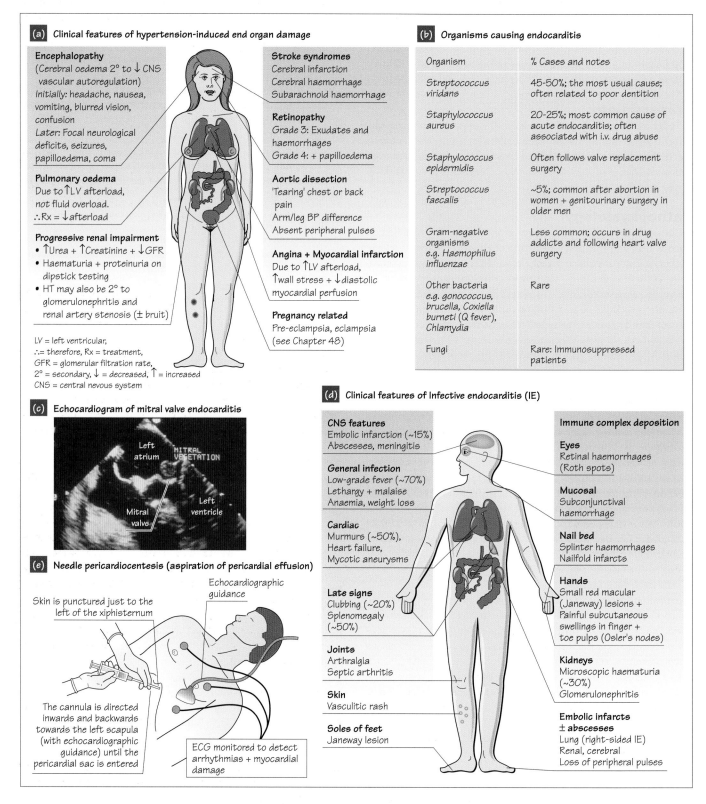

(a) Clinical features of hypertension-induced end organ damage

Encephalopathy
(Cerebral oedema 2° to ↓ CNS vascular autoregulation)
Initially: headache, nausea, vomiting, blurred vision, confusion
Later: Focal neurological deficits, seizures, papilloedema, coma

Pulmonary oedema
Due to ↑LV afterload, not fluid overload.
∴.Rx = ↓afterload

Progressive renal impairment
- ↑Urea + ↑Creatinine + ↓GFR
- Haematuria + proteinuria on dipstick testing
- HT may also be 2° to glomerulonephritis and renal artery stenosis (± bruit)

LV = left ventricular,
∴.= therefore, Rx = treatment,
GFR = glomerular filtration rate,
2° = secondary, ↓ = decreased, ↑ = increased
CNS = central nevous system

Stroke syndromes
Cerebral infarction
Cerebral haemorrhage
Subarachnoid haemorrhage

Retinopathy
Grade 3: Exudates and haemorrhages
Grade 4: + papilloedema

Aortic dissection
'Tearing' chest or back pain
Arm/leg BP difference
Absent peripheral pulses

Angina + Myocardial infarction
Due to ↑LV afterload,
↑wall stress + ↓diastolic myocardial perfusion

Pregnancy related
Pre-eclampsia, eclampsia (see Chapter 48)

(b) Organisms causing endocarditis

Organism	% Cases and notes
Streptococcus viridans	45-50%; the most usual cause; often related to poor dentition
Staphylococcus aureus	20-25%; most common cause of acute endocarditis; often associated with i.v. drug abuse
Staphylococcus epidermidis	Often follows valve replacement surgery
Streptococcus faecalis	~5%; common after abortion in women + genitourinary surgery in older men
Gram-negative organisms e.g. Haemophilus influenzae	Less common; occurs in drug addicts and following heart valve surgery
Other bacteria e.g. gonococcus, brucella, Coxiella burneti (Q fever), Chlamydia	Rare
Fungi	Rare: Immunosuppressed patients

(c) Echocardiogram of mitral valve endocarditis

Left atrium
MITRAL VEGETATION
Mitral valve
Left ventricle

(d) Clinical features of Infective endocarditis (IE)

CNS features
Embolic infarction (~15%)
Abscesses, meningitis

General infection
Low-grade fever (~70%)
Lethargy + malaise
Anaemia, weight loss

Cardiac
Murmurs (~50%),
Heart failure,
Mycotic aneurysms

Late signs
Clubbing (~20%)
Splenomegaly (~50%)

Joints
Arthralgia
Septic arthritis

Skin
Vasculitic rash

Soles of feet
Janeway lesion

Immune complex deposition

Eyes
Retinal haemorrhages (Roth spots)

Mucosal
Subconjunctival haemorrhage

Nail bed
Splinter haemorrhages
Nailfold infarcts

Hands
Small red macular (Janeway) lesions +
Painful subcutaneous swellings in finger + toe pulps (Osler's nodes)

Kidneys
Microscopic haematuria (~30%)
Glomerulonephritis

Embolic infarcts ± abscesses
Lung (right-sided IE)
Renal, cerebral
Loss of peripheral pulses

(e) Needle pericardiocentesis (aspiration of pericardial effusion)

Echocardiographic guidance

Skin is punctured just to the left of the xiphisternum

The cannula is directed inwards and backwards towards the left scapula (with echocardiographic guidance) until the pericardial sac is entered

ECG monitored to detect arrhythmias + myocardial damage

Hypertensive emergencies

- *Definition* Severe hypertension (HT) is a systolic blood pressure (BP) >220–240 mmHg or a diastolic BP >120–140 mmHg. In the past, hypertensive emergencies (HEs) were termed either 'accelerated' or 'malignant' HT; the latter associated with more advanced retinopathy (±organ damage). Current HE classification is based on the presence or absence of **life-threatening organ damage** (LTOD), which determines the urgency for treatment. When LTOD is present (e.g. aortic dissection), BP is reduced to safe levels (diastolic BP ~100–110 mmHg) within <1–2 hours. However, caution is required as rapid falls in BP can cause strokes, accelerated renal failure and myocardial ischaemia. Therefore, in the absence of LTOD, gradual reduction of BP over >6–72 hours is preferred.

• *Aetiology* The commonest cause of HE is inadequate or discontinued therapy for benign essential HT. However, in young (<30 years) or black patients, >50% have a secondary cause including renovascular disease, phaeochromocytoma, endocrine syndromes (Chapter 41) or drug-induced catecholamine release (e.g. cocaine). Pregnancy-related HT is discussed in Chapter 56. **Pathophysiology:** most organ damage is due to arteriolar necrotizing vasculitis and loss of vascular autoregulation.

• *Clinical features* of HT-induced organ damage are illustrated in Fig. (a). **Prognosis**: the 1-year mortality is >90% if severe HT with LTOD is untreated.

Management

• *Severe HT with LTOD* is a medical emergency requiring admission for close monitoring. *Rarely*, immediate BP reduction is required (e.g. dissecting aneurysm) using potent, titratable, vasodilator infusions. In these circumstances, arterial BP monitoring is mandatory. **Intravenous therapies** include: (i) **Sodium nitroprusside,** a rapidly reversible, arteriovenous dilator, always administered by infusion pump to avoid hypotensive episodes. Prolonged use can cause cyanide poisoning. (ii) **Glycerol trinitrate,** an arteriovenous dilator, particularly effective when myocardial ischaemia or pulmonary oedema co-exist. (iii) **Labetalol,** an α + β-blocker, is valuable for hypertensive encephalopathy but may exacerbate asthma, heart failure and heart block. **(d) Rarely used agents,** include hydralazine and diazoxide which are difficult to titrate due to their prolonged action. Angiotensin-converting enzyme (ACE) inhibitors can cause severe hypotension and are best avoided.

• *Severe HT in the absence of LTOD* (i.e. renal failure) rarely presents the same therapeutic crisis. Whenever possible **oral** regimes are used to lower diastolic BP to ~100 mmHg over ~24–72 hours. Sublingual **nifedipine** is popular as it has a rapid onset of action, short half-life and is titratable. Oral beta-blockers, ACE inhibitors and calcium antagonists are introduced as normal.

Infective endocarditis

Infection of heart valves or endocardium is usually **subacute** and causes a chronic illness when due to non-virulent organisms (e.g. *Streptococcus viridans*). However, it can be **acute** with a fulminant course when due to virulent organisms (e.g. *Staphylococcus*). Figure (b) lists organisms that cause infective endocarditis.

• *Aetiology* It is most common in elderly people with degenerative aortic and mitral valve disease but also affects patients with prosthetic valves, rheumatic or congenital heart disease. Abnormal valves are more susceptible to infection following dental or surgical procedures. Normal valves are occasionally infected by virulent organisms (e.g. staphylococcal valve infection following intravenous drug abuse).

• *Clinical features* are illustrated in Fig. (d). **Systemic embolization:** causes splenic, lung, renal and cerebral infarcts (± abscesses). **Immune complex deposition:** produces nail bed splinter haemorrhages, retinal haemorrhage (Roth spots), mucosal haemorrhage (e.g. subconjunctival) and painful nodular lesions in finger pulps (Osler's nodes). Microscopic haematuria and splenomegaly are common.

• *Diagnosis* is initially clinical and should be suspected in any patient with fever, anaemia, raised ESR/CRP, microscopic haematuria, new heart murmurs, flu-like symptoms or weight loss. Repeatedly positive blood cultures (~50–80%) and echocardiography confirm the diagnosis. Transthoracic echocardiography (Fig. c) detects <50% of vegetations. Transoesophageal studies are more sensitive.

• *Management* Look for and treat underlying infection (e.g. dental abscesses). Empiric antibiotic therapy is started with benzylpenicillin and an aminoglycoside and adjusted when the results of blood cultures and antibiotic sensitivities are available. Treatment is usually for 3–6 weeks. Severely damaged native valves (± heart failure) and infected prosthetic valves often require surgical replacement.

• *Prognosis* In developed countries, the high mortality (~15%) is due to prosthetic valve infection. **Prophylactic antibiotics** are often given to patients with valvular heart disease before dental or potentially septic procedures (e.g. cystoscopy)

Pericardial emergencies

Acute pericarditis

Acute pericarditis is due to infection (mostly viral), MI, uraemia, connective tissue disease, trauma, TB and neoplasia. An immunologically mediated febrile pleuropericarditis (Dressler's syndrome) can occur 2–6 weeks after MI (~2%).

• *Clinical features* include severe, positional (i.e. relief sitting forward), retrosternal chest pain and pericardial rub on auscultation.

• *Investigation* ECG shows concave ST-segment elevation in all leads. Cardiac enzymes may be elevated with myocarditis.

• *Management* Anti-inflammatory drugs (e.g. aspirin) relieve discomfort. Steroids are required occasionally (e.g. Dressler's syndrome).

Pericardial effusion

Pericardial effusion is due to infection (e.g. TB), uraemia, MI, aortic dissection, myxoedema, neoplasia and radiotherapy.

• *Clinical features* are due to cardiac tamponade which occurs when pericardial fluid impairs ventricular filling, reducing CO. Breathlessness and pericarditic pain often precede acute cardiovascular collapse. Examination may reveal a raised JVP which increases on inspiration (Kussmaul's sign), hypotension with a paradoxical pulse (i.e. BP falls > 15 mmHg during inspiration) and distant heart sounds.

• *Investigation* ECG (reduced voltage), CXR (globular cardiomegaly) and echocardiography (pericardial fluid and tamponade-induced right ventricular diastolic collapse) are diagnostic.

• *Management* Echocardiography-directed, pericardial drainage is required for tamponade (Fig. e).

Constrictive pericarditis

Progressive pericardial fibrotic constriction may cause pericardial tamponade. Surgical removal of the pericardium may be necessary.

Other cardiac emergencies

Acute valve lesions, type A ascending aorta dissection, trauma (Chapter 52), myocarditis and congenital heart disease may also present as cardiac emergencies.

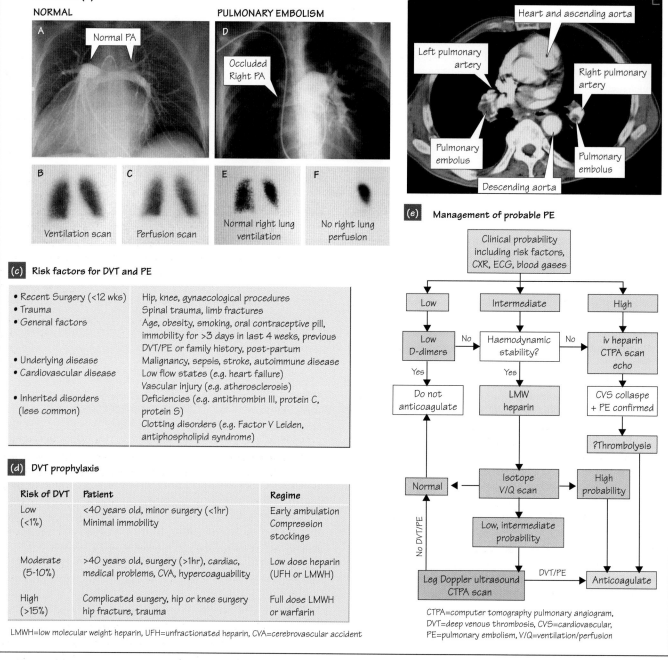

(a) Pulmonary angiograms (A,D) and V/Q scans (B,E = ventilation scans, C,F = perfusion scans) in a normal patient and a patient with a massive right-sided pulmonary embolism. The angiogram (D) shows complete occlusion of the right pulmonary artery. On the V/Q scan there is loss of right lung perfusion (F) but normal ventilation (E)

NORMAL

PULMONARY EMBOLISM

Normal PA

Occluded Right PA

Ventilation scan

Perfusion scan

Normal right lung ventilation

No right lung perfusion

(b) Contrast CT scan showing contrast in the heart and pulmonary arteries (PA). Both the right and left PA show irregular defects consistent with pulmonary emboli

Heart and ascending aorta

Left pulmonary artery

Right pulmonary artery

Pulmonary embolus

Pulmonary embolus

Descending aorta

(c) Risk factors for DVT and PE

• Recent Surgery (<12 wks)	Hip, knee, gynaecological procedures
• Trauma	Spinal trauma, limb fractures
• General factors	Age, obesity, smoking, oral contraceptive pill, immobility for >3 days in last 4 weeks, previous DVT/PE or family history, post-partum
• Underlying disease	Malignancy, sepsis, stroke, autoimmune disease
• Cardiovascular disease	Low flow states (e.g. heart failure) Vascular injury (e.g. atherosclerosis)
• Inherited disorders (less common)	Deficiencies (e.g. antithrombin III, protein C, protein S) Clotting disorders (e.g. Factor V Leiden, antiphospholipid syndrome)

(d) DVT prophylaxis

Risk of DVT	Patient	Regime
Low (<1%)	<40 years old, minor surgery (<1hr) Minimal immobility	Early ambulation Compression stockings
Moderate (5-10%)	>40 years old, surgery (>1hr), cardiac, medical problems, CVA, hypercoagulability	Low dose heparin (UFH or LMWH)
High (>15%)	Complicated surgery, hip or knee surgery hip fracture, trauma	Full dose LMWH or warfarin

LMWH=low molecular weight heparin, UFH=unfractionated heparin, CVA=cerebrovascular accident

(e) Management of probable PE

Clinical probability including risk factors, CXR, ECG, blood gases

Low — Intermediate — High

Low → No → Haemodynamic → No → iv heparin
D-dimers ← stability? ← CTPA scan echo

Yes ↓ — Yes ↓ — CVS collaspe + PE confirmed

Do not anticoagulate — LMW heparin — ?Thrombolysis

Normal — Isotope V/Q scan — High probability

Low, intermediate probability

Leg Doppler ultrasound CTPA scan — DVT/PE — Anticoagulate

No DVT/PE

CTPA=computer tomography pulmonary angiogram, DVT=deep venous thrombosis, CVS=cardiovascular, PE=pulmonary embolism, V/Q=ventilation/perfusion

Venous stasis, hypercoagulability and vascular injury (Virchow's triad) predispose to deep venous thrombosis (DVT) of which pulmonary embolism (PE) is the most significant complication. Appropriate clinical suspicion and a systematic approach to investigation reduce frequently missed diagnoses. **Risk factors** for venous thromboembolism (VTE) are listed in Fig. (c). Up to 70% of high risk patients without prophylaxis develop DVT (e.g. hip replacement surgery). **Epidemiology:** VTE affects ~$70/10^6$ population/yr; a third with PE and two-thirds DVT alone.

Deep venous thrombosis

Most clinically significant PE (~90%) arise from DVTs that originate in the calves and propagate above the knees. Clots confined to the calves (~65%) are of little importance, but half of the 15–25% that extend into the femoral and iliac veins release PE. Occasional axillary or subclavian DVT are due to central lines or surgery but associated emboli are small and less serious. The risk of PE is greatest during early clot proliferation and decreases once thrombus has organised.

- **Clinical features:** are non-specific including mild fever and calf swelling, tenderness, erythema and warmth. *Homan's sign* (calf pain on forced foot dorsiflexion) may dislodge thrombus and is best avoided. Clinical examination fails to detect >50% of DVT.
- **Diagnosis:** D-dimers are fibrin degradation products created when fibrin is lysed by plasmin. **D-dimers assays** are sensitive but not specific for DVT. They increase with infection, inflammation and malignancy. Consequently a negative D-dimer excludes but a raised level cannot confirm VTE. A compression **Doppler ultrasound scan (USS)** is performed if the D-dimer is raised or clinical probability high but may fail to detect ~30% of proximal DVTs. Venography is rarely necessary
- **Prevention:** stop smoking and contraceptive pills, lose weight and treat infection or heart failure before elective surgery. Prophylaxis is essential after surgery and in high risk patients and depends on the level of risk (Fig. c, d). It includes pneumatic compression devices, regular leg exercises and early mobilization. Unfractionated heparin (UFH) and low molecular weight heparin (LMWH) reduce post-operative DVTs by ~50% and PEs by ~65–75%.
- **Treatment:** LMWH is as effective as UFH for prevention of clot extension and PE in DVT. Subsequent oral anticoagulation with warfarin is required for at least 6 weeks.

Pulmonary embolism

PE occurs when thrombus, usually from an iliac or femoral DVT, passes through the venous system and right heart and suddenly occludes a pulmonary artery (PA) with respiratory or circulatory consequences. Hypoxaemia is mainly due to V/Q mismatch and increased ventilatory dead-space necessitates increased minute ventilation to maintain a normal $P_a\text{CO}_2$. Reduced surfactant in affected areas causes atelectasis. Circulatory collapse occurs with >50% PA obstruction. Pre-existing heart failure, rate of onset and degree of PA obliteration determine clinical and cardiovascular responses. **Massive PE** due to large central PA emboli may cause catastrophic circulatory collapse and hypoxaemia. **Multiple small PEs** with extensive segmental PA occlusions causes breathlessness, hypoxia and right ventricular (RV) failure but may be well tolerated due to adaptive responses. A **single small PE** occluding a segmental PA causes mild dyspnoea, haemoptysis and pleuritic pain due to pulmonary infarction (<25% cases). Small emboli can be fatal with co-existing lung or heart disease.

Clinical presentation

PE present with pleuritic pain and haemoptysis in ~65%, isolated dyspnoea in ~25% and circulatory collapse in ~10% of cases. Dyspnoea does not occur in ~30% of confirmed PE cases. Other non-specific features include apprehension, tachypnoea, tachycardia, cough, sweating and syncope. RV failure with hypotension and elevated JVP occurs in severe PE. **CXR** abnormalities are non-specific (e.g. atelectasis) but other causes (e.g. pneumonia) can be excluded. **ECGs** shows non-specific ST segment changes and rarely, following a large PE, RV strain with an $S_1Q_3T_3$ pattern, right axis deviation and right bundle branch block. **Arterial blood gas** abnormalities include a widened A-a gradient, hypoxaemia and hypocapnia (despite increased dead space). PE should be considered in all hypoxaemic patients with a normal CXR.

Diagnosis

Figure (e) illustrates management of suspected PE.

- **Isotope V/Q scans:** have significant limitations but are often the initial investigation (Fig. a). A negative perfusion scan effectively rules out PE and a 'high probability' scan (segmental perfusion defects with normal ventilation) has a >85% probability of PE. A high clinical suspicion, with a 'high probability' V/Q scan has a positive predictive value >95%. Unfortunately, most V/Q scans are not diagnostic or indeterminate with a 15–50% likelihood of PE, necessitating further imaging.
- **Doppler USS:** confirmation of lower limb DVT precludes the need for further investigation as treatment is required. Absence of a DVT combined with a low probability V/Q scan permits withholding treatment whereas a negative USS with an intermediate probability V/Q scan (or cardiopulmonary disease) necessitates CT scanning.
- **Spiral CT scans** (Fig. b): are replacing V/Q scans as the investigation of choice. They are sensitive (70–95%; highest for proximal emboli) and specific (>90%) for PE and are useful when parenchymal disease (e.g. COPD) limits V/Q scan interpretation.
- **Transthoracic and transoesophageal echocardiography:** may reveal RV dysfunction and main PA emboli (but not lobar/segmental emboli) respectively.
- **Pulmonary angiography:** the diagnostic standard but infrequently used.

Treatment

Therapy is similar to that for established DVT.

- **Anticoagulation (AC):** stops propagation of DVT and allows organization. Immediate therapy may prevent further life-threatening emboli in those at high risk. **Heparin (UFH *or* LMWH)** for 5–7 days followed by warfarin for 3–6 months is standard therapy. Monitor UFH and warfarin as subtherapeutic levels increase the risk of recurrent VTE. LMWH is more bioavailable and does not require monitoring. Patients with inherited or acquired hypercoagulability may require lifelong AC (Chapter 49). If contraindications prevent AC (e.g. surgery, haemorrhagic stroke, CNS metastases) or recurrent PE occur whilst anticoagulated, insertion of an **inferior vena cava filter** may prevent further PE.
- **Thrombolytic therapy:** hastens clot breakdown, corrects perfusion defects and alleviates RV dysfunction. Prognosis was not improved in patients without massive PE despite increased bleeding complications, including a 0.3–1.5% risk of intra-cerebral haemorrhage. Consequently, thrombolysis is only recommended in life-threatening PE with compromised haemodynamics.

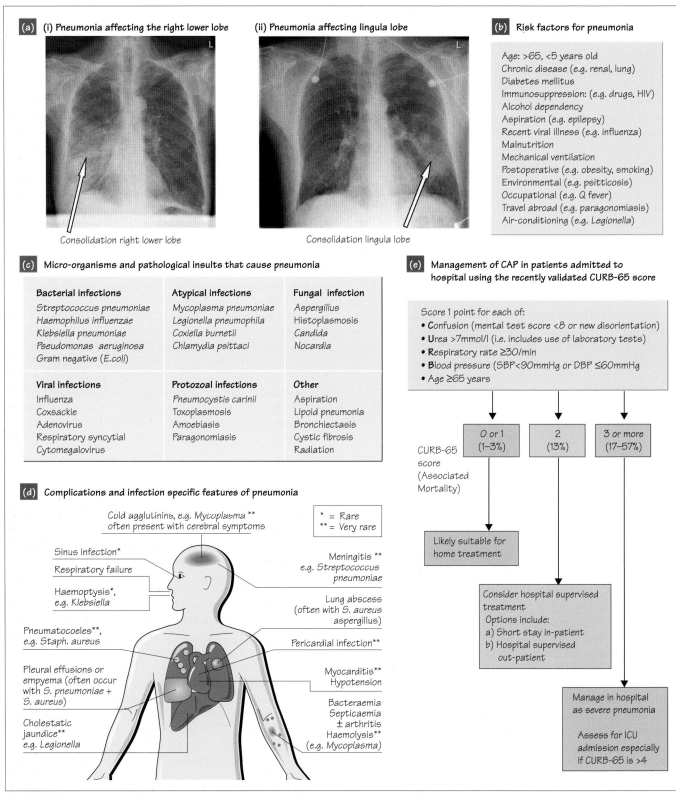

(a)

(i) Pneumonia affecting the right lower lobe

Consolidation right lower lobe

(ii) Pneumonia affecting lingula lobe

Consolidation lingula lobe

(b) Risk factors for pneumonia

Age: >65, <5 years old
Chronic disease (e.g. renal, lung)
Diabetes mellitus
Immunosuppression: (e.g. drugs, HIV)
Alcohol dependency
Aspiration (e.g. epilepsy)
Recent viral illness (e.g. influenza)
Malnutrition
Mechanical ventilation
Postoperative (e.g. obesity, smoking)
Environmental (e.g. psitticosis)
Occupational (e.g. Q fever)
Travel abroad (e.g. paragonomiasis)
Air-conditioning (e.g. Legionella)

(c) Micro-organisms and pathological insults that cause pneumonia

Bacterial infections	Atypical infections	Fungal infection
Streptococcus pneumoniae	Mycoplasma pneumoniae	Aspergillus
Haemophilus influenzae	Legionella pneumophila	Histoplasmosis
Klebsiella pneumoniae	Coxiella burnetii	Candida
Pseudomonas aeruginosa	Chlamydia psittaci	Nocardia
Gram negative (E.coli)		

Viral infections	Protozoal infections	Other
Influenza	Pneumocystis carinii	Aspiration
Coxsackie	Toxoplasmosis	Lipoid pneumonia
Adenovirus	Amoebiasis	Bronchiectasis
Respiratory syncytial	Paragonomiasis	Cystic fibrosis
Cytomegalovirus		Radiation

(d) Complications and infection specific features of pneumonia

Cold agglutinins, e.g. Mycoplasma **
often present with cerebral symptoms

* = Rare
** = Very rare

Sinus infection*
Respiratory failure
Haemoptysis*,
e.g. Klebsiella

Meningitis **
e.g. Streptococcus
pneumoniae

Lung abscess
(often with S. aureus
aspergillus)

Pneumatocoeles**,
e.g. Staph. aureus

Pericardial infection**

Pleural effusions or
empyema (often occur
with S. pneumoniae +
S. aureus)

Myocarditis**
Hypotension

Bacteraemia
Septicaemia
± arthritis
Haemolysis**
(e.g. Mycoplasma)

Cholestatic
jaundice**
e.g. Legionella

(e) Management of CAP in patients admitted to hospital using the recently validated CURB-65 score

Score 1 point for each of:
• **C**onfusion (mental test score <8 or new disorientation)
• **U**rea >7mmol/l (i.e. includes use of laboratory tests)
• **R**espiratory rate ≥30/min
• **B**lood pressure (SBP<90mmHg or DBP ≤60mmHg
• Age **≥65** years

CURB-65 score (Associated Mortality)

0 or 1 (1–3%)	2 (13%)	3 or more (17–57%)

Likely suitable for home treatment

Consider hospital supervised treatment
Options include:
a) Short stay in-patient
b) Hospital supervised out-patient

Manage in hospital as severe pneumonia

Assess for ICU admission especially if CURB-65 is >4

Definition

Pneumonia is an **acute lower respiratory tract (LRT) illness**, usually due to **infection**, associated with **fever, focal chest symptoms** (**± signs**) and **new shadowing on CXR** (Fig. a). Figure (c) lists micro-organisms and pathological insults that cause pneumonia.

Classification

In the clinical situation, **microbiological classification** of pneumonia is not practical as causative organisms may not be identified or diagnosis takes several days. Likewise **anatomical** (radiographic) appearance (e.g. lobar- (affecting one lobe) or broncho-pneumonia (widespread, patchy involvement)) gives little information about cause. The following classification is widely accepted:

• **Community-acquired pneumonia (CAP):** describes LRT infections occurring before or within 48 hours of hospital admission in patients who have not been hospitalized for >14 days. The most frequently identified organisms are *Streptococcus pneumoniae* (20–75%). *Mycoplasma pneumoniae, Chlamydia pneumoniae* and *Legionella* spp., the 'atypical' bacterial pathogens (2–25%) and viral infections (8–12%) are relatively common causes. *Haemophilus influenzae* and *Mycobacterium catarrhalis* are associated with COPD exacerbations and staphylococcal infection may follow influenza. Alcoholic, diabetic, heart failure and nursing-home patients are prone to staphylococcal, anaerobic and gram-negative organisms.

• **Hospital-acquired (nosocomial) pneumonia (Chapter 32):** LRT infections developing >2 days after hospital admission. Likely organisms are gram-negative bacilli (~65%) or staphylococcus (~15%).

• **Aspiration/anaerobic pneumonia:** follows aspiration of oropharyngeal contents due to impaired consciousness or laryngeal incompetence. Causative organisms include bacteroides and other anaerobes.

• **Opportunistic pneumonia (Chapter 51):** occurs in immunosuppressed patients (e.g. chemotherapy, HIV) who are susceptible to viral, fungal, mycobacterial and unusual bacterial infections.

• **Recurrent pneumonia:** is due to aerobic and anaerobic organisms in cystic fibrosis and bronchiectasis.

Epidemiology

• **Annual CAP incidence:** 5–11 cases per 1000 adult population; 15–45% require hospitalization (1–4 cases per 1000) of whom 5–10% are treated in ICU. Incidence is highest in the very young and elderly. **Mortality:** is 5–12% in hospitalized and 25–50% in ICU patients. **Seasonal variation:** (e.g. mycoplasma in autumn, staphylococcus in spring) and annual cycles (e.g. 4-yearly mycoplasma epidemics) occur. Frequent viral infections increase CAP in winter.

Risk factors

Factors associated with increased risk of CAP are listed in Fig. (b). **Specific risk factors** include **age** (e.g. mycoplasma in young adults), **occupation** (e.g. brucellosis in abattoir workers, Q fever in sheep workers), **environment** (e.g. psittacosis with pet birds, ehrlichiosis due to tick bites) or **geographical** (e.g. coccidomycosis in southwest USA). Epidemics of *Coxiella burnetii* (Q fever) or *Legionella pneumophila* may be localized (e.g. legionnaires' disease often involves a specific hotel due to air-conditioner contamination).

Diagnosis

The aims are to establish the **diagnosis**, identify **complications**, assess **severity** and determine **classification** to aid antibiotic choice.

Clinical features

These are inaccurate without a CXR and cannot predict causative organisms (i.e. 'atypical' pathogens do not have characteristic presentations). **Symptoms** may be general (e.g. malaise, fever, myalgia) or chest specific (e.g. dyspnoea, pleurisy, cough, haemoptysis). **Signs** include cyanosis, tachycardia and tachypnoea; with focal dullness, crepitations, bronchial breathing and pleuritic rub on chest examination. In young or old patients and those with atypical pneumonias (e.g. mycoplasma) **non-respiratory features** (e.g. headache, confusion, diarrhoea) may predominate. **Complications** are shown in Fig. (d).

Investigations

Routine blood tests: white cell count (WCC) and C-reactive protein confirm infection; haemolysis and cold agglutinins occur in ~50% of mycoplasma infection; abnormal liver function tests suggest legionella or mycoplasma infection. **Blood gases:** identify respiratory failure. **Microbiology:** no micro-organism is isolated in ~33-50% of patients due to previous antibiotic therapy or inadequate specimen collection. Blood cultures in severe CAP, and sputum, pleural fluid and bronchoalveolar lavage samples, with appropriate staining (e.g. Gram stain), culture and assessment of antibiotic sensitivity may determine the pathogen and effective therapy. **Serology:** identifies mycoplasma infection but long processing times limit clinical value. Rapid antigen detection tests for legionella (e.g. urine) and pneumococcus (e.g. serum, pleural fluid) are more useful. **Radiology:** CXR (Fig. a) and CT scans aid diagnosis, indicate severity and detect complications.

Severity assessment

The following features are associated with increased mortality and indicate the need for monitoring in HDU; **(a) Clinical:** age >60 years, respiratory rate >30/min, diastolic blood pressure <60 mmHg, new atrial fibrillation, confusion, multilobar involvement and coexisting illness. **(b) Laboratory:** urea >7 mmol/L, albumin <35 g/L, hypoxaemia $Po_2 < 8$ kPa, leucopenia (WCC $< 4 \times 10^9$/L), leucocytosis (WCC $> 20 \times 10^9$/L) and bacteraemia. **Severity scoring:** the CURB-65 score allocates points for **C**onfusion; **U**rea >7 mmol/l; **R**espiratory rate >30/min; low systolic (<90 mmHg) or diastolic (<60 mmHg); **B**lood pressure and age >**65** years, to stratify patients into mortality groups suitable for different management pathways (Fig. c).

Management

• **Supportive measures:** include oxygen to maintain P_aO_2 >8 kPa (S_aO_2 <90%) and intravenous fluid (± inotrope) resuscitation to ensure haemodynamic stability. **Ventilatory support:** non-invasive or mechanical ventilation may be required in respiratory failure (Chapters 11, 16). **Physiotherapy and bronchoscopy:** aid sputum clearance.

• **Initial antibiotic therapy:** represents the 'best guess', according to pneumonia classification and likely organisms, as microbiological results are not available for 12–72 hours. Therapy is adjusted when results and antibiotic sensitivities are available. The American and British Thoracic Societies (ATS, BTS) recommend the following initial antibiotic protocols for CAP:

  • **Non-hospitalized patients:** usually respond to oral therapy with amoxicillin (BTS) or a macrolide (e.g. clarithromycin) or doxycycline (ATS). Patients with severe symptoms or at risk for drug-resistant *S. pneumoniae* (e.g. recent antibiotics, comorbidity) are treated with a beta-lactam plus a macrolide or doxycycline; or an antipneumococcal fluoroquinolone (e.g. moxifloxacin) alone.

  • **Hospitalized patients,** therapy must cover 'atypical' organisms and *S. pneumoniae* at admission. An intravenous macrolide is combined with a beta-lactam or an antipneumococcal fluoroquinolone (ATS/BTS) or cefuroxime (BTS). If not severe, combined ampicillin and macrolide (oral) is adequate. Staphylococcal infection after influenza or *H. influenzae* in COPD should be covered.

32 Hospital-acquired (nosocomial) pneumonia

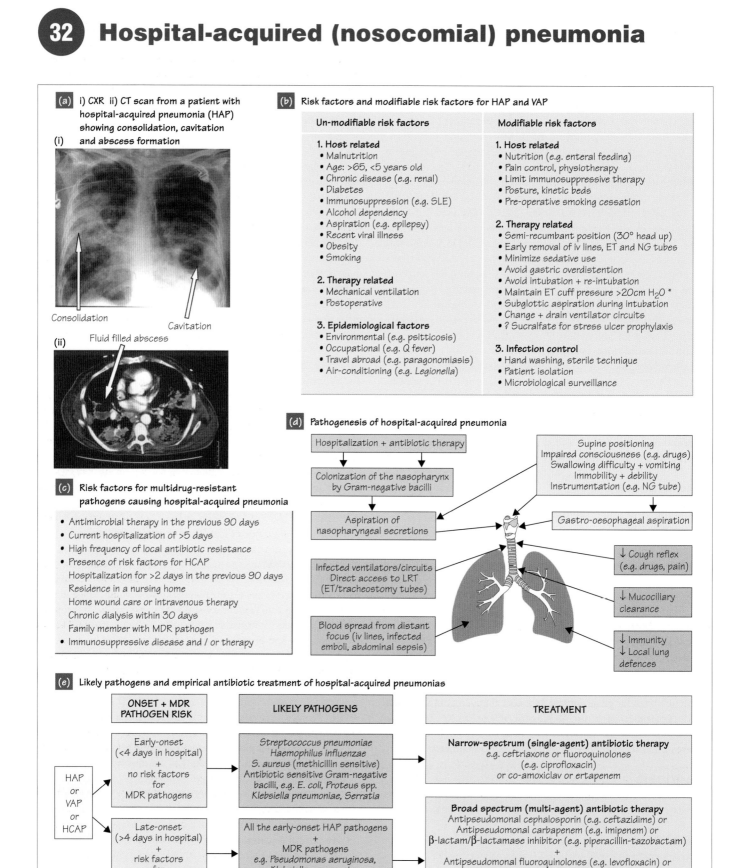

(a) i) CXR ii) CT scan from a patient with hospital-acquired pneumonia (HAP) showing consolidation, cavitation and abscess formation

(i)

Consolidation   Cavitation

(ii) Fluid filled abscess

(b) Risk factors and modifiable risk factors for HAP and VAP

Un-modifiable risk factors	Modifiable risk factors
1. Host related • Malnutrition • Age: >65, <5 years old • Chronic disease (e.g. renal) • Diabetes • Immunosuppression (e.g. SLE) • Alcohol dependency • Aspiration (e.g. epilepsy) • Recent viral illness • Obesity • Smoking **2. Therapy related** • Mechanical ventilation • Postoperative **3. Epidemiological factors** • Environmental (e.g. psitticosis) • Occupational (e.g. Q fever) • Travel abroad (e.g. paragonomiasis) • Air-conditioning (e.g. Legionella)	**1. Host related** • Nutrition (e.g. enteral feeding) • Pain control, physiotherapy • Limit immunosuppressive therapy • Posture, kinetic beds • Pre-operative smoking cessation **2. Therapy related** • Semi-recumbant position (30° head up) • Early removal of iv lines, ET and NG tubes • Minimize sedative use • Avoid gastric overdistention • Avoid intubation + re-intubation • Maintain ET cuff pressure >20cm H_2O * • Subglottic aspiration during intubation • Change + drain ventilator circuits • ? Sucralfate for stress ulcer prophylaxis **3. Infection control** • Hand washing, sterile technique • Patient isolation • Microbiological surveillance

(c) Risk factors for multidrug-resistant pathogens causing hospital-acquired pneumonia

• Antimicrobial therapy in the previous 90 days
• Current hospitalization of >5 days
• High frequency of local antibiotic resistance
• Presence of risk factors for HCAP
  Hospitalization for >2 days in the previous 90 days
  Residence in a nursing home
  Home wound care or intravenous therapy
  Chronic dialysis within 30 days
  Family member with MDR pathogen
• Immunosuppressive disease and / or therapy

(d) Pathogenesis of hospital-acquired pneumonia

Hospitalization + antibiotic therapy → Colonization of the nasopharynx by Gram-negative bacilli → Aspiration of nasopharyngeal secretions

Supine positioning
Impaired consciousness (e.g. drugs)
Swallowing difficulty + vomiting
Immobility + debility
Instrumentation (e.g. NG tube)

Gastro-oesophageal aspiration

Infected ventilators/circuits Direct access to LRT (ET/tracheostomy tubes)

↓ Cough reflex (e.g. drugs, pain)

↓ Mucociliary clearance

Blood spread from distant focus (iv lines, infected emboli, abdominal sepsis)

↓ Immunity ↓ Local lung defences

(e) Likely pathogens and empirical antibiotic treatment of hospital-acquired pneumonias

ONSET + MDR PATHOGEN RISK	LIKELY PATHOGENS	TREATMENT
Early-onset (<4 days in hospital) + no risk factors for MDR pathogens	*Streptococcus pneumoniae* *Haemophilus influenzae* *S. aureus* (methicillin sensitive) Antibiotic sensitive Gram-negative bacilli, e.g. *E. coli, Proteus spp.* *Klebsiella pneumoniae, Serratia*	**Narrow-spectrum (single-agent) antibiotic therapy** e.g. ceftriaxone or fluoroquinolones (e.g. ciprofloxacin) or co-amoxiclav or ertapenem
Late-onset (>4 days in hospital) + risk factors for MDR pathogens	All the early-onset HAP pathogens + MDR pathogens e.g. *Pseudomonas aeruginosa, Klebsiella pneumoniae, Acinetobacter spp.*, MRSA, *Legionella pneumophila*	**Broad spectrum (multi-agent) antibiotic therapy** Antipseudomonal cephalosporin (e.g. ceftazidime) or Antipseudomonal carbapenem (e.g. imipenem) or β-lactam/β-lactamase inhibitor (e.g. piperacillin-tazobactam) + Antipseudomonal fluoroquinolones (e.g. levofloxacin) or Aminoglycoside (e.g. amikacin, gentamicin) + Vancomycin or linezolid (if risk factors for MRSA)

HAP or VAP or HCAP

Hospital-acquired (nosocomial) pneumonia (HAP) including **ventilator-associated pneumonia** (VAP) and **health-care associated pneumonia** (HCAP) affects 0.5–2% of hospital patients and is a leading cause of nosocomial infection (i.e. with wound and urinary tract infection). Pathogenesis, causative organisms and outcome differ from community-acquired pneumonia (CAP). Preventative measures and early antibiotic therapy, guided by awareness of the role of multidrug resistant (MDR) pathogens, improves outcome.

Definitions

HAP Pulmonary infection developing >48 hours after hospital admission which was not incubating at the time of admission. **VAP:** pneumonia developing >48–72 hours after endotracheal intubation. **HCAP:** includes any patient admitted to hospital for >2 days within 90 days of the infection, residing in a nursing home, receiving therapy (e.g. wound care, intravenous therapy) within 30 days of the current infection, or attending a hospital or haemodialysis clinic.

Epidemiology

Incidence: varies between 5 and 10 episodes per 1000 discharges and is highest on surgical and ICU wards and in teaching hospitals. It lengthens hospital stay by between 3 and 14 days per patient. The risk of HAP increases 6- to 20-fold during mechanical ventilation (MV) and in ICU, it accounts for 25% of infections and ~50% of prescribed antibiotics. VAP accounts for >80% of all HAP and occurs in 9–27% of intubated patients. **Risk factors:** include those that predispose to CAP and factors associated with HAP pathogenesis, some of which can be **prevented** (Fig. b). **Mortality:** is between 30 and 70%. **Early-onset HAP/VAP** (<4 days in hospital) is usually caused by antibiotic-sensitive bacteria and carries a better prognosis than **late-onset HAP/VAP** (>4 days in hospital), which is associated with MDR pathogens. In early onset HAP/VAP, prior antibiotic therapy or hospitalization predisposes to MDR pathogens and is treated as late onset HAP/VAP. Bacteraemia, medical rather than surgical illness, VAP and late or ineffective antibiotic therapy also increases mortality.

Pathogenesis (Fig. d)

Oropharyngeal colonization with enteric gram-negative bacteria occurs in most hospital patients due to immobility, impaired consciousness, instrumentation (e.g. nasogastric tubes), poor hygiene or inhibition of gastric acid secretion. Subsequent aspiration of nasopharyngeal secretions (± gastric contents) causes HAP.

Aetiology

Time of onset (early/late) and risk factors for infection with MDR organisms (Fig. c) determine potential pathogens (Fig. e). Aerobic gram-negative bacilli (e.g. *Klebsiella pneumoniae, Pseudomonas aeruginosa, Escherichia coli, Acinetobacter* species) cause ~60–70% of infections and *Staphylococcus aureus* ~10–15%. *Streptococcus pneumoniae* and *Haemophilus influenza* may be isolated in early-onset HAP/VAP. In ICU, >50% *S. aureus* infections are methicillin-resistant (MRSA). *S. aureus* is more common in diabetics and ICU patients.

Diagnosis

Requires both *clinical* and *microbiological* assessment. It may be difficult as (i) clinical features are non-specific or confused with concurrent illness (e.g. ARDS) and (ii) previous antibiotics limit microbiological evaluation. **Clinical:** HAP is suspected when new radiographic infiltrates occur with features suggestive of infection (e.g. fever >38°C, purulent sputum, leukocytosis, hypoxaemia). **Diagnostic tests:** confirm infection and determine the causative organism (± antibiotic sensitivity). They include routine blood counts, blood gases, serology, blood cultures, pleural fluid aspiration, sputum, endotracheal aspirate and bronchioalveolar lavage microbiology and CXR. CT scanning (Fig. a) aids diagnosis and detects **complications** (e.g. cavitation, abscesses).

Management

Early diagnosis and treatment improves morbidity and mortality and requires constant vigilance in hospital patients. Antibiotic therapy must not be delayed whilst awaiting microbiological results.

Supportive therapy

This includes supplemental **oxygen** to maintain $P_aO_2 > 8\,kPa$ ($S_aO_2 < 90\%$), **intravenous fluids** (± **vasopressors/inotropes**) for haemodynamic stability and **ventilatory support** (e.g. CPAP, MV) in respiratory failure. **Physiotherapy** and **analgesia** aid sputum clearance post-operatively and in the immobilized patient. **Semi-recumbent** (i.e. 30° bed-head elevation) nursing of bed-bound patients reduces aspiration risk. Strict glycaemic control and attention to other modifiable risk factors (Fig. b) may improve outcome

Antibiotic therapy

This is empirical whilst awaiting microbiological guidance. The key decision is whether the patient has risk factors for MDR organisms. Figure (e) illustrates the American Thoracic Society guidelines for initial, empiric, intravenous antibiotic therapy. Local patterns of bacterial antibiotic resistance are used to modify these protocols.

• In **early-onset HAP/VAP** with no risk factors for MDR organisms, **monotherapy** with a β-lactam/β-lactamase, third generation cephalosporin or fluoroquinolone antibiotic is advised.

• In **late-onset HAP/VAP** or with risk factors for MDR pathogens (Fig. c), **combination therapy**, with broad-spectrum antibiotics to cover MDR gram-negative bacilli and MRSA (e.g. vancomycin) is required (Fig. e). Adjunctive therapy with inhaled aminoglycosides or polymyxin is considered in patients not improving with systemic therapy. A short course of therapy (e.g. 7 days) is appropriate, if the clinical response is good. Aggressive or resistant pathogens (e.g. *Pseudomonas aeruginosa, S. aureus*) may require 14–21 days treatment. Therapy is focused on causative organisms when culture data is available and unnecessary antibiotics withdrawn. Sterile cultures (in the absence of new antibiotics for >72 hours) virtually rules out HAP.

Other pneumonias

• **Aspiration/anaerobic pneumonia:** *Bacteroides* and other anaerobic infections follow aspiration of oropharyngeal contents due to laryngeal incompetence or reduced consciousness (e.g. CVA, drugs). Lung abscesses are common. Antibiotic therapy should include anaerobic coverage (e.g. metronidazole).

• **Pneumonia during immunosuppression (Chapter 51):** HIV, transplant and chemotherapy patients are susceptible to viral (e.g. cytomegalovirus), fungal (e.g. *Aspergillus*) and mycobacterial infections, in addition to the normal range of organisms. HIV patients with CD4 counts <200/mm^3, also develop opportunistic infections such as *Pneumocystis jirovecii (carinii)* pneumonia (PCP) or toxoplasma. Severely immunocompromised patients require broad-spectrum antibiotic, antifungal and anti-viral regimes. PCP is treated with steroids and high dose co-trimoxazole.

33 Asthma

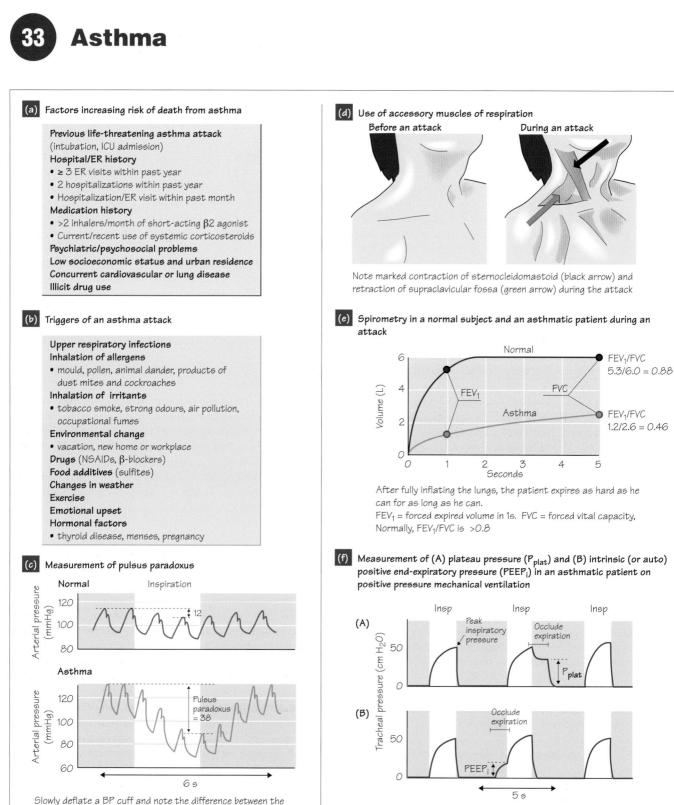

(a) Factors increasing risk of death from asthma

Previous life-threatening asthma attack
(intubation, ICU admission)
Hospital/ER history
- ≥ 3 ER visits within past year
- 2 hospitalizations within past year
- Hospitalization/ER visit within past month

Medication history
- >2 inhalers/month of short-acting β2 agonist
- Current/recent use of systemic corticosteroids

Psychiatric/psychosocial problems
Low socioeconomic status and urban residence
Concurrent cardiovascular or lung disease
Illicit drug use

(b) Triggers of an asthma attack

Upper respiratory infections
Inhalation of allergens
- mould, pollen, animal dander, products of dust mites and cockroaches

Inhalation of irritants
- tobacco smoke, strong odours, air pollution, occupational fumes

Environmental change
- vacation, new home or workplace

Drugs (NSAIDs, β-blockers)
Food additives (sulfites)
Changes in weather
Exercise
Emotional upset
Hormonal factors
- thyroid disease, menses, pregnancy

(c) Measurement of pulsus paradoxus

Slowly deflate a BP cuff and note the difference between the highest pressure at end inspiration and the rest of the respiratory cycle

(d) Use of accessory muscles of respiration

Before an attack   During an attack

Note marked contraction of sternocleidomastoid (black arrow) and retraction of supraclavicular fossa (green arrow) during the attack

(e) Spirometry in a normal subject and an asthmatic patient during an attack

FEV$_1$/FVC
5.3/6.0 = 0.88

FEV$_1$/FVC
1.2/2.6 = 0.46

After fully inflating the lungs, the patient expires as hard as he can for as long as he can.
FEV$_1$ = forced expired volume in 1s. FVC = forced vital capacity,
Normally, FEV$_1$/FVC is >0.8

(f) Measurement of (A) plateau pressure (P$_{plat}$) and (B) intrinsic (or auto) positive end-expiratory pressure (PEEP$_i$) in an asthmatic patient on positive pressure mechanical ventilation

P$_{plat}$ and PEEP$_i$ reflect alveolar pressures at end-inspiration and end-expiration, respectively, assuming the patient's muscles are relaxed

Asthma is **reversible obstruction** of inflamed, hyperreactive airways manifested by recurrent episodes of wheezing, coughing, and dyspnoea. It affects 5–10% of the population. **Prevalence** is increasing, particularly in children. Although **mortality is low** (2 deaths/year/100,000), it has increased for 20 years and is higher in blacks. Factors increasing risk of death are shown in Fig. (a).

Pathogenesis

Airway inflammation, usually allergic, is central to pathogenesis and may derive from predominance of type 2, over type 1, T-helper lymphocytes due to genetic-environmental interactions in childhood. Characteristic airway changes include inflammatory cell accumulation, mediator release, epithelial denudation, oedema and submucosal fibrosis, goblet cell hyperplasia, mucous hypersecretion and hypertrophied hyperresponsive smooth muscle.

Pathophysiology Acute airway obstruction can be triggered by many factors (Fig. b). During an attack, the patient struggles to keep obstructed airways open by breathing at high lung volumes, using accessory muscles (Fig. d). Work of breathing increases due to high airways resistance, decreased lung compliance and reduced muscle efficiency. Heroic efforts sufficient to increase alveolar ventilation and lower P_aCO_2 despite increasing deadspace fail to maintain airway patency, resulting in hypoxaemia due to regional hypoventilation (i.e. low ventilation/perfusion ratio). Hypoxic vasoconstriction and pulmonary capillary compression cause pulmonary hypertension, increased RV afterload and right heart failure. Increased RV filling pressures may push the interventricular septum into the LV cavity, decreasing LV end-diastolic volume. During inspiration marked falls in pleural pressure impair LV emptying reducing systolic volume and causing abnormal reductions (≥ 15 mmHg) in systolic blood pressure (pulsus paradoxus (Fig. c)). If the attack does not abate, respiratory muscles become exhausted, leading to respiratory arrest and death.

Clinical features

Onset of asthma is usually gradual but may be sudden. Episodic wheeze, cough and nocturnal waking with breathlessness are typical. The history may reveal a seasonal pattern, precipitating causes (Fig. b) and risk factors for death (Fig. a). **Physical examination:** detects wheeze with prolonged expiration on chest auscultation and signs of hyperinflation (e.g. hyperresonance).
- **Severe asthma:** characterized by a peak expiratory flow rate (PEFR) <50% of predicted, agitation, difficulty completing sentences, respiratory rate >25/min, sweating, accessory muscle use and pulsus paradoxus (Fig. c).
- **Features of life-threatening asthma** that indicate respiratory failure (± impending arrest) include confusion and drowsiness, silent chest, PEFR <33% predicted, paradoxical thoracoabdominal excursions (outward abdominal and inward sternal movement during inspiration), bradycardia, hypotension, pulsus paradoxus and hypercapnia (± hypoxaemia).

Investigation

Initially **arterial blood gases** demonstrate hypoxaemia (or normoxia), hypocapnia and alkalosis. A rise in P_aCO_2 suggests impending respiratory failure. **Chest radiography** excludes other pathology (e.g.

pneumothorax). **Electrocardiography** may exhibit signs of right ventricular strain. FEV_1 (Fig. e) or **PEFR** are measured to assess severity and monitor therapy.

Initial management
- **Primary pharmacological therapy:** is essential in all patients and includes inhaled short-acting β_2-**adrenergic agonists** (e.g. albuterol, salbutamol) and **intravenous (i.v.) corticosteroids** which are given until sustained improvement is achieved. Systemic β_2-adrenergic agonists (e.g. salbutamol) have no proven advantage over inhaled therapy. Failure to improve within 6–24 hours warrants addition of **secondary pharmacological therapy** although evidence of benefit is limited. Inhaled **ipratropium bromide** reduces airways obstruction caused by cholinergic mechanisms. Although i.v. **magnesium sulphate** may improve severe asthma, it should not be used in renal failure or heart block. Use of i.v. **aminophylline** is controversial. It dilates airway and pulmonary vascular smooth muscle and increases contractility of respiratory and cardiac muscle by inhibiting phosphodiesterases; however, close monitoring of serum levels is required to avoid serious toxic effects (e.g. seizures).
- **Respiratory therapy** aims to establish adequate oxygenation and relieve dyspnoea. All patients should receive high dose (~60%) **supplemental oxygen** (Chapter 12) to correct hypoxaemia. **Non-invasive positive pressure ventilation** (Chapter 14) may alleviate fatigue and improve gas exchange. Using tight-fitting facemasks, modest levels of positive pressure are administered during expiration (5–10 cmH$_2$O) and inspiration (10–15 cmH$_2$O) to reduce the effort required to initiate and sustain airflow into hyperinflated lungs, where end-expiratory alveolar pressure may exceed atmospheric pressure (intrinsic or auto-PEEP). *Risks* include worsened hyperinflation, agitation and aspiration. Occasionally, removing mucus plugs by **bronchoalveolar lavage** may relieve obstruction.

Management of deteriorating asthma
- **HDU/ICU admission** is indicated if severe asthma deteriorates during initial therapy, fails to improve after ≥ 6 hours' treatment, if respiratory arrest is imminent or complications (e.g. pneumothorax, arrhythmia) occur.
- **Mechanical ventilation** is required in ventilatory failure, coma or cardiopulmonary arrest (Chapter 16). Deep **sedation** allows **controlled hypoventilation**, a strategy which reduces hyperinflation by increasing expiratory time. Resulting CO$_2$ retention, due to reduced ventilation, is termed '**permissive hypercapnia**' and associated respiratory acidosis (pH < 7.2) may require correction with sodium bicarbonate. Paralytic agents interact with corticosteroids to cause post-paralytic myopathy (Chapter 48) but cannot always be avoided. Volume-control ventilation is used in patients making little respiratory effort or intermittent mandatory ventilation if respiratory effort is not reduced by sedation. In both modes, the rate (≤ 10/min) and volume of ventilator breaths (≤ 6 ml/kg) should be minimized. Inspiratory flow should be rapid (≥ 100 L/min) but the associated increase in peak inspiratory pressure (usually ≥ 50 cmH$_2$0) should not cause this strategy to be abandoned. Better indicators of lung volume are plateau pressure (P_{plat}) and the level of intrinsic or auto-PEEP (PEEP$_i$), measured as shown in Fig. (f) to estimate alveolar pressure at end-inspiration and end-expiration, respectively. Safe levels are unknown, but P_{plat} < 30 and PEEP$_i$ < 10 cmH$_2$O are likely to reduce risks. Intubated patients who deteriorate may respond to a trial of **general anaesthesia with halothane or isoflurane**.

(34) Chronic obstructive pulmonary disease

(a) Risk factors for COPD

Smoking
Age >50 years old; prevalence ~5–10%
Male gender
Childhood chest infections
Airways hyperreactivity
• asthma/atopy
Low socioeconomic status
α_1-Antitrypsin deficiency
Heavy metal exposure
• cadmium
Atmospheric pollution

(c) Spirometry. FEV_1/FVC ratio decreases in COPD

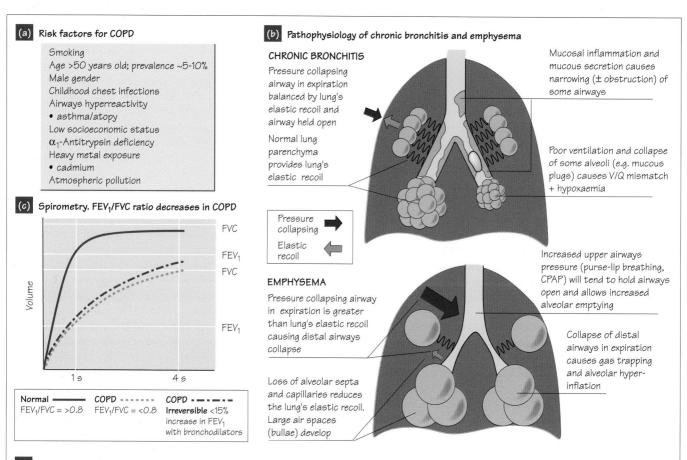

Normal —	COPD ⋯⋯	COPD –·–·–
FEV_1/FVC = >0.8	FEV_1/FVC = <0.8	**Irreversible** <15% increase in FEV_1 with bronchodilators

(b) Pathophysiology of chronic bronchitis and emphysema

CHRONIC BRONCHITIS

Pressure collapsing airway in expiration balanced by lung's elastic recoil and airway held open

Normal lung parenchyma provides lung's elastic recoil

Mucosal inflammation and mucous secretion causes narrowing (± obstruction) of some airways

Poor ventilation and collapse of some alveoli (e.g. mucous plugs) causes V/Q mismatch + hypoxaemia

Pressure collapsing ➡
Elastic recoil ⬅

EMPHYSEMA

Pressure collapsing airway in expiration is greater than lung's elastic recoil causing distal airways collapse

Loss of alveolar septa and capillaries reduces the lung's elastic recoil. Large air spaces (bullae) develop

Increased upper airways pressure (purse-lip breathing, CPAP) will tend to hold airways open and allows increased alveolar emptying

Collapse of distal airways in expiration causes gas trapping and alveolar hyper-inflation

(d) Mechanical ventilation in COPD requires an adequate inspiratory time to ensure alveolar inflation (i); increased expiratory time to prevent gas trapping (ii); ± ventilator (extrinsic) PEEP to balance auto-PEEP and reduce gas trapping and work of breathing (iii)

(i) Adequate inspiratory time
A short inspiratory time results in incomplete inflation of alveoli with narrowed airways causing V/Q mismatching and hypoxaemia

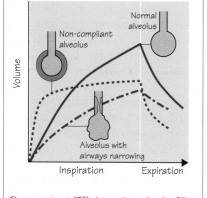

Time constant (TC) determines alveolar filling
Time constant = compliance x resistance
• Non-compliant alveoli have short TC
• Alveoli with narrowed airways have long TC

(ii) Increased expiratory time
A long expiratory time is required to prevent gas trapping because the rate of alveolar deflation is decreased due to:
1. Airways obstruction: which slows expiration. A short expiratory time causes incomplete alveolar emptying (gas trapping)

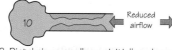

Reduced airflow

2. Distal airways collapse: initially reduces airflow and then causes gas trapping (Fig b)

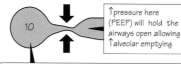

↑pressure here (PEEP) will hold the airways open allowing ↑alveolar emptying

The pressure of the trapped gas (intrinsic (or auto) PEEP) can be measured at end expiration by occluding the expiratory limb of the ventilator

A reduction in breath rate (8–10/min) increases both inspiratory and expiratory times

(iii) Reduced work of breathing (WoB)
Hyperinflation increases WoB which can be reduced by bronchodilation, ↑expiratory time (i.e. ↓ breath rate) and ventilator (extrinsic) PEEP matched to auto-PEEP

No PEEP added

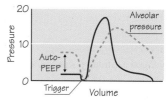

Auto-PEEP represents an end-expiratory alveolar pressure that must be overcome by respiratory effort before the ventilator can be triggered or spontaneous breathing can begin

5cm H_2O PEEP added

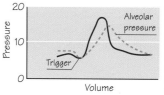

PEEP similar to the auto-PEEP added downstream from the site of flow limitation does not significantly slow expiratory airflow but reduces the inspiratory work of breathing

 Acute and Critical Care Medicine at a Glance, 2e. By R. Leach. Published 2009 by Blackwell Publishing. ISBN 978-1-4051-6139-8.

Chronic obstructive pulmonary disease (COPD) is characterized by irreversible, expiratory airflow obstruction, hyperinflation, mucous hypersecretion and increased work of breathing (WoB). Typically, smoking and other risk factors (Fig. a) accelerate the normal age-related decline in expiratory airflow and cause chronic respiratory symptoms, disability and respiratory failure punctuated by intermittent acute exacerbations (AEs).

Pathophysiology

In COPD, emphysema and chronic bronchitis often co-exist but are different processes (Fig. b). **Emphysema** destroys **alveolar septa and capillaries** and may be due to inadequate anti-protease defences. Smoking causes *centrilobular* emphysema with mainly upper lobes involvement, whereas α_1-antitrypsin deficiency causes *panacinar* emphysema which affects the lower lobes. Lung tissue loss results in bullae, reduced elastic recoil and impaired diffusion capacity. Airways obstruction is caused by distal airways collapse during expiration due to loss of 'elastic' radial traction from normal lung tissue (Fig. b). Resulting hyperinflation enhances expiratory airflow but inspiratory muscles work at a mechanical disadvantage. **Chronic bronchitic** airways obstruction is due to **chronic mucosal inflammation**, mucous gland hypertrophy with **mucous hypersecretion** and **bronchospasm** (Fig. b). Lung parenchyma is unaffected.

Diagnosis

Spirometry (Fig. c) demonstrates airflow obstruction (**FEV$_1$/FVC ratio <0.7**) which is largely irreversible with bronchodilator or steroid therapy (i.e. <15% increase in FEV$_1$). In **emphysema** resting arterial blood gases (ABGs) are usually normal because alveolar septa and capillaries are destroyed in proportion. Exercise desaturation and increased ventilation are due to reduced diffusion capacity. Lung function tests confirm impaired diffusion (D$_L$CO, KCO) and increased lung volumes (TLC, FRC, residual volume). CXR reveals hyperinflation (e.g. flat diaphragms), narrow mediastinum, bullae and reduced vascular markings. In **bronchitis** diffusion capacity and lung volumes are normal but V/Q mismatching may cause hypoxaemia. CXR shows increased vascular markings but normal lung volumes.

Clinical features

The concept of emphysematous '**pink puffers**' and bronchitic '**blue bloaters**' is unreliable as most patients have elements of both. **Emphysematous patients** tend to be **thin, breathless** and **tachypnoeic**, with signs of hyperinflation (e.g. barrel chest, purse-lipped breathing, accessory muscle use). Chest auscultation reveals distant breath sounds and prolonged expiratory wheeze. **Chronic bronchitis** is clinically defined as daily morning cough and mucus production for 3 months over 2 successive years. These patients are often less breathless despite potential **hypoxaemia** (± polycythaemia). Reduced respiratory drive leads to **CO$_2$ retention** with associated bounding pulse, vasodilation, confusion, headache, flapping tremor and papilloedema. Hypoxaemia-induced renal fluid retention (i.e. not right heart failure) causes **cor pulmonale** (i.e. hepatomegaly, ankle oedema, raised CVP). **Pulmonary hypertension** is a late feature due to hypoxic pulmonary vasoconstriction and/or extensive capillary loss.

Management

Established COPD is irreversible but symptoms, AEs and disease progression can be reduced by **smoking cessation. Pharmacological therapy:** inhaled β-agonists (e.g. salbutamol) and anticholinergics (e.g. tiotropium bromide) alleviate symptoms and improve lung function, with additive effects when combined. Theophyllines improve exercise tolerance and ABGs but do not alter spirometry. Inhaled corticosteroids are recommended in severe COPD (FEV$_1$ < 50% predicted; or >2 steroid requiring AEs/yr). Long-term oral corticosteroids are best avoided as they benefit <25% of patients and cause significant side-effects. Mucolytics assist a few patients with excessive sputum production. **Pulmonary rehabilitation** strengthens respiratory muscles, increases exercise tolerance, improves quality of life and reduces hospitalizations but spirometry is unchanged. **Home oxygen therapy** for >15 hours/day improves survival in chronically hypoxaemic (P_aO_2 < 7.5 kPa) patients. **Prophylaxis:** pneumococcal and influenza vaccinations reduce AEs. **Surgery:** lung volume reduction or transplantation may occasionally benefit carefully selected advanced COPD patients.

Prognosis Yearly mortality is ~25% when FEV$_1$ is <0.8 L. This is increased by co-existing cor pulmonale, hypercapnia and weight loss.

Acute exacerbations

The cause is often unknown but infection, pulmonary embolism, pneumothorax, IHD, arrhythmias, drugs and metabolic disturbances can precipitate AEs.

• **General measures:** fluid management is difficult, especially in cor pulmonale, and requires careful monitoring. Nutrition and electrolyte correction (e.g. hypokalaemia) improve respiratory muscle strength. Thromboembolic prophylaxis is essential. **Oxygen therapy (OT)** relieves life-threatening hypoxia and the small P_aCO_2 increase that occurs in most cases is of no consequence. In a few patients with reduced hypoxic respiratory drive (± hypercapnia) OT causes hypoventilation and further CO_2 retention. However, on the steep part of the oxyhaemoglobin dissociation curve, small P_aO_2 increases do not cause much CO_2 retention but significantly increase arterial oxygen content. Monitor OT with serial ABGs to achieve a P_aO_2 > 8 kPa without a substantial rise in P_aCO_2 (Chapters 11, 12). **Pharmacological therapy:** high dose, aerosolized β-agonists and anticholinergic bronchodilators improve symptoms and gas-exchange. Short courses of oral corticosteroids (i.e. 30 mg/day for 10 days) improve lung function and hasten recovery. Antibiotic therapy is directed at likely organisms (e.g. *H. influenza*) and adjusted according to microbiological results. **Respiratory therapy:** may aid sputum clearance (Chapter 17). Timely **NIV**, as discussed in Chapter 14, may reverse early respiratory failure.

• **Mechanical ventilation (MV)** can be lifesaving but may be associated with prolonged weaning (Chapter 17) and complications (e.g. pneumothorax). Dynamic hyperinflation, raised intrathoracic pressure and patient-ventilator dysynchrony are treated with bronchodilators, increased expiratory time, decreased minute ventilation and by setting ventilator PEEP at auto-PEEP levels (Fig. d). Avoid over-ventilating patients with CO_2 retention as this causes metabolic alkalosis. In end-stage COPD it may be appropriate to limit ventilatory support to NIV (Chapters 14, 16).

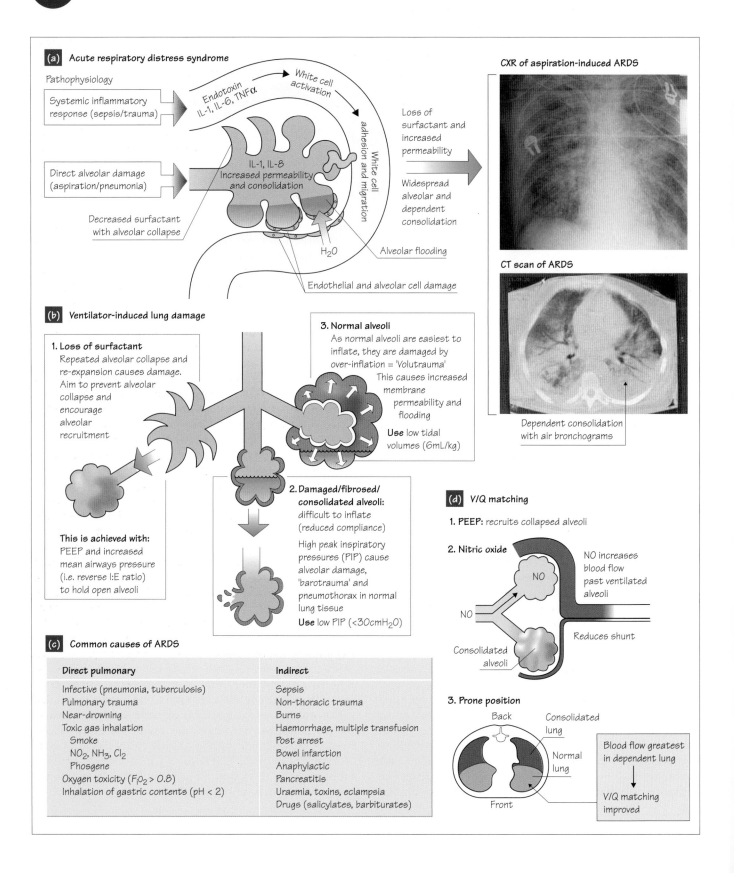

(a) Acute respiratory distress syndrome

Pathophysiology

Systemic inflammatory response (sepsis/trauma) → Endotoxin IL-1, IL-6, TNFα → White cell activation

Direct alveolar damage (aspiration/pneumonia)

White cell adhesion and migration

IL-1, IL-8 Increased permeability and consolidation

Decreased surfactant with alveolar collapse

H_2O

Alveolar flooding

Endothelial and alveolar cell damage

Loss of surfactant and increased permeability

Widespread alveolar and dependent consolidation

CXR of aspiration-induced ARDS

CT scan of ARDS

Dependent consolidation with air bronchograms

(b) Ventilator-induced lung damage

1. Loss of surfactant
Repeated alveolar collapse and re-expansion causes damage. Aim to prevent alveolar collapse and encourage alveolar recruitment

This is achieved with:
PEEP and increased mean airways pressure (i.e. reverse I:E ratio) to hold open alveoli

3. Normal alveoli
As normal alveoli are easiest to inflate, they are damaged by over-inflation = 'Volutrauma' This causes increased membrane permeability and flooding
Use low tidal volumes (6mL/kg)

2. Damaged/fibrosed/ consolidated alveoli:
difficult to inflate (reduced compliance)
High peak inspiratory pressures (PIP) cause alveolar damage, 'barotrauma' and pneumothorax in normal lung tissue
Use low PIP (<30cmH$_2$O)

(d) V/Q matching

1. PEEP: recruits collapsed alveoli

2. Nitric oxide
NO
NO
Consolidated alveoli
NO increases blood flow past ventilated alveoli
Reduces shunt

3. Prone position
Back
Consolidated lung
Normal lung
Front
Blood flow greatest in dependent lung
↓
V/Q matching improved

(c) Common causes of ARDS

Direct pulmonary	Indirect
Infective (pneumonia, tuberculosis)	Sepsis
Pulmonary trauma	Non-thoracic trauma
Near-drowning	Burns
Toxic gas inhalation	Haemorrhage, multiple transfusion
Smoke	Post arrest
NO_2, NH_3, Cl_2	Bowel infarction
Phosgene	Anaphylactic
Oxygen toxicity ($F_iO_2 > 0.8$)	Pancreatitis
Inhalation of gastric contents (pH < 2)	Uraemia, toxins, eclampsia
	Drugs (salicylates, barbiturates)

ARDS is most simply defined as 'leaky lung syndrome' or 'low pressure (i.e. non-cardiogenic) pulmonary oedema'. It describes acute inflammatory lung injury, often in previously health lungs, mediated by a uniform pulmonary pathological process (Fig. a) in response to a variety of direct (i.e. inhaled) or indirect (i.e. blood borne) insults (Fig. c). During the **acute inflammatory phase** of ARDS (Fig. a), cytokine-activated neutrophils and monocytes adhere to alveolar epithelium or pulmonary endothelium, releasing inflammatory mediators and proteolytic enzymes. These damage the integrity of the alveolar–capillary membrane, increase permeability and cause alveolar oedema. Reduced surfactant production causes alveolar collapse and hyaline membrane formation. Progressive hypoxaemia and respiratory failure result from loss of functioning alveoli and V/Q mismatch. The later **healing, fibroproliferative phase** causes progressive pulmonary fibrosis and associated pulmonary hypertension.

Diagnosis

The internationally agreed criteria for the diagnosis of ARDS are:
- **Severe hypoxaemia:** $P_aO_2/F_iO_2 < 200$ (regardless of PEEP); for example, if P_aO_2 is 80 mmHg on 80% inspired oxygen; $P_aO_2/F_iO_2 = 80/0.8 = 100$.
- **Bilateral diffuse pulmonary infiltrates on CXR.**
- **Normal or only slightly elevated left atrial pressure:** (pulmonary artery occlusion pressure <18 mmHg; Chapter 3).

Acute lung injury (ALI) is the precursor to ARDS. Apart from a lesser degree of hypoxaemia ($P_aO_2/F_iO_2 < 300$), the criteria for diagnosis are the same.

Epidemiology and prognosis

The incidence of ARDS is ~2–8 cases/100,000/population/year but its precursor ALI is much more common. Overall **mortality** is high (~40%) but is determined by the precipitating condition (trauma <35%, sepsis ~50%, aspiration pneumonia ~80%) and increased by age (>60 years old) and associated sepsis. The cause of death is multi-organ failure (MOF) and <20% die from hypoxaemia alone.

Clinical features

The **acute inflammatory phase** lasts 3–10 days and results in hypoxaemia and MOF. It presents with progressive breathlessness, tachypnoea, cyanosis, hypoxic confusion and lung crepitations. These features are not diagnostic and frequently misinterpreted as heart failure. During the **healing, fibroproliferative phase**, lung scarring and pneumothoraces are common. Secondary chest and systemic infections are common in both phases.

Investigation and monitoring

Routine measurements include temperature, respiratory rate, S_aO_2 and urine output. Haemodynamic monitoring of central venous pressure, cardiac output (CO) and occasionally left atrial pressure using a pulmonary artery catheter, ensure appropriate fluid balance and adequate tissue oxygen delivery. Serial arterial blood gases measurement and occasionally capnography (Chapter 3) are used to monitor gas exchange. Regular microbiological samples (e.g. bronchial lavage) identify secondary infection early. **Radiology** (Fig.a): serial CXRs detect progression of diffuse bilateral pulmonary infiltrates. Early CT scans often demonstrate dependent consolidation and later scans pneumothoraces, pneumatocoeles and fibrosis.

Management

Initially identify and treat the precipitating cause. In mild disease (e.g. ALI) oxygen therapy, diuretics and physiotherapy maintain gas exchange. If respiratory failure progresses, non-invasive ventilation (Chapter 14) with CPAP improves oxygenation and may avoid the need for MV. However, in severe disease, MV with high-inspired oxygen concentrations is necessary. Due to reduced lung compliance, high PIPs are required to achieve normal tidal volumes (T_v). These high pressures cause lung damage termed 'barotrauma' (e.g. pneumothorax). 'Volutrauma' describes damage to healthy alveoli due to over-distention (Fig. b).
- **Mechanical ventilation:** aims to avoid oxygen toxicity (i.e. $F_iO_2 < 80\%$), limit pressure-induced lung damage and volutrauma, optimize alveolar recruitment and oxygenation, and avoid circulatory compromise due to high intrathoracic pressures. A **'protective' lung ventilation strategy** of low T_v (6 ml/kg) and low PIP (<30 cmH_2O) prevent lung damage (Chapter 17) whilst high positive end expiratory pressures (PEEP; >10 cmH_2O) and long inspiratory to expiratory (I : E) times (i.e. 2 : 1 instead of the normal 1 : 2) recruit collapsed alveoli. No ventilatory mode is proven to be superior, although pressure-controlled modes (Chapter 16) are generally favoured. The CO_2 retention, termed 'permissive hypercapnia', resulting from this low T_v strategy is usually tolerated with adequate sedation.
- **Avoid excessive fluid loading:** which causes alveolar oedema due to increase alveolar permeability. Aim to maintain adequate CO and organ perfusion at the lowest LAP by using inotropes or vasoactive drugs rather than aggressive fluid filling. In the acute phase, diuretics reduce pulmonary oedema and may improve oxygenation
- **General measures:** include good nursing care, physiotherapy, nutrition, sedation and infection control. Minimize metabolic demand by preventing fever and shivering and controlling agitation with sedatives. No drug therapy including steroids, anti-inflammatory agents or surfactant has been consistently beneficial in clinical trials of adult ARDS. High dose steroid therapy to reduce the development of pulmonary fibrosis, 7–10 days after ARDS onset, remains controversial.
- **Additional measures** include: **inhaled nitric oxide** which increases perfusion of ventilated alveoli by vasodilating surrounding vessels, improving V/Q matching and reducing overall shunt fraction (Fig. d). Unfortunately, the initial P_aO_2 improvement is not sustained and there is no survival benefit. **Prone positioning:** as consolidation is usually dependent and blood flow is greatest in the dependent areas, improved V/Q matching can be achieved by turning the patient prone so that non-consolidated, ventilated lung is dependent (Fig. d). **Bronchoscopy:** improves ventilation and V/Q matching by removing sputum plugs and secretions. **Extracorporeal membrane oxygenation (ECMO):** techniques to oxygenate blood or remove CO_2 are effective in children but the benefit in adults has not been established. **Chest drainage:** pneumothorax and pneumatocoeles are common during the late fibroproliferative phase and may be difficult to detect on CXR. The importance of CT scanning to localize and drain these has only recently been appreciated (Chapter 37).

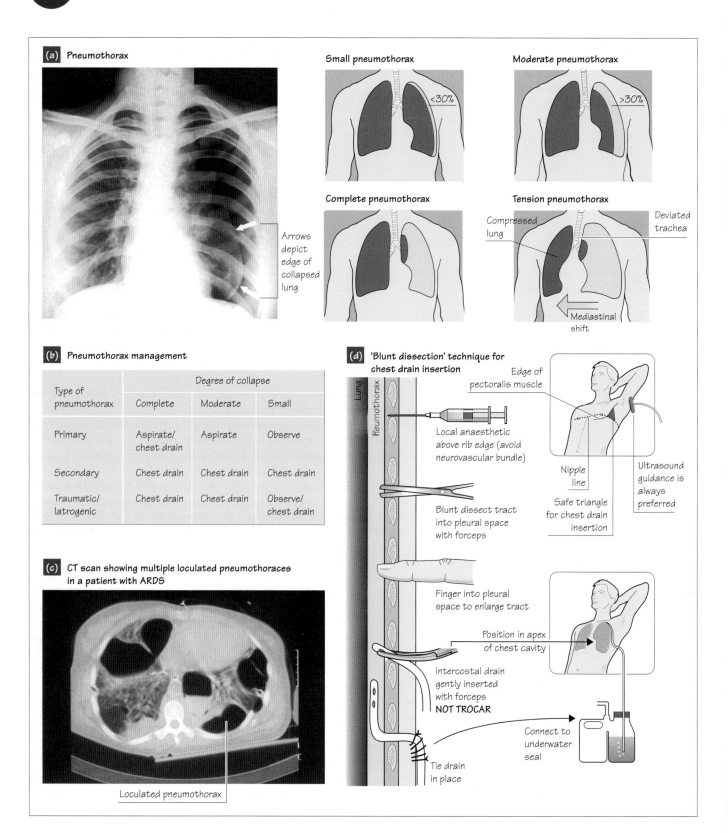

(a) Pneumothorax

Arrows depict edge of collapsed lung

Small pneumothorax — <30%

Moderate pneumothorax — >30%

Complete pneumothorax

Tension pneumothorax — Compressed lung, Deviated trachea, Mediastinal shift

(b) Pneumothorax management

Type of pneumothorax	Degree of collapse		
	Complete	Moderate	Small
Primary	Aspirate/chest drain	Aspirate	Observe
Secondary	Chest drain	Chest drain	Chest drain
Traumatic/Iatrogenic	Chest drain	Chest drain	Observe/chest drain

(c) CT scan showing multiple loculated pneumothoraces in a patient with ARDS

Loculated pneumothorax

(d) 'Blunt dissection' technique for chest drain insertion

Lung

Pneumothorax

Local anaesthetic above rib edge (avoid neurovascular bundle)

Blunt dissect tract into pleural space with forceps

Finger into pleural space to enlarge tract

Intercostal drain gently inserted with forceps NOT TROCAR

Tie drain in place

Edge of pectoralis muscle

Nipple line

Safe triangle for chest drain insertion

Ultrasound guidance is always preferred

Position in apex of chest cavity

Connect to underwater seal

Pneumothorax (i.e. a collection of air between the visceral and parietal pleura causing a real rather than potential pleural space) and air leaks are common in acute and critical illnesses. Recognition and early drainage can be life saving. Predisposing and precipitating factors include necrotizing lung disease, chest trauma, ventilator-associated lung injury and cardiothoracic surgery.

Pneumothorax classification

1 Primary spontaneous pneumothorax (PSP) is the commonest type of pneumothorax. It is caused by rupture of apical subpleural air-cysts ('blebs') and rarely associated with significant physiological disturbance. PSP usually affects tall, 20- to 40-year-old men (M:F 5:1) without underlying lung disease (prevalence $8/10^5$/year, rising to $200/10^5$/year in subjects >1.9 m in height). Recurrence is >60% following a second PSP and pleurodesis is recommended to fuse the visceral and parietal pleura using either medical (e.g. pleural insertion of talc) or surgical (e.g. abrasion of the pleural lining) techniques.

2 Secondary pneumothorax (SP) is associated with respiratory diseases that damage lung architecture; most commonly obstructive (e.g. COPD), fibrotic or infective (e.g. pneumonia), and occasionally rare or inherited disorders (e.g. Marfan's, cystic fibrosis). The incidence of SP increases with age and the severity of the underlying lung disease. These patients usually require hospital admission as even a small SP in a patient with reduced respiratory reserve may have more serious implications than a large PSP. Mechanically ventilated (MV) patients with lung disease are at particular risk of SP due to associated high pressures ('barotrauma') and alveolar overdistention ('volutrauma'). 'Protective' ventilation strategies using low-pressure, limited-volume ventilation reduces this risk (Chapters 16, 17, 35).

3 Traumatic (iatrogenic) pneumothorax (TP) follows blunt (e.g. road traffic accidents) or penetrating (e.g. stab wounds) chest trauma (Chapter 54). Therapeutic procedures (e.g. line insertion, chest surgery) are common causes of iatrogenic pneumothorax.

A **tension pneumothorax** may complicate PSP or SP but is most common in MV patients and following TP. It occurs when air accumulates in the pleural cavity faster than it can be removed. Increased intrathoracic pressure causes mediastinal shift, lung compression, impaired venous return and shock due to reduced CO. It is a medical emergency and fatal if not rapidly relieved by drainage. Detection is a clinical diagnosis; awaiting CXR confirmation may be life-threatening. Immediate drainage with a 14G needle in the second intercostal space in the midclavicular line is essential. A characteristic 'hiss' of escaping gas confirms the diagnosis. A chest drain is then inserted.

Clinical assessment Pneumothorax is graded and treated according to Figs (a) and (b). Sudden breathlessness and/or sharp pleuritic pain suggest a pneumothorax. Most PSPs are small (<30%), and cause few symptoms other than pain. Clinical signs can be surprisingly difficult to detect, but in large pneumothoraces reduced air entry and hyper-resonant percussion over one hemithorax are characteristic and may be associated with tachypnoea and cyanosis. Cardiorespiratory compromise can develop rapidly in a tension pneumothorax or in MV patients and requires immediate drainage. **Monitoring** reveals tachycardia, hypotension and desaturation. **Blood gases** may demonstrate respiratory failure. **Chest X-ray (CXR)** confirms the diagnosis (Fig. a). **CT scan** may detect localized pneumothoraces following trauma or MV (Fig. c).

Management Immediate supportive therapy includes supplemental oxygen and analgesia. Treatment is dependent on the cause, size and symptoms.
• A tension pneumothorax must be drained immediately. A small PSP (<30%) is simply observed and spontaneous reabsorption is confirmed on serial outpatient CXR. A PSP > 30% may be aspirated, under ultrasound (US) guidance, through a 16G needle using a 50-ml syringe connected to a three-way tap and underwater seal. Following overnight observation successful aspiration is confirmed by lung re-expansion on repeat CXR. Occasionally intercostal chest drainage is required if aspiration fails or in large PSP with respiratory failure.
• In general, SP and TP **always** require hospital admission and US-guided intercostal chest drain insertion. Although the 'Seldinger' technique (i.e. chest drain inserted over a guide wire) is popular, complications have been reported (e.g. lung trauma) and recent recommendations advise daytime insertion under mandatory US guidance. Figure (d) illustrates chest drain insertion using the relatively safe 'blunt dissection' technique. Multiple chest drains may be needed to ensure adequate lung re-expansion in patients with loculated pneumothoraces (Fig. c). During MV high airways pressures and alveolar recruitment (e.g. PEEP) encourage persistent leaks. 'Protective' ventilation and the lowest airway pressures compatible with adequate gas exchange should be used (Chapter 17).
• Persistent drain leakage suggests development of a bronchopleural fistula (BPF). High flow, wall suction with pressures of 5–30 cmH$_2$O may oppose visceral and parietal pleura allowing spontaneous pleurodesis but early surgical advice is essential. Video-assisted thoracoscopy is as effective as thoracotomy at correcting BPF but causes less respiratory dysfunction.
• Chest drains are removed when CXR confirms lung expansion and there has been no air leakage through the drain for >24 hours. Drains should not be clamped before removal. Following adequate analgesia, the drain is pulled out during inspiration and the drain site secured with 'purse string' sutures.

Air leaks

Pneumomediastinum describes air in the mediastinal-pleural reflection, outlining the heart and great vessels on CXR. Air may also dissect along perivascular sheaths into the neck causing **subcutaneous emphysema (SE)** or around the heart with **pneumopericardium**, which may cause tamponade. Air leaks follow ventilator-induced barotrauma or traumatic damage to the trachea (e.g. tracheostomy), bronchus and oesophagus (Chapter 54). SE may cause localized (e.g. neck, chest) or grotesque facial and body swelling. It has a characteristic crackling sensation on palpation. The voice may have a nasal quality and auscultation over the precordium may reveal a 'crunch' with each heart beat (Homan's sign). Management includes good drainage of pneumothorax and 'protective' ventilation strategies (Chapters 16, 17). Failure of spontaneous resolution should prompt investigation (e.g. bronchoscopy) to detect unrecognized air leaks and problems that decrease chest drain efficiency.

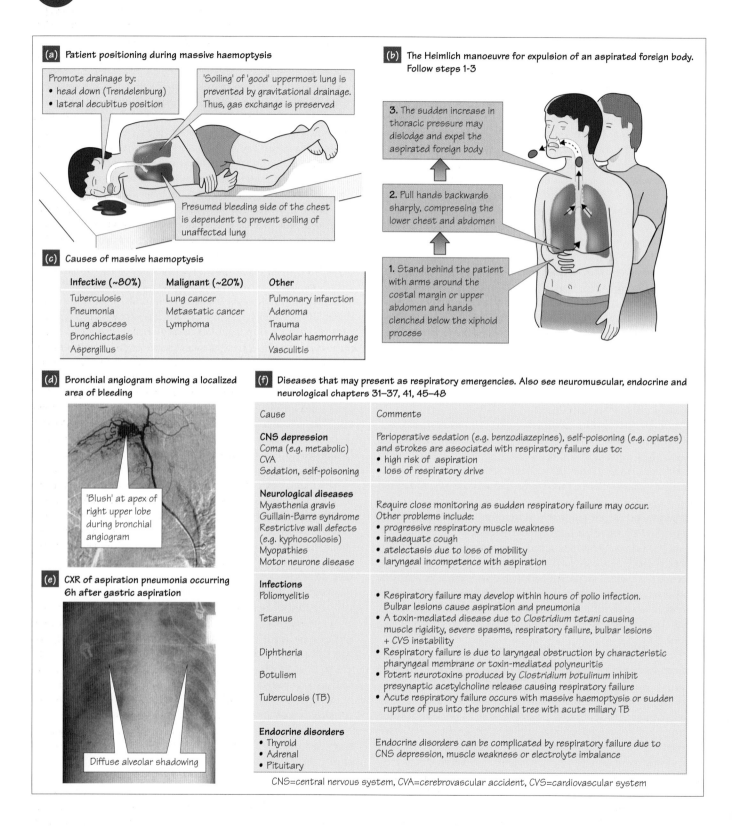

(a) Patient positioning during massive haemoptysis

Promote drainage by:
- head down (Trendelenburg)
- lateral decubitus position

'Soiling' of 'good' uppermost lung is prevented by gravitational drainage. Thus, gas exchange is preserved

Presumed bleeding side of the chest is dependent to prevent soiling of unaffected lung

(b) The Heimlich manoeuvre for expulsion of an aspirated foreign body. Follow steps 1-3

3. The sudden increase in thoracic pressure may dislodge and expel the aspirated foreign body

2. Pull hands backwards sharply, compressing the lower chest and abdomen

1. Stand behind the patient with arms around the costal margin or upper abdomen and hands clenched below the xiphoid process

(c) Causes of massive haemoptysis

Infective (~80%)	Malignant (~20%)	Other
Tuberculosis	Lung cancer	Pulmonary infarction
Pneumonia	Metastatic cancer	Adenoma
Lung abscess	Lymphoma	Trauma
Bronchiectasis		Alveolar haemorrhage
Aspergillus		Vasculitis

(d) Bronchial angiogram showing a localized area of bleeding

'Blush' at apex of right upper lobe during bronchial angiogram

(e) CXR of aspiration pneumonia occurring 6h after gastric aspiration

Diffuse alveolar shadowing

(f) Diseases that may present as respiratory emergencies. Also see neuromuscular, endocrine and neurological chapters 31–37, 41, 45–48

Cause	Comments
CNS depression Coma (e.g. metabolic) CVA Sedation, self-poisoning	Perioperative sedation (e.g. benzodiazepines), self-poisoning (e.g. opiates) and strokes are associated with respiratory failure due to: • high risk of aspiration • loss of respiratory drive
Neurological diseases Myasthenia gravis Guillain-Barre syndrome Restrictive wall defects (e.g. kyphoscoliosis) Myopathies Motor neurone disease	Require close monitoring as sudden respiratory failure may occur. Other problems include: • progressive respiratory muscle weakness • inadequate cough • atelectasis due to loss of mobility • laryngeal incompetence with aspiration
Infections Poliomyelitis Tetanus Diphtheria Botulism Tuberculosis (TB)	• Respiratory failure may develop within hours of polio infection. Bulbar lesions cause aspiration and pneumonia • A toxin-mediated disease due to *Clostridium tetani* causing muscle rigidity, severe spasms, respiratory failure, bulbar lesions + CVS instability • Respiratory failure is due to laryngeal obstruction by characteristic pharyngeal membrane or toxin-mediated polyneuritis • Potent neurotoxins produced by *Clostridium botulinum* inhibit presynaptic acetylcholine release causing respiratory failure • Acute respiratory failure occurs with massive haemoptysis or sudden rupture of pus into the bronchial tree with acute miliary TB
Endocrine disorders • Thyroid • Adrenal • Pituitary	Endocrine disorders can be complicated by respiratory failure due to CNS depression, muscle weakness or electrolyte imbalance

CNS=central nervous system, CVA=cerebrovascular accident, CVS=cardiovascular system

Massive haemoptysis

Definition Expectoration of >600 ml of blood in 24 hours.

Causes Infection causes ~80% of cases (Fig. c).

Prognosis Death is usually due to asphyxia, not blood loss, and is related to pathology, lung function and rate of bleeding (i.e. 600 ml in <4 hours or >16 hours, causes 70% or 5% mortality, respectively).

Clinical evaluation Haematemesis and nose bleeds must be distinguished from haemoptysis. Food particles suggest haematemesis; purulent secretions bronchiectasis or lung abscesses; CXR apical cavities, TB or mycetoma; and haematuria, alveolar haemorrhage syndromes. Localization of the bleeding site may be difficult as blood aspiration results in diffuse clinical (e.g. crepitations) and radiological signs. **Investigations** include serology, blood gases, clotting profile, CXR and sputum microbiology (e.g. acid fast bacilli).

Management involves:

1 Airways protection: assess bleeding severity and prevent asphyxia (e.g. secretion clearance, oxygen therapy). **Promote airways drainage** by placing the patient slightly head down in the lateral decubitus position (Fig. a). This prevents alveolar 'soiling' of the 'good' lung. Cough suppression (e.g. codeine) and withholding physiotherapy reduces bleeding. Consider mechanical ventilation (MV) when overwhelming haemoptysis causes respiratory failure. The unaffected lung can be independently ventilated by placing the endotracheal tube (ETT) in the corresponding main bronchus or by using a double lumen tube until bleeding is controlled.

2 Determine the site and cause of bleeding: early fibreoptic bronchoscopy allows examination of upper lobes and subsegmental bronchi, which account for ~80% of bleeding sites. Rigid bronchoscopy enhances suctioning in torrential haemorrhage but limits inspection. CT scans identify structural abnormalities (e.g. tumours) and bronchial arteriography, pulmonary angiography or nuclear scans may detect active bleeding (Fig. d).

3 Control of bleeding: immediate measures include bronchoscopic iced-saline (± epinephrine) lavages, topical fibrin or tamponade of affected bronchi using balloon catheters.

- **Bronchial artery embolization** is initially successful in >70% of cases, especially those with dilated bronchial arteries (e.g. bronchiectasis). However, re-bleeding occurs in >50% within 3 months. Serious complications include paraplegia following anterior spinal artery thrombosis (~5%).
- **Surgical therapy** has the best long-term outcomes but only medical management is possible in diffuse or end-stage disease (e.g. cancer, FEV_1 < 40% predicted).

4 General measures: include fluid replacement, antibiotics and bronchodilators.

Aspiration syndromes

High risk groups for aspiration include those with depressed conscious level (e.g. drug overdose), laryngeal incompetence (e.g. bulbar syndromes) and critically ill patients. The clinical scenario depends on the type and volume of aspiration. Thus, peri-anaesthetic aspiration of large volumes of gastric contents rapidly progresses to ARDS, whereas repeated microaspiration (e.g. bulbar palsy) causes pneumonia. A high index of suspicion is required as aspiration is not always witnessed.

- **Solid particulate matter:** including peanuts, coins and teeth can be aspirated. Partially masticated food is most common giving rise to the '*café-coronary*' syndrome. **Partial obstruction** causes stridor, cough, wheeze, atelectasis and recurrent pneumonia. **Complete obstruction** prevents breathing and speech with rapidly developing cyanosis, coma and death. If a sharp blow to the back of the chest fails to dislodge the particle the Heimlich manoeuvre is attempted (Fig. b). If this fails, an emergency cricothyroidectomy is performed by inserting a large bore needle or sharp implement through the cricothyroid membrane (Chapter 17). Urgent bronchoscopy follows to remove the obstruction.
- **Fluid aspiration:** gastric contents (pH < 2) are most frequently aspirated and large volumes rapidly cause respiratory failure, pulmonary oedema and ARDS. The right main bronchus is the most direct path of aspiration and right lower lobe involvement is common (~60%). CXR shows pulmonary infiltrates in ~90% of cases (Fig. e). **Prevention is essential** (i.e. nasogastric (NG) tube, preoperative fasting) as treatment is largely supportive including airways clearance, oxygen therapy, bronchodilators, antibiotics, CPAP or MV. Neither steroid therapy nor bronchoscopy is beneficial. Preventing pneumonia due to microaspiration (e.g. post CVA) is difficult and includes the use of thickened feeds, upright posture and long-term NG feeding.
- **Near-drowning:** is a common cause of accidental death and is often associated with alcohol consumption or a primary medical event (e.g. MI). Although more frequent in rivers, sea or lakeside areas, deaths may occur at home in small volumes of water (e.g. bath). **Freshwater aspiration** affects pulmonary surfactant causing atelectasis, pulmonary shunt and hypoxaemia. Rapid pulmonary absorption of hypotonic freshwater causes initial hypervolaemia, haemolysis and hyperkalaemia. Hypertonic **seawater aspiration** pulls fluid into alveoli causing hypovolaemia, shunting and hypoxaemia. Profound hypothermia (<30°C) is common in near-drowning and predisposes to resistant arrhythmias particularly during rough handling or cardiopulmonary resuscitation (CPR). The Heimlich manoeuvre is not recommended as gravitational drainage of aspirated water is just as effective, without risking arrhythmias. Hypothermic patients must be rewarmed before terminating CPR (Chapter 5). Treatment is largely supportive and overnight observation is recommended as late (>12 hours) pulmonary oedema can occur. The degree of hypoxic brain damage determines outcome (Chapter 53). Mortality is similar in fresh or seawater.

Upper airways obstruction

Causes include aspirated particulate matter, inhaled toxic gases and burns (Chapter 57), trauma (Chapter 54), anaphylaxis, laryngeal oedema, laryngospasm and large airway stenoses. Obstruction by the tongue should be excluded and prevented with a pharyngeal airway (Chapter 13). Extubation can be associated with laryngospasm due to oedema or irritation during ETT removal. **Treatment:** Severe respiratory distress requires immediate intubation. In less critical situations nebulized epinephrine (± salbutamol) with intravenous steroids may reduce oedema and spasm sufficiently to avoid intubation. Helium and oxygen mixtures may improve gas flow through obstructed airways.

Other respiratory emergencies

There is an extensive list of infective, neuromuscular and endocrine diseases (Chapters 31–37, 41, 45–48) that predispose to rapid respiratory impairment (Fig. f). Although rare in countries with advanced public health programmes, poliomyelitis, tetanus, diphtheria and TB remain relatively common causes of respiratory emergencies in the developing world.

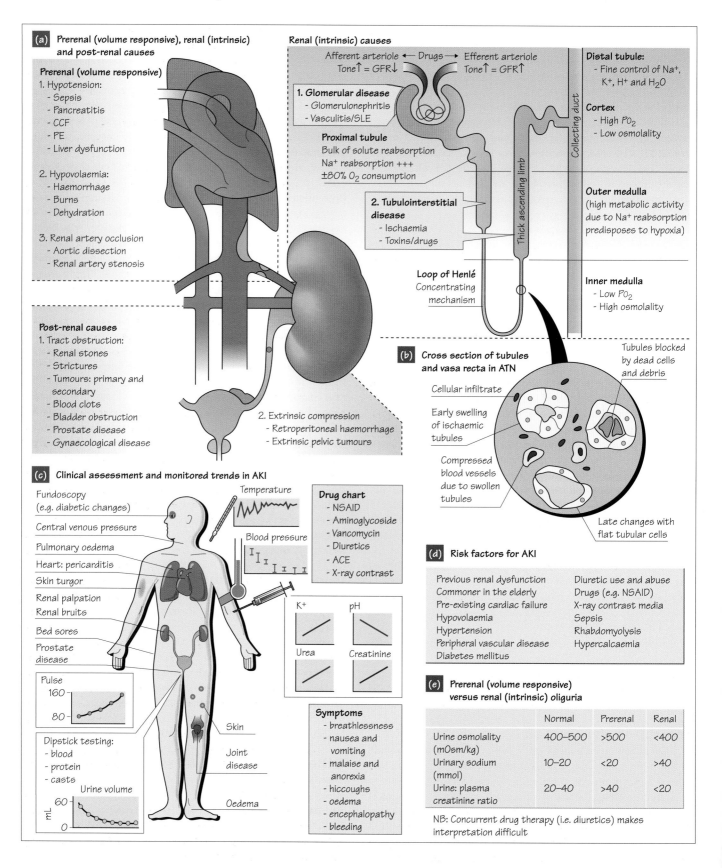

(a) Prerenal (volume responsive), renal (intrinsic) and post-renal causes

Prerenal (volume responsive)

1. Hypotension:
   - Sepsis
   - Pancreatitis
   - CCF
   - PE
   - Liver dysfunction

2. Hypovolaemia:
   - Haemorrhage
   - Burns
   - Dehydration

3. Renal artery occlusion
   - Aortic dissection
   - Renal artery stenosis

Post-renal causes

1. Tract obstruction:
   - Renal stones
   - Strictures
   - Tumours: primary and secondary
   - Blood clots
   - Bladder obstruction
   - Prostate disease
   - Gynaecological disease

2. Extrinsic compression
   - Retroperitoneal haemorrhage
   - Extrinsic pelvic tumours

Renal (intrinsic) causes

Afferent arteriole ← Drugs → Efferent arteriole
Tone↑ = GFR↓   Tone↑ = GFR↑

1. Glomerular disease
- Glomerulonephritis
- Vasculitis/SLE

Proximal tubule
Bulk of solute reabsorption
Na^+ reabsorption +++
±80% O_2 consumption

2. Tubulointerstitial disease
- Ischaemia
- Toxins/drugs

Loop of Henlé
Concentrating mechanism

Thick ascending limb

Collecting duct

Distal tubule:
- Fine control of Na^+, K^+, H^+ and H_2O

Cortex
- High P_{O_2}
- Low osmolality

Outer medulla
(high metabolic activity due to Na^+ reabsorption predisposes to hypoxia)

Inner medulla
- Low P_{O_2}
- High osmolality

(b) Cross section of tubules and vasa recta in ATN

Cellular infiltrate
Early swelling of ischaemic tubules
Compressed blood vessels due to swollen tubules
Tubules blocked by dead cells and debris
Late changes with flat tubular cells

(c) Clinical assessment and monitored trends in AKI

Fundoscopy (e.g. diabetic changes)
Central venous pressure
Pulmonary oedema
Heart: pericarditis
Skin turgor
Renal palpation
Renal bruits
Bed sores
Prostate disease

Temperature
Blood pressure

Drug chart
- NSAID
- Aminoglycoside
- Vancomycin
- Diuretics
- ACE
- X-ray contrast

K^+ pH
Urea   Creatinine

Pulse
160
80

Dipstick testing:
- blood
- protein
- casts

Urine volume
60
0
mL

Skin
Joint disease
Oedema

Symptoms
- breathlessness
- nausea and vomiting
- malaise and anorexia
- hiccoughs
- oedema
- encephalopathy
- bleeding

(d) Risk factors for AKI

Previous renal dysfunction	Diuretic use and abuse
Commoner in the elderly	Drugs (e.g. NSAID)
Pre-existing cardiac failure	X-ray contrast media
Hypovolaemia	Sepsis
Hypertension	Rhabdomyolysis
Peripheral vascular disease	Hypercalcaemia
Diabetes mellitus	

(e) Prerenal (volume responsive) versus renal (intrinsic) oliguria

	Normal	Prerenal	Renal
Urine osmolality (mOsm/kg)	400–500	>500	<400
Urinary sodium (mmol)	10–20	<20	>40
Urine: plasma creatinine ratio	20–40	>40	<20

NB: Concurrent drug therapy (i.e. diuretics) makes interpretation difficult

Acute kidney injury network definition 2008

Acute kidney injury (AKI) is an abrupt (<48 hour) reduction in kidney function defined as an increase in serum creatinine (SCr) of ≥26.4 μmol/L; or SCr ≥150% (1.5-fold) of baseline; or a documented reduction in urine output (UO; <0.5 ml/kg/h for >6 h). AKI severity (Appendix 2) is classified as:

- **Stage I:** SCr increase ≥26.4 μmol/L (0.3 mg/dl) **or** SCr ≥150% of baseline **or** UO <0.5 ml/kg/h for >6 hours.
- **Stage II:** SCr increase >200–300% from baseline; **or** UO <0.5 ml/kg/h for >12 hours.
- **Stage III:** SCr increase ≥354 μmol/L (4.0 mg/dl) **or** SCr ≥300% of baseline **or** use of renal replacement therapy (RRT); **or** UO <0.3 ml/kg/h for >24 hours **or** anuria for 12 hours.

Classification of acute kidney injury
(Fig. a)

1 Pre-renal (volume responsive) AKI (~55%): inadequate renal perfusion (e.g. hypotension, haemorrhage, dehydration, renal vascular obstruction) causes ischaemia and potential acute tubular necrosis (ATN).

2 Renal (intrinsic) AKI (~30%): causes include:
- **Glomerular** – glomerulonephritis, vasculitis (e.g. Goodpasture's syndrome).
- **Acute tubular necrosis and tubulointerstitial disease (TID)** – are caused by ischaemia, toxicity (e.g. drugs, heavy metals, contrast media) and free haemoglobin or myoglobin. Haemoglobin is released during haemolysis (e.g. haemolytic-uraemic syndrome) and myoglobin during rhabdomyolysis (e.g. trauma). AKI also follows tubular precipitation of calcium in acute hypercalcaemia or 'light chains' in myeloma.
- **Drugs and toxins** – NSAIDs cause renal arteriolar vasoconstriction by inhibiting normal prostaglandin-induced vasodilation. In hypovolaemic patients this seriously reduces renal blood flow (RBF) and glomerular filtration rate (GFR). NSAIDs also precipitate AKI in chronic kidney disease (CKD) and those using diuretics (e.g. cirrhosis). Radiocontrasts, ciclosporin and amphotericin cause vasoconstriction, whereas aminoglycosides and cephalosporins are direct tubular toxins. ACE inhibitors block the angiotensin-mediated efferent arteriolar vasodilation that maintains GFR. Many drugs may cause TID (e.g. antibiotics, diuretics)

3 Post-renal (~15%): due to urinary tract obstruction (Fig. a). Resulting back-pressure inhibits GFR and causes ischaemia. AKI only occurs if both kidneys are obstructed.

Pathophysiology

Renal ischaemia contributes to most cases of AKI due to failure of complex vascular control mechanisms. BP is a poor indicator of renal hypoperfusion as local autoregulatory feedback mechanisms act to maintain GFR and the renal renin-angiotensin mechanism raises BP despite hypovolaemia. The juxta-medullary region (i.e. proximal tubule and thick ascending limb of the loop of Henlé) is particularly susceptible to ischaemia because: (i) active sodium absorption in this region accounts for 80% of renal oxygen consumption and (ii) most RBF (normally ~30% cardiac output) is directed to the cortex, whilst medullary blood flow is limited to maintain the concentration gradient of osmolality. Reduced RBF (± sepsis, toxicity) causes ATN and tubular cell death in this region due to this combination of high oxygen demand and poor blood supply. Subsequent tubular blockage reduces GFR and swelling further compromises medullary perfusion (Fig. b).

Clinical features

There are two characteristic clinical presentations:
- Most AKI occurs in critically ill patients (ICU incidence ~5–20%) and after surgery, trauma or burns as part of the multiple organ dysfunction syndrome ('**critical-illness AKI**'). Although renal ischaemia (i.e. hypotension) is the main cause, aetiology is often multifactorial (i.e. sepsis, drugs). Presentation with oliguria and progressive increases in SCr and urea (±metabolic acidosis, hyperkalaemia) is typical. Mortality is high (>50%) but >65% of survivors recover renal function and discontinue RRT.
- Single organ AKI occurring on general wards due to specific renal disease (e.g. glomerulonephritis) is less common ('**medical AKI**'). It often presents as a failure to excrete nitrogenous waste rather than oliguria. Although mortality is low (<10%), it can progresses to CKD requiring RRT.

Clinical assessment (Fig. c)

The history identifies factors which predispose to AKI (Fig. d). Recent throat or skin infections and haematuria suggest glomerulonephritis. Haemoptysis is associated with Goodpasture's syndrome. Renal colic or male prostatism (e.g. frequency, poor stream) indicates post-renal obstruction. The past medical history may suggest possible associations (e.g. malignancy and hypercalcaemia) and potential sites of chronic infection (e.g. endocarditis).

Examination

Assess fluid status (i.e. is there hypovolaemia?), cardiovascular function (i.e. is there tissue hypoperfusion?) and exclude renal bruits. Fundoscopy identifies diabetic or hypertensive changes. Sites of sepsis and features of multisystem disease (e.g. arthritis) must be sought. Cardiac auscultation may reveal uraemic pericarditis or valve disease. Upper airways are examined for signs of Wegener's granulomatosis and the chest for pulmonary oedema. Abdominal examination may detect polycystic kidneys, pelvic disease and bladder or prostatic enlargement.
- **Monitor** trends in: (i) **vital signs:** pulse, BP, CVP, UO, fever and weight; (ii) **biochemical parameters:** potassium, urea, SCr, calcium and pH. Creatine kinase indicates severity of rhabdomyolysis.
- **Investigations** include: **haematology** to assess anaemia and haemolysis; **Reagent strip urinalysis** is always required to detect blood, protein, glucose and ketones. Haematuria occurs in renal and post-renal disease; haemoglobin indicates haemolysis; proteinuria suggests glomerulonephritis, CKD or myeloma and myoglobin, rhabdomyolysis; **urine biochemistry** is of limited value but may differentiate between pre-renal and renal failure (Fig. e). It is not performed routinely. **Urine microscopy:** red cell casts confirm glomerulonephritis, granular casts occur in ATN and urinary eosinophils suggest interstitial nephritis. **Microbiology:** assesses urine, blood, chest and wound infections. **Immunology:** antinuclear antibodies are high in SLE. Antiglomerular basement membrane antibody indicates Goodpasture's syndrome and antineutrophil cytoplasmic antibodies (ANCA) suggest vasculitis (e.g. Wegener's). Low complement levels occur in SLE and postinfective glomerulonephritis. **Radiology:** ultrasonography should be performed within 24 hours to assess kidney size and exclude renal tract obstruction. Small kidneys indicate CKD. Radioisotope studies and angiography evaluate renal perfusion. **Histology:** renal biopsy may be required to establish the cause.

39 Acute kidney injury: management and renal replacement therapy

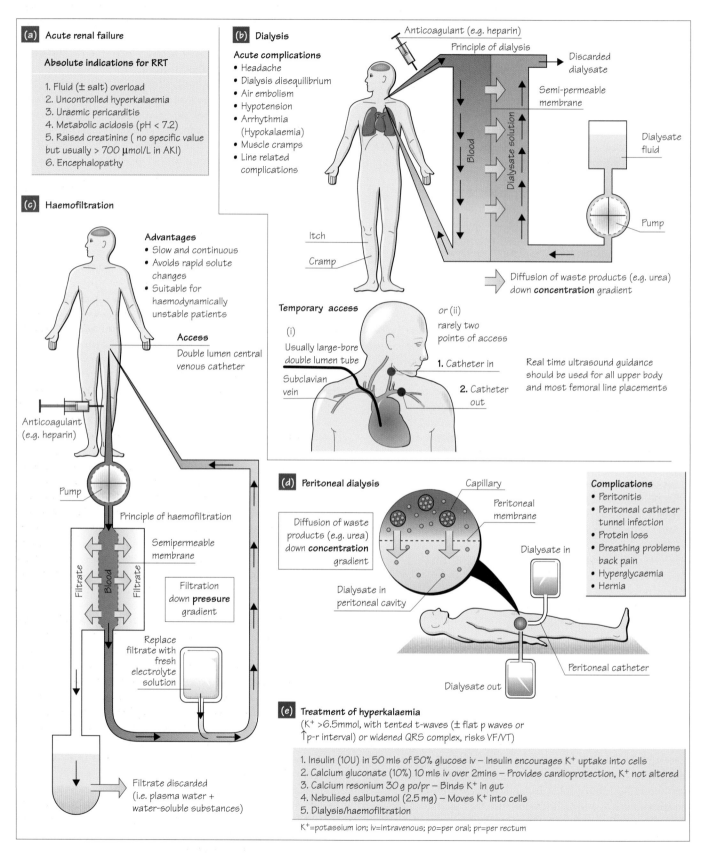

(a) Acute renal failure

Absolute indications for RRT

1. Fluid (± salt) overload
2. Uncontrolled hyperkalaemia
3. Uraemic pericarditis
4. Metabolic acidosis (pH < 7.2)
5. Raised creatinine (no specific value but usually > 700 μmol/L in AKI)
6. Encephalopathy

(c) Haemofiltration

Advantages
- Slow and continuous
- Avoids rapid solute changes
- Suitable for haemodynamically unstable patients

Access
Double lumen central venous catheter

Anticoagulant (e.g. heparin)

Pump

Principle of haemofiltration

Semipermeable membrane

Filtrate

Blood

Filtrate

Filtration down **pressure** gradient

Replace filtrate with fresh electrolyte solution

Filtrate discarded (i.e. plasma water + water-soluble substances)

(b) Dialysis

Acute complications
- Headache
- Dialysis disequilibrium
- Air embolism
- Hypotension
- Arrhythmia (Hypokalaemia)
- Muscle cramps
- Line related complications

Anticoagulant (e.g. heparin)

Principle of dialysis

Discarded dialysate

Semi-permeable membrane

Blood

Dialysate solution

Dialysate fluid

Pump

Itch

Cramp

Diffusion of waste products (e.g. urea) down **concentration** gradient

Temporary access

(i)
Usually large-bore double lumen tube

Subclavian vein

or (ii) rarely two points of access

1. Catheter in
2. Catheter out

Real time ultrasound guidance should be used for all upper body and most femoral line placements

(d) Peritoneal dialysis

Capillary

Peritoneal membrane

Diffusion of waste products (e.g. urea) down **concentration** gradient

Dialysate in peritoneal cavity

Dialysate in

Complications
- Peritonitis
- Peritoneal catheter tunnel infection
- Protein loss
- Breathing problems back pain
- Hyperglycaemia
- Hernia

Peritoneal catheter

Dialysate out

(e) Treatment of hyperkalaemia
(K^+ >6.5mmol, with tented t-waves (± flat p waves or ↑p-r interval) or widened QRS complex, risks VF/VT)

1. Insulin (10U) in 50 mls of 50% glucose iv – Insulin encourages K^+ uptake into cells
2. Calcium gluconate (10%) 10 mls iv over 2mins – Provides cardioprotection, K^+ not altered
3. Calcium resonium 30 g po/pr – Binds K^+ in gut
4. Nebulised salbutamol (2.5 mg) – Moves K^+ into cells
5. Dialysis/haemofiltration

K^+=potassium ion; iv=intravenous; po=per oral; pr=per rectum

Prevention of acute kidney injury

Acute kidney injury (AKI) is preventable in 30% of cases and many more can be corrected with simple measures including volume repletion, discontinuing or avoiding nephrotoxins and early recognition of oliguria and renal dysfunction.

1 Identify and treat the cause: including pre-renal, renal and post-renal pathology (e.g. steroids for vasculitis).

2 Fluid management: regular assessment of fluid and electrolyte balance is essential (Chapters 8, 9). Fluid intake, urine output and daily weight are monitored. A central venous catheter may be required to measure CVP. Volume replacement should match daily and insensible losses with an additional 0.5 L/°C of fever. Inadequate perfusion and renal ischaemia (e.g. hypovolaemia, hypotension) are the commonest cause of AKI and *must be corrected immediately*. If oliguria or renal dysfunction (i.e. rising urea or SCr concentrations) develop consider the following:

- **Fluid challenge** (~0.5–1 L crystalloid over 30–60 mins) – particularly if examination (± urinalysis) suggests a pre-renal cause. The aim is to raise CVP, BP and GFR. Increased urine output supports the diagnosis. Further fluid challenges are guided by CVP assessment. In established AKI oliguria persists and further fluid challenges risk pulmonary oedema.
- **Diuretics** – although loop diuretics (e.g. furosemide (frusemide)), given as boluses or continuous infusions, are often recommended for their putative tubuloprotective effects (i.e. inhibition of sodium absorption in the loop of Henlé, reduces energy requirements and potentially alleviates ischaemia), there is no evidence that they prevent or treat AKI. In fact, they may cause harm (e.g. nephro-/ototoxicity) or potentiate drug toxicity (e.g. aminoglycosides) in hypovolaemic patients. Their only role is to induce diuresis in patients with fluid overload. In rhabdomyolysis, osmotic diuresis with mannitol will not prevent AKI but fluid resuscitation, high urinary flows and cautious urine alkalinization (pH > 6.5) with sodium bicarbonate (1.2%) solution are recommended. **Low dose 'renal' dopamine** has no role in the treatment or prophylaxis of AKI despite its diuretic effects and may be harmful (e.g. arrhythmias).
- **Inotropes** (e.g. epinephrine (adrenaline)) – maintain GFR by increasing CO and MAP (i.e. >70 mmHg) if fluid resuscitation is unsuccessful.

3 Oxygenation: optimize gas exchange (Chapter 12).

4 Sepsis: must be identified and treated (e.g. antibiotics ± surgical intervention).

5 Monitor biochemistry and drug levels: correct electrolyte imbalance/acidosis and adjust prescriptions.

6 Renal protection during imaging includes prophylactic fluid therapy (normal saline 1 ml/kg/h for 12 hours pre- and post-procedure), iso-osmolar contrast media and temporary discontinuation of nephrotoxic drugs (e.g. ACE inhibitors, metformin). Prophylactic *N*-acetylcysteine may be protective.

Established acute kidney injury

Once AKI is established, treatment is supportive. Management aims to: (i) prevent fluid overload; (ii) maintain electrolyte and acid–base balance; and (iii) limit accumulation of toxic metabolic waste by nutritional control and RRT. In >65% of patients with ATN, renal function recovers after ~2–60 days and is heralded by a diuretic phase. AKI due to other causes may progress to CKD and the need for ongoing RRT.

General management

- **Fluid balance:** during anuric or oliguric periods, fluid replacement is restricted to insensible loss (~0.5–1 L/day). If pulmonary oedema occurs due to fluid overload (Chapter 28), it is treated with oxygen and pulmonary vasodilators (e.g. nitrates) whilst RRT is arranged to remove fluid. Diuretics, CPAP and venesection may help. During the diuretic phase of ATN recovery, fluid losses and electrolyte imbalance must be corrected.
- **Electrolytes:** are monitored daily and sodium and potassium intake restricted. Calcium exchange resins, insulin with dextrose or RRT may be required to treat hyperkalaemia (Fig. e). During AKI, SCr rises by ~80–100 μmol/L/day but depends on muscle mass, metabolic rate and tissue damage. The rate of rise of urea is more variable. Uraemic complications (e.g. pericarditis, seizures) develop above 50 mmol/L.
- **Nutritional support:** improves outcome and early referral to a dietician is recommended. AKI patients should receive 20–35 kcal/kg/day and up to a maximum of 1.7 g amino acids/kg/day if hypercatabolic and receiving RRT. Vitamin supplements may be required.
- **Metabolic acidosis:** ideally RRT commences before respiratory distress or myocardial instability occurs.
- **Uraemic bleeding:** is usually due to platelet dysfunction. Treatment with clotting factors is ineffective but DDAVP (i.v.) may restore platelet function.
- **General factors:** modify drug doses, control hypertension and prevent infection (e.g. line sepsis). Remove urinary catheters in anuric patients.

Renal replacement therapy

Absolute indications for RRT are listed in Fig. (a). Three main methods of fluid and solute removal are used in AKI. In haemodynamically unstable patients continuous forms of RRT are better tolerated.

- **Dialysis** (Fig. b): blood flows on one side and a solution of crystalloids (dialysis fluid) is pumped in the opposite direction along the other side of a semipermeable membrane. Small molecules and toxic waste diffuse across the membrane according to imposed concentration gradients. Dialysis fluid composition is designed to normalize plasma. Small molecules such as urea (60 Da) are efficiently removed, larger molecules like creatinine (113 Da) less so. Hyperphosphataemia occurs due to poor clearance of phosphate ions. Dialysis corrects biochemical abnormalities and rapidly removes excess extracellular fluid (~2–4 hours) but may cause hypokalaemia or intravascular hypovolaemia. In unstable patients, life-threatening hypotension or cardiac arrhythmias may occur.
- **Haemofiltration** (Fig. c): plasma water and water soluble substances (<50 kDa) pass across a highly permeable membrane by convective flow (e.g. glomerular filtration). Unlike dialysis, urea, creatinine and phosphate are cleared at similar rates. Hypophosphataemia may occur if phosphate is not supplemented. Molecules like heparin are also efficiently cleared. The filtrate is discarded and replaced by a physiological solution. Low flow rates make haemofiltration less efficient at removing uraemic toxins but continuous use allows clearance of any amount of fluid and nitrogenous waste. Haemofiltration's advantage is its relative ease of use in haemodynamically unstable patients.
- **Peritoneal dialysis** (Fig. d): uses hypertonic dialysate to draw fluid and solutes across the peritoneum following insertion of a peritoneal catheter. The dialysate (1–3 L) dwells in the abdominal cavity for ~4–5 hours before drainage. Abdominal pathology, infection risks and interference with ventilation limit use.

40 Diabetic emergencies

(a) Causes of hypoglycaemia

1. Usually related to diabetic therapy
Inadequate food intake, excessive exercise, accidental or deliberate overdose, prolonged drug effect (e.g. long-acting oral hypoglycaemics; chlorpropamide), poor clearance in renal failure (e.g. insulin)

2. General causes
Starvation, rebound hypoglycaemia after a large meal, alcohol, renal and liver disease, systemic diseases (e.g. sepsis, infection, hypothermia), endocrine disease (e.g. hypopituitarism, adrenal failure), poisoning or drug therapy (e.g. salicylate) and rare insulin secreting tumours (e.g. insulinomas) or insulin-like growth factor II producing tumours (e.g. pleural fibromas)

(b) Clinical features of hypoglycaemia

Early warning signs*
Poor concentration
Anxiety/aggression
Faintness
Vague/glazed appearance

Sweating*

Palpitations*

Tremor*

Nausea
Lip tingling
Hunger
Slurred speech
Personality change

Late features
Impaired consciousness
Seizures
Coma
Irreversible brain damage

Pupillary dilation

Neurological signs e.g. altered reflexes, extensor plantar responses

* Early adrenergic signs may be lost in long-standing DM

(c) Ketogenesis in DKA

Adipose tissue

Triglycerides from breakdown of fat

Plasma
Free fatty acid

Liver
Free fatty CoA → Glucose
→ Acetyl CoA
Ketone bodies
Acetoacetate
β-hydroxybutyrate
Acetone

(d) Initial management of DKA

Confirm diagnosis (investigations)
↓
Immediate, rapid fluid replacement with normal saline
↓
Start insulin therapy (bolus 4–8U iv), then sliding scale insulin infusion
↓
Beware K+
↓
Monitor / replace electrolytes
↓
Insulin rapidly corrects acidosis but consider bicarbonate if pH <7.1 with cardiovascular instability
↓
Assess co-existing problems and treat cause

(e) Clinical features of DKA and investigations

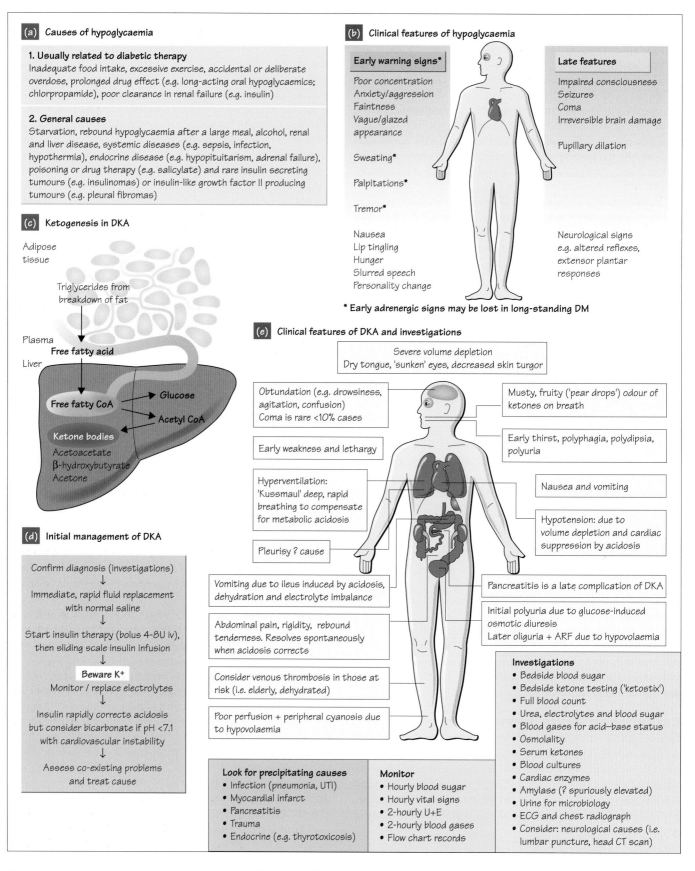

Severe volume depletion
Dry tongue, 'sunken' eyes, decreased skin turgor

Obtundation (e.g. drowsiness, agitation, confusion) Coma is rare <10% cases

Musty, fruity ('pear drops') odour of ketones on breath

Early weakness and lethargy

Early thirst, polyphagia, polydipsia, polyuria

Hyperventilation: 'Kussmaul' deep, rapid breathing to compensate for metabolic acidosis

Nausea and vomiting

Pleurisy ? cause

Hypotension: due to volume depletion and cardiac suppression by acidosis

Vomiting due to ileus induced by acidosis, dehydration and electrolyte imbalance

Pancreatitis is a late complication of DKA

Abdominal pain, rigidity, rebound tenderness. Resolves spontaneously when acidosis corrects

Initial polyuria due to glucose-induced osmotic diuresis
Later oliguria + ARF due to hypovolaemia

Consider venous thrombosis in those at risk (i.e. elderly, dehydrated)

Poor perfusion + peripheral cyanosis due to hypovolaemia

Investigations
- Bedside blood sugar
- Bedside ketone testing ('ketostix')
- Full blood count
- Urea, electrolytes and blood sugar
- Blood gases for acid–base status
- Osmolality
- Serum ketones
- Blood cultures
- Cardiac enzymes
- Amylase (? spuriously elevated)
- Urine for microbiology
- ECG and chest radiograph
- Consider: neurological causes (i.e. lumbar puncture, head CT scan)

Look for precipitating causes
- Infection (pneumonia, UTI)
- Myocardial infarct
- Pancreatitis
- Trauma
- Endocrine (e.g. thyrotoxicosis)

Monitor
- Hourly blood sugar
- Hourly vital signs
- 2-hourly U+E
- 2-hourly blood gases
- Flow chart records

Diabetes mellitus (DM) is a metabolic disorder characterized by hyperglycaemia (fasting blood sugar (BS) >7 mmol/L or >11.1 mmol/L 2 hours after a glucose challenge) due to insulin deficiency or resistance.

- **Type I DM:** is rare (2/1000 population) and presents in young people (<30 years). Genetic (HLA-linked), autoimmune and viral factors contribute to pancreatic β-islet cell destruction and insulin deficiency. Hyperglycaemic symptoms (e.g. polyuria, weight loss, fatigue) progress to ketoacidosis if insulin therapy is not commenced.
- **Type II DM:** occurs in older adults (>40 years) mainly due to insulin resistance (± deficiency). There is a strong genetic association but diet and obesity determine age of onset. Treatment is with diet ± oral hypoglycaemic agents including biguanides (e.g. metformin) and/or sulphonylureas (e.g. gliclazide). Insulin therapy is required if BS control is poor and during intercurrent illness.
- **Other causes of DM:** include malnutrition, rare genetic and secondary DM (e.g. pancreatitis, endocrine disease, steroids).
- **Stress-induced hyperglycaemia:** occurs during acute illness. Tight glycaemic control with insulin may improve outcome.

DM can also present with end-organ damage (e.g. nephropathy) or life-threatening diabetic emergencies (see below).

Hypoglycaemia

Symptoms occur when BS is <2.2 mmol/L but the threshold varies (i.e. higher in poorly controlled DM). It must be suspected in patients with sudden changes in mental state or neurological function. **Causes** are listed in Fig. (a). Problems with diabetic therapy are most common. **Clinical features** (Fig. b) include early 'adrenergic' symptoms (e.g. tremor, sweating), followed by progressive anxiety, confusion and seizures. Coma and neurological damage rapidly follow due to the brain's dependence on glucose metabolism.

Management Bedside BS measurement confirms hypoglycaemia. A glucose drink or 'carbohydrate snack' is given to conscious patients and intravenous (i.v.) glucose (e.g. 50 ml 20% dextrose) if the conscious level is depressed. Severe or refractory hypoglycaemia (e.g. sulphonylurea overdose) may require glucagon (1 mg i.v./i.m.) or hydrocortisone therapy. These patients must be admitted for BS monitoring (± glucose infusions). When BS measurement is unavailable, glucose may have to be given empirically. Supplemental thiamine prevents Wernicke's encephalopathy (i.e. eye movement paralysis, ataxia, confusion) in malnourished patients (e.g. alcoholics).

Diabetic ketoacidosis (DKA)

DKA occurs in type I DM due to insulin deficiency. Precipitants include infection (~30%), MI, surgery, pancreatitis and non-compliance. No cause is found in ~25%. **Pathogenesis:** insulin deficiency and stress hormones accelerate hepatic glucose production and prevent cellular glucose uptake. Resulting hyperglycaemia (BS >20 mmol/L) exceeds the renal glucose threshold and glycosuria causes an osmotic diuresis with water and electrolyte loss. Dehydration occurs when nausea and vomiting prevent adequate fluid intake. Insulin deficiency promotes intracellular lipolysis and hepatic metabolism of released fatty acids results in ketone production (e.g. β-hydroxybutyrate) and metabolic acidosis (Fig. c). **Mortality** is ~5%.

Clinical presentation (Fig. e) ~10% of type I DM presents as DKA. Nausea, lethargy, thirst and polyuria often precede DKA which may develop within hours. Presenting features are due to **severe volume depletion** (e.g. hypotension) and **metabolic acidosis** (e.g. hyperventilation).

Investigation (Fig. e) Bedside BS testing, arterial blood gases and urinary ketones are usually diagnostic. Laboratory tests assess dehydration, electrolyte imbalance and acidosis. The precipitating cause and co-existing problems (e.g. renal failure) must be established.

Management (Fig. d) Haemodynamic instability due to severe volume depletion, acidosis and rapid ion fluxes during initial therapy (particularly K⁺), is potentially lethal.

- **Fluid replacement:** with ~3–5 L normal saline (NS) in <6 hours (i.e. 1 L in 30 min, then 1 L over 1 hour, etc.) rapidly corrects hypovolaemia and restores cardiovascular stability. Total fluid deficits of ~5–10 L and sodium losses of ~400 mmol are replaced over 48 hours. Monitor CVP if pulmonary oedema is a risk.
- **Insulin:** is given as a bolus (6–10 U i.v.), followed by an infusion (~6 U/h). BS often corrects before the acidosis but insulin must be continued until the acidosis has resolved by replacing the NS with a 10% dextrose infusion to maintain BS (monitored hourly) at 6–10 mmol/L. As osmotic shifts during rapid BS correction can cause cerebral oedema, aim to reduce the BS by ~3–5 mmol/h.
- **Electrolyte replacement:** diuresis (± vomiting) cause severe potassium (K⁺) depletion. However, initial serum K⁺ levels are high due to acidosis-induced K⁺ movement out of cells. Insulin therapy and correction of acidosis stimulates cellular K⁺ uptake and a rapid fall in serum K⁺. Hourly monitoring and K⁺ supplements prevent profound hypokalaemia (± cardiac arrest). Correct hypomagnesaemia to prevent insulin resistance and arrhythmias. Phosphate supplementation maintains tissue oxygenation.
- **Sodium bicarbonate therapy:** is controversial. It may reduce oxygen delivery and cause hypokalaemia. However, in severe acidosis (pH < 7.1) with myocardial depression treatment may be unavoidable.
- **General measures:** include antibiotics, heparin, oxygen (± nasogastric tube for vomiting or coma).
- **The post-resuscitation phase:** is often poorly managed and a diabetic specialist should be involved. When BS is <15 mmol/L, a dextrose infusion is commenced. Regular insulin regimes restart when ketoacidosis has resolved and nutrition is normal.

Hyperosmolar non-ketotic coma (HONK)

HONK is less common than DKA but mortality is ~40%. It occurs in elderly type II DM with sufficient insulin production to prevent ketogenesis but not hyperglycaemia. Osmotic diuresis leads to severe dehydration and hyperosmolality. Significant metabolic acidosis does not occur.

- **Clinical features:** anorexia, malaise, polyuria and weakness progress slowly to confusion, seizures and coma. Diagnosis is based on BS (>40 mmol/L) and hyperosmolality (>330 mosm/L). Serum sodium is often >160 mmol/L.
- **Management:** despite severe fluid deficits (>10 L), slow rehydration with normal saline and gradual sodium and BS reductions (e.g. insulin 1 U/h) are essential to avoid sudden osmotic and electrolyte shifts, which may precipitate cerebral oedema and central pontine demyelinolysis. Anticoagulation prevents dehydration-induced thromboembolic events.

Lactic acidosis

This is a rare complication of type II DM (e.g. metformin use, sepsis). It presents with hyperventilation, vomiting, drowsiness and coma. A high anion gap acidosis with normal glucose and no ketones is characteristic. Despite supportive and bicarbonate therapy, prognosis is poor.

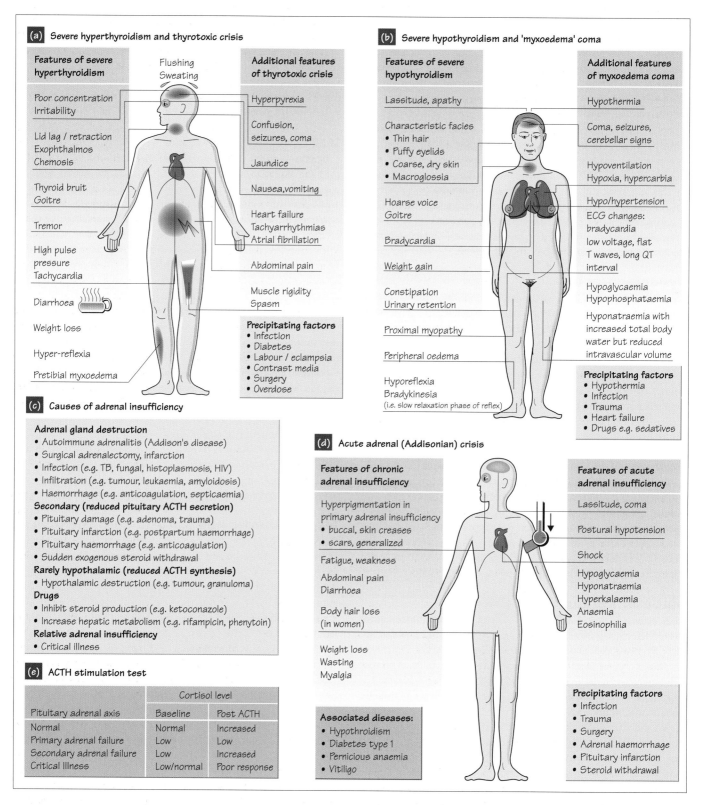

(a) Severe hyperthyroidism and thyrotoxic crisis

Features of severe hyperthyroidism		Additional features of thyrotoxic crisis
Poor concentration Irritability	Flushing Sweating	Hyperpyrexia
Lid lag / retraction Exophthalmos Chemosis		Confusion, seizures, coma
Thyroid bruit Goitre		Jaundice
Tremor		Nausea, vomiting
High pulse pressure Tachycardia		Heart failure Tachyarrhythmias Atrial fibrillation
Diarrhoea		Abdominal pain
Weight loss		Muscle rigidity Spasm
Hyper-reflexia		
Pretibial myxoedema		

Precipitating factors
- Infection
- Diabetes
- Labour / eclampsia
- Contrast media
- Surgery
- Overdose

(b) Severe hypothyroidism and 'myxoedema' coma

Features of severe hypothyroidism	Additional features of myxoedema coma
Lassitude, apathy	Hypothermia
Characteristic facies • Thin hair • Puffy eyelids • Coarse, dry skin • Macroglossia	Coma, seizures, cerebellar signs
Hoarse voice Goitre	Hypoventilation Hypoxia, hypercarbia
Bradycardia	Hypo/hypertension
Weight gain	ECG changes: bradycardia low voltage, flat T waves, long QT interval
Constipation Urinary retention	Hypoglycaemia Hypophosphataemia
Proximal myopathy	Hyponatraemia with increased total body water but reduced intravascular volume
Peripheral oedema	
Hyporeflexia Bradykinesia (i.e. slow relaxation phase of reflex)	

Precipitating factors
- Hypothermia
- Infection
- Trauma
- Heart failure
- Drugs e.g. sedatives

(c) Causes of adrenal insufficiency

Adrenal gland destruction
- Autoimmune adrenalitis (Addison's disease)
- Surgical adrenalectomy, infarction
- Infection (e.g. TB, fungal, histoplasmosis, HIV)
- Infiltration (e.g. tumour, leukaemia, amyloidosis)
- Haemorrhage (e.g. anticoagulation, septicaemia)

Secondary (reduced pituitary ACTH secretion)
- Pituitary damage (e.g. adenoma, trauma)
- Pituitary infarction (e.g. postpartum haemorrhage)
- Pituitary haemorrhage (e.g. anticoagulation)
- Sudden exogenous steroid withdrawal

Rarely hypothalamic (reduced ACTH synthesis)
- Hypothalamic destruction (e.g. tumour, granuloma)

Drugs
- Inhibit steroid production (e.g. ketoconazole)
- Increase hepatic metabolism (e.g. rifampicin, phenytoin)

Relative adrenal insufficiency
- Critical illness

(d) Acute adrenal (Addisonian) crisis

Features of chronic adrenal insufficiency	Features of acute adrenal insufficiency
Hyperpigmentation in primary adrenal insufficiency • buccal, skin creases • scars, generalized	Lassitude, coma
Fatigue, weakness	Postural hypotension
Abdominal pain Diarrhoea	Shock
Body hair loss (in women)	Hypoglycaemia Hyponatraemia Hyperkalaemia Anaemia Eosinophilia
Weight loss Wasting Myalgia	

Associated diseases:
- Hypothroidism
- Diabetes type 1
- Pernicious anaemia
- Vitiligo

Precipitating factors
- Infection
- Trauma
- Surgery
- Adrenal haemorrhage
- Pituitary infarction
- Steroid withdrawal

(e) ACTH stimulation test

Pituitary adrenal axis	Cortisol level	
	Baseline	Post ACTH
Normal	Normal	Increased
Primary adrenal failure	Low	Low
Secondary adrenal failure	Low	Increased
Critical Illness	Low/normal	Poor response

Thyroid emergencies

Thyrotoxic crisis (thyroid storm) is a life-threatening hypermetabolic emergency (mortality rate 20%) which affects <2% of thyrotoxic patients. Precipitants include infection, surgery, diabetes, labour, radioiodine therapy and iodinated contrast media. Thyroxine overdose and eclampsia are rare causes.

- **Clinical features:** include those of severe hyperthyroidism (Fig. a) with fever, anxiety, weight loss (>15 kg in ~50%), confusion and tachycardia. High output cardiac failure complicates ~50% of cases. Differential diagnosis includes sepsis, phaeochromocytoma, drug abuse and malignant hyperthermia.
- **Treatment:** may be required before diagnostic confirmation (i.e. T3, T4 levels). Admit to ICU/HDU.
  - **General management** – treat the precipitating cause and correct dehydration (which may be severe), electrolyte disturbances and hypoglycaemia (common). Institute cooling but avoid aspirin (displaces T4 from binding protein). Sedation reduces agitation and dantrolene reduces pyrexia due to extreme muscle activity (Chapter 21).
  - **High dose beta-blockers** (e.g. propranolol) are the mainstay of therapy. They inhibit the peripheral effects of thyroid hormone reducing heart rate, hypertension, fever and tremor.
  - **Immediate antithyroid drugs** block T4 synthesis. Propylthiouracil is preferred because it blocks T4 to T3 conversion but must be given enterally (e.g. NG tube). Carbimazole is metabolized to methimazole, has a slow onset but long duration of action and can be given by rectal suppository. White cell suppression occurs with both drugs and therapy is stopped if sore throat develops.
  - **Hydrocortisone** (100 mg/6 h i.v.) inhibits T4 to T3 conversion.
  - **Iodine** (e.g. Lugol's solution), or lithium in allergic patients, prevent T4 release from the thyroid gland. Antithyroid drugs must be given 2 hours before iodine which inhibits their thyroid uptake.

Severe hypothyroidism (myxoedema coma) occurs when intercurrent illness (infection) or drugs (sedatives) complicate pre-existing hypothyroidism causing hypothermia, coma and hypotension. It often affects elderly females with unrecognized hypothyroidism or patients who fail to take thyroxine replacement. It should be suspected in any patient with hypothermia and coma. Mortality is >50%.
- **Clinical features** are those of severe hypothyroidism (Fig. b).
- **Investigation** may reveal anaemia, hypoglycaemia, hyponatraemia and ECG changes (Fig. b). In primary hypothyroidism, thyroid stimulating hormone (TSH) is raised and T3/T4 is low. In pituitary failure (suspect when Na+ low) both TSH and T3/T4 are low.
- **Management** includes rewarming, respiratory support and correction of hypoglycaemia. Immediate treatment with T3 (5–20 μg i.v. slowly as IHD can be unmasked; 6 hourly) may be required. Corticosteroid therapy is given until concurrent pituitary or adrenal insufficiency has been excluded.

Sick euthyroid syndrome occurs in severe illness. It is not due to a thyroid disorder and should not be treated. Low T4 binding protein and altered T4 metabolism results in abnormal thyroid function tests (e.g. low total T4, normal free T4, low T3 and normal TSH).

Adrenal emergencies

Adrenocortical insufficiency (AI) describes reduced cortisol (± aldosterone) production by the adrenal cortex. **Causes** are listed in Fig. (c). Primary adrenal insufficiency (PAI) follows adrenal damage (e.g. autoimmune adrenalitis; 'Addison's disease'). Secondary adrenal insufficiency (SAI) due to adrenocorticotrophic hormone (ACTH) deficiency follows pituitary or hypothalamic damage. Abrupt withdrawal of therapeutic steroids also presents as adrenal insufficiency because ACTH secretion remains depressed after clearance of exogenous steroid.

- **Clinical presentation** (Fig. d): is either acute or chronic.
- **Acute (Addisonian) crisis** can be precipitated by stress (e.g. surgery) in patients with unrecognized, chronic AI. It follows sepsis or adrenal haemorrhage in critical illness and pituitary infarction after postpartum haemorrhage (Sheehan's syndrome). Acute AI should always be suspected in shock with hyponatraemia (± hyperkalaemia and hypoglycaemia) if the cause is not apparent. Other characteristic features include apathy, postural hypotension and coma. In critical illness, relative AI is common and steroid supplementation may be beneficial.
- **Chronic deficiency** (e.g. autoimmune adrenalitis) presents with fatigue, weakness, weight loss, fever and nausea. In PAI hyperpigmentation is caused by excess pituitary melanocyte-stimulating hormone. Body hair loss in females is due to reduced adrenal androgen production.
- **Investigation:** hyponatraemia and hyperkalaemia are features of aldosterone reduction in PAI. Hypoglycaemia, hypercalcaemia, eosinophilia and volume depletion with raised blood urea occur in all forms of AI. Immunology may reveal autoantibodies. **Adrenal function tests** must not delay cortisol replacement. A low baseline cortisol confirms adrenal insufficiency. Cortisol levels taken at 30 and 60 minutes after i.v. ACTH injection (short Synacthen test) rapidly indicate the cause (Fig. e). ACTH is high in PAI and low in SAI.
- **Treatment:** of shock (Chapters 6, 7) may require aggressive fluid therapy (e.g. 4–5 L NS over 24 hours) and inotropic support. Stress can increase cortisol levels tenfold and high dose hydrocortisone (or dexamethasone which does not interfere with serum cortisol assays) is needed. Hyperkalaemia corrects rapidly with fluid and steroids and hypoglycaemia with glucose supplements. Treat infection with antibiotics. Mineralocorticoid replacement (e.g. fludrocortisone) is only needed in PAI.

Adrenocortical excess Cortisol is increased in Cushing's syndrome (e.g. steroid therapy, adrenal tumours) and Cushing's disease (e.g. ACTH secreting pituitary tumour). Characteristic features include a moon face, thin easily bruised skin, hypertension (~50%), diabetes (~10%), osteoporosis (~50%), central obesity and hypokalaemia (e.g. arrhythmias, muscle weakness). Excess aldosterone secretion from an adrenal adenoma (Conn's syndrome) causes hypokalaemia, muscle weakness (e.g. post-operative ventilatory impairment) and hypertension.

Other endocrine emergencies

Hypopituitary crisis follows pituitary trauma, infiltration (e.g. tumour), haemorrhage or infarction. Reduced anterior pituitary hormone secretion causes adrenal and thyroid insufficiency (see above) and hypogonadism. Failure of posterior pituitary antidiuretic hormone release causes diabetes insipidus with thirst, dehydration and severe polyuria. Detailed assessment of the pituitary-adrenal axis and hormone replacement therapy are required.

Phaeochromocytomas are rare, benign (~90%), adrenal (~90%) tumours that release catecholamines. They are often familial and associated with other tumours (e.g. multiple endocrine neoplasia). Crises can be precipitated by drugs, surgery and foods (e.g. cheese). Features include headaches, sweating, flushing and arrhythmias. Hypertension may be sustained or labile. Raised plasma catecholamines or 24-hour urinary vanillyl mandelic acid (VMA) confirm the diagnosis. Treatment is with alpha-blockers (e.g. phenoxybenzamine), beta-blockers and surgery.

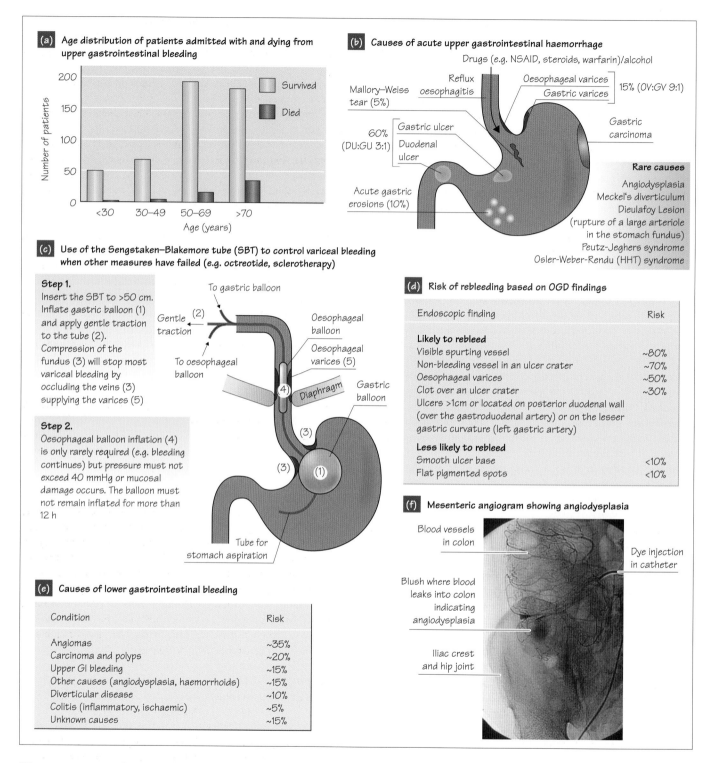

(a) Age distribution of patients admitted with and dying from upper gastrointestinal bleeding

Number of patients (y-axis: 0, 50, 100, 150, 200)
Age (years) (x-axis: <30, 30–49, 50–69, >70)
Survived / Died

(b) Causes of acute upper gastrointestinal haemorrhage

Drugs (e.g. NSAID, steroids, warfarin)/alcohol
Reflux oesophagitis
Mallory–Weiss tear (5%)
Oesophageal varices
Gastric varices
15% (OV:GV 9:1)
Gastric carcinoma
60% (DU:GU 3:1)
Gastric ulcer
Duodenal ulcer
Acute gastric erosions (10%)

Rare causes
Angiodysplasia
Meckel's diverticulum
Dieulafoy Lesion
(rupture of a large arteriole in the stomach fundus)
Peutz-Jeghers syndrome
Osler-Weber-Rendu (HHT) syndrome

(c) Use of the Sengstaken–Blakemore tube (SBT) to control variceal bleeding when other measures have failed (e.g. octreotide, sclerotherapy)

Step 1.
Insert the SBT to >50 cm. Inflate gastric balloon (1) and apply gentle traction to the tube (2). Compression of the fundus (3) will stop most variceal bleeding by occluding the veins (3) supplying the varices (5)

Step 2.
Oesophageal balloon inflation (4) is only rarely required (e.g. bleeding continues) but pressure must not exceed 40 mmHg or mucosal damage occurs. The balloon must not remain inflated for more than 12 h

To gastric balloon
Gentle traction (2)
To oesophageal balloon
Oesophageal balloon
Oesophageal varices (5)
Diaphragm
Gastric balloon
Tube for stomach aspiration

(d) Risk of rebleeding based on OGD findings

Endoscopic finding	Risk
Likely to rebleed	
Visible spurting vessel	~80%
Non-bleeding vessel in an ulcer crater	~70%
Oesophageal varices	~50%
Clot over an ulcer crater	~30%
Ulcers >1cm or located on posterior duodenal wall (over the gastroduodenal artery) or on the lesser gastric curvature (left gastric artery)	
Less likely to rebleed	
Smooth ulcer base	<10%
Flat pigmented spots	<10%

(f) Mesenteric angiogram showing angiodysplasia

Blood vessels in colon
Dye injection in catheter
Blush where blood leaks into colon indicating angiodysplasia
Iliac crest and hip joint

(e) Causes of lower gastrointestinal bleeding

Condition	Risk
Angiomas	~35%
Carcinoma and polyps	~20%
Upper GI bleeding	~15%
Other causes (angiodysplasia, haemorrhoids)	~15%
Diverticular disease	~10%
Colitis (inflammatory, ischaemic)	~5%
Unknown causes	~15%

Upper gastrointestinal (GI) haemorrhage

Incidence Acute upper GI bleeding occurs in ~1/1000 population. It is most common in patients >50 years old (Fig. a). Stress-induced ulceration and bleeding occurs in <10% of acutely ill patients. **Causes** (Fig. b): include peptic ulceration (~60%), gastritis/oesophagitis (10%) and oesophageal varices (15%). No cause is found in ~20%.

Aspirin and NSAID cause ~33% of gastritis and ulceration. Cirrhosis is the main cause of portal hypertension (PrHT) and oesophageal (± gastric, rectal, umbilical) varices develop when portal pressure is >12 mmHg. Acute variceal bleeding occurs in ~30% and causes >70% of upper GI bleeds in cirrhotics.

Clinical features

Common presentations include haematemesis (i.e. vomited fresh or altered blood; ~50–65%), melaena (i.e. black 'tarry' stool; ~65%) and shock (Chapter 6). Rectal blood clots may be seen in massive bleeds. Epigastric discomfort suggests peptic ulceration. Stigmata of chronic liver disease (CLD), hepatosplenomegaly, mucocutaneous changes (e.g. hereditary haemorrhagic telangiectasia (HHT), Peutz–Jegher's syndrome) and bleeding disorders must be sought. Angiodysplasia is common in chronic renal failure (CRF). Previous retching or vomiting raises the possibility of a gastro-oesophageal tear (Mallory–Weiss syndrome). Anorexia, weight loss, lymph nodes and an epigastric mass suggest gastric carcinoma. An aortoenteric fistula may occur following aortic surgery. A drug history is essential (e.g. NSAID).

Investigation

- **Blood tests:** initial haemoglobin levels are normal as haemodilution occurs over many hours. A microcytic anaemia suggests previous chronic bleeding. A raised urea, due to the blood protein load, suggests upper rather than lower GI bleeding. Liver function and coagulation tests assess liver damage, synthetic function (e.g. albumin) and clotting function.
- **Diagnostic imaging:** air beneath the diaphragm on chest or abdominal radiography indicates viscus perforation. **Upper GI endoscopy**, performed within 12 hours, establishes the diagnosis, predicts rebleeding risk and treats bleeding lesions endoscopically. **Angiography** is indicated when endoscopy fails to locate the bleeding site (~20%).
- **Exploratory laparotomy:** is required in life-threatening bleeding when investigations are negative.

Management of upper GI bleeding

- **Prophylaxis** to reduce the risk of upper GI bleeding includes enteral nutrition, gastric acid suppression (e.g. omeprazole) and gastric mucosal coatings (e.g. sucralphate).
- **General management**: liaise with specialists early (e.g. gastroenterologists, surgeons). The priorities are:

  1 Resuscitation – protect the airway and give oxygen therapy. Immediate plasma expanders are followed by blood transfusion (Chapter 8). Monitor BP, CVP, ABG and urine output to guide ongoing resuscitation. Insert a nasogastric tube except in patients with varices.

  2 Identification and control of active bleeding – correct clotting abnormalities (e.g. FFP, platelets, vitamin K), arrange urgent/early endoscopy and treat the cause (see below).

  3 Prevent recurrence – identify patients at risk of rebleeding (Fig. d).

Peptic ulcer management

Proton pump inhibitors (PPI; e.g. pantoprazole) and H₂ receptor antagonists reduce gastric acid secretion and promote ulcer healing. Intravenous PPI also reduces rebleeding after endoscopic therapy. Eradication therapy is indicated if *Helicobacter pylori* is detected. The value of tranexamic acid, antifibrinolytic agents and octreotide is not established.
- **Endoscopic therapy.** Thermal coagulation (e.g. electrocautery) or epinephrine (adrenaline) injection around a bleeding ulcer achieves haemostasis in >90%. It reduces rebleeding, mortality and the need for emergency surgery.
- **Surgery** is required in exsanguinating haemorrhage or perforation despite the associated mortality (~20%). Bleeding gastric ulcers require a Billroth I gastrectomy and duodenal ulcers are oversewn (± vagotomy and pyloroplasty). In high risk patients, arterial embolization controls bleeding in ~50% but risks necrosis.

Management of oesophageal varices

Treat the underlying cause (e.g. cirrhosis) and associated liver failure (Chapter 43), which determine prognosis and the risk of variceal bleeding (Appendix 4).
- **Sclerotherapy:** is the treatment of choice. Endoscopic injection of a sclerosant (e.g. alcohol, ethanolamine) thromboses varices and controls bleeding in >90%. Complications include ulceration and stricture formation.
- **Endoscopic variceal ligation (banding):** is equally effective.
- **Pharmacotherapy:** terlipressin, a vasopressin analogue and splanchnic vasoconstrictor, lowers PrHT and controls variceal bleeding in >50% but may cause cardiac ischaemia. Somatostatin and octreotide are also effective. Beta-blockade reduces PrHT and is used as prophylaxis.
- **Balloon tamponade** (e.g. Sengstaken-Blakemore tube; Fig. c): is an effective temporizing measure to control massive bleeding.
- **Transjugular intrahepatic portal stents (TIPS):** if medical therapy fails the portal system is decompressed by placing a self-expanding stent over a wire passed from the hepatic vein (transjugular approach), through liver substance into the portal vein. Encephalopathy may ensue.
- **Surgery:** variceal ligation (e.g. transoesophageal stapling) or portocaval shunting are occasionally required.

Prognosis

About 70% of upper GI bleeding stops spontaneously regardless of the cause. Recently mortality has fallen from 10% to 5%. Poor prognostic factors and risk factors for rebleeding (Rockall Score; Appendix 3) include age >60 years, oesophageal varices (mortality ~30%), coexisting disease and persistent bleeding.

Lower gastrointestinal bleeding

Causes are listed in Fig. (e). Lower GI bleeding presents with either frank rectal bleeding or melaena (± shock). Abdominal examination may reveal a mass (e.g. neoplasia) or tenderness. A bruit suggests ischaemia. Angiodysplasia occurs in CRF, aortic stenosis and inherited vascular conditions like HHT. Initial investigation is as for upper GI bleeding but sequential diagnostic imaging includes sigmoidoscopy, colonoscopy if oesophagogastroduodenoscopy (OGD) is negative, mesenteric arteriography (Fig. f), labelled red cell isotope scans or small bowel barium studies. Exploratory laparotomy may be necessary if profuse undiagnosed bleeding persists.

Management

Most bleeding stops spontaneously (~80%) but recurs in ~25%.
- **General management:** is as for upper GI bleeding.
- **Specific measures:** include **colonoscopy** with electrocoagulation or laser therapy which stops bleeding from polyps, angiodysplasia, telangectasia and colorectal carcinomas. **Elective surgery** is often required for lower GI bleeding. Severe, persistent but undiagnosed bleeding due to presumed angiodysplasia may require a right hemicolectomy although this is an unsatisfactory compromise. **Arterial embolization** may be used for vascular malformations including angiodysplasia (Fig. f).

43 Acute liver failure

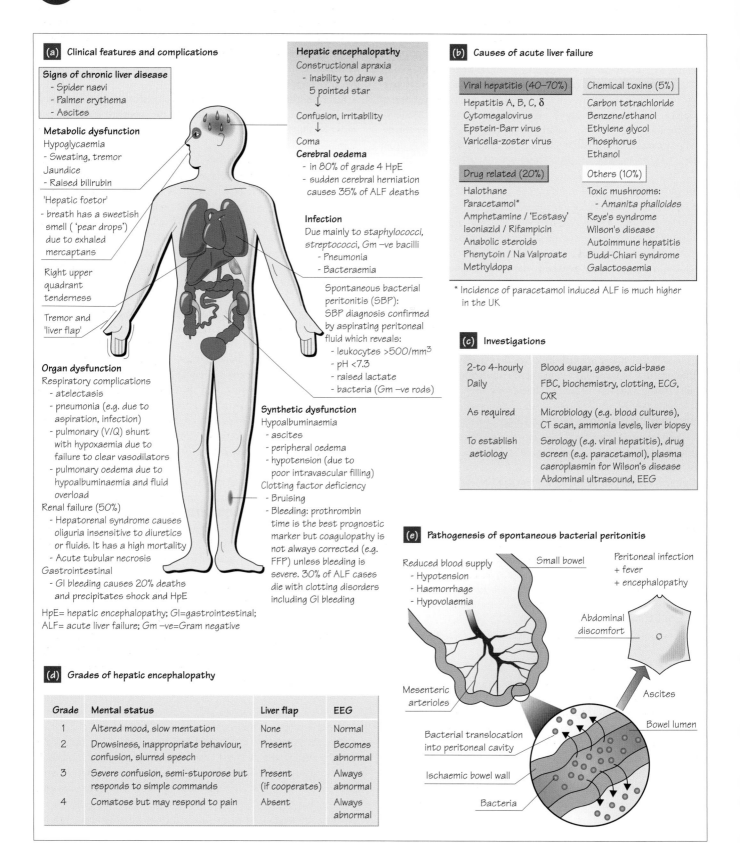

(a) Clinical features and complications

Signs of chronic liver disease
- Spider naevi
- Palmer erythema
- Ascites

Metabolic dysfunction
Hypoglycaemia
- Sweating, tremor
Jaundice
- Raised bilirubin

'Hepatic foetor'
- breath has a sweetish smell ('pear drops') due to exhaled mercaptans

Right upper quadrant tenderness

Tremor and 'liver flap'

Organ dysfunction
Respiratory complications
- atelectasis
- pneumonia (e.g. due to aspiration, infection)
- pulmonary (V/Q) shunt with hypoxaemia due to failure to clear vasodilators
- pulmonary oedema due to hypoalbuminaemia and fluid overload
Renal failure (50%)
- Hepatorenal syndrome causes oliguria insensitive to diuretics or fluids. It has a high mortality
- Acute tubular necrosis
Gastrointestinal
- GI bleeding causes 20% deaths and precipitates shock and HpE

HpE= hepatic encephalopathy; GI=gastrointestinal; ALF= acute liver failure; Gm –ve=Gram negative

Hepatic encephalopathy
Constructional apraxia
- inability to draw a 5 pointed star
↓
Confusion, irritability
↓
Coma
Cerebral oedema
- in 80% of grade 4 HpE
- sudden cerebral herniation causes 35% of ALF deaths

Infection
Due mainly to staphylococci, streptococci, Gm –ve bacilli
- Pneumonia
- Bacteraemia

Spontaneous bacterial peritonitis (SBP):
SBP diagnosis confirmed by aspirating peritoneal fluid which reveals:
- leukocytes >500/mm^3
- pH <7.3
- raised lactate
- bacteria (Gm –ve rods)

Synthetic dysfunction
Hypoalbuminaemia
- ascites
- peripheral oedema
- hypotension (due to poor intravascular filling)
Clotting factor deficiency
- Bruising
- Bleeding: prothrombin time is the best prognostic marker but coagulopathy is not always corrected (e.g. FFP) unless bleeding is severe. 30% of ALF cases die with clotting disorders including GI bleeding

(b) Causes of acute liver failure

Viral hepatitis (40–70%)
Hepatitis A, B, C, δ
Cytomegalovirus
Epstein-Barr virus
Varicella-zoster virus

Chemical toxins (5%)
Carbon tetrachloride
Benzene/ethanol
Ethylene glycol
Phosphorus
Ethanol

Drug related (20%)
Halothane
Paracetamol*
Amphetamine / 'Ecstasy'
Isoniazid / Rifampicin
Anabolic steroids
Phenytoin / Na Valproate
Methyldopa

Others (10%)
Toxic mushrooms:
- Amanita phalloides
Reye's syndrome
Wilson's disease
Autoimmune hepatitis
Budd-Chiari syndrome
Galactosaemia

* Incidence of paracetamol induced ALF is much higher in the UK

(c) Investigations

2-to 4-hourly	Blood sugar, gases, acid-base
Daily	FBC, biochemistry, clotting, ECG, CXR
As required	Microbiology (e.g. blood cultures), CT scan, ammonia levels, liver biopsy
To establish aetiology	Serology (e.g. viral hepatitis), drug screen (e.g. paracetamol), plasma caeroplasmin for Wilson's disease Abdominal ultrasound, EEG

(e) Pathogenesis of spontaneous bacterial peritonitis

Reduced blood supply
- Hypotension
- Haemorrhage
- Hypovolaemia

Small bowel

Peritoneal infection
+ fever
+ encephalopathy

Abdominal discomfort

Ascites

Bowel lumen

Mesenteric arterioles

Bacterial translocation into peritoneal cavity

Ischaemic bowel wall

Bacteria

(d) Grades of hepatic encephalopathy

Grade	Mental status	Liver flap	EEG
1	Altered mood, slow mentation	None	Normal
2	Drowsiness, inappropriate behaviour, confusion, slurred speech	Present	Becomes abnormal
3	Severe confusion, semi-stuporose but responds to simple commands	Present (if cooperates)	Always abnormal
4	Comatose but may respond to pain	Absent	Always abnormal

 Acute and Critical Care Medicine at a Glance, 2e. By R. Leach. Published 2009 by Blackwell Publishing. ISBN 978-1-4051-6139-8.

Classification

• **Primary ALF (fulminant hepatic failure):** is defined as potentially reversible liver injury with hepatic encephalopathy (HpE), coagulopathy and jaundice developing within 4 weeks in a previously healthy person. Hyperacute liver failure describes encephalopathy within 7 days of jaundice. It is fatal in 40–85% of cases. The commonest causes (Fig. b) are viral hepatitis (40–70%) and paracetamol toxicity (5–40%). Hepatitis A (5–30%) and B (25–75%) are the main viral causes but the risk of developing ALF in viral hepatitis is <1%. Paracetamol poisoning is discussed in Chapter 50.

• **Secondary ALF:** is more frequent and occurs when acute illness causes decompensation in pre-existing chronic liver disease (CLD; e.g. cirrhosis). Potential precipitants include ischaemia (e.g. shock, sepsis, thrombosis) and liver toxins (e.g. drugs, TPN).

Clinical features

Biochemical and CNS dysfunction are the hallmarks of ALF. Figure (a) illustrates these features (and those of CLD), which are due to:

• **Metabolic dysfunction:** reduced hepatic gluconeogenesis and raised insulin levels cause hypoglycaemia in ~40%. Inadequate lactate metabolism causes lactic acidosis in ~50% of late ALF. **Liver function tests** (e.g. bilirubin, serum aminotransferase >2000 IU/L) and ammonia levels are usually raised. Clinically 'hepatic foetor' and jaundice are detected. **Electrolyte disturbances** (e.g. hyponatraemia, hypokalaemia) and secondary hyperaldosteronism are common.

• **Synthetic dysfunction:** includes hypoalbuminaemia and clotting factor deficiencies. Gastrointestinal (GI) bleeding causes ~20% of deaths (Chapter 42), and often precipitates shock and HpE.

• **Reduced immunity:** although fever and leukocytosis only affects ~30%, phagocytic dysfunction leads to severe infection (e.g. pneumonia) in ~80% and fatal bacteraemia in ~15% of ALF cases.

• **Spontaneous bacterial peritonitis (SBP)** is due to splanchnic hypoperfusion, which impairs bowel wall integrity, allowing bacterial translocation and peritoneal infection (Fig. e). Characteristic features are fever, abdominal discomfort and encephalopathy. Sudden renal impairment, weight gain or ascites also suggest SBP. The diagnosis is confirmed if aspirated peritoneal fluid reveals bacteria, typically gram-negative rods (e.g. *E. coli*), but a leukocyte count >500/mm³, pH < 7.3 or raised lactate are also indications for treatment. Blood cultures are positive in ~50%. Untreated SBP is fatal in 70–90%.

• **Organ dysfunction** (Fig. a): including respiratory complications (e.g. pneumonia, shunt, oedema), renal failure (e.g. hepatorenal syndrome, ATN) and cerebral oedema may progress to multi-organ failure.

• **Hepatic encephalopathy (HpE):** arises when toxin-laden portal blood bypasses the liver and is shunted into the systemic circulation. It is the commonest cause of death.

• **Precipitating factors** include: (i) upper GI bleeding which increases gut protein (i.e. blood) and allied bacterial ammonia formation; (ii) intravascular volume depletion, which reduces hepatic perfusion (e.g. diuretics); (iii) renal failure which impairs toxin/drug clearance; and (iv) infection.

• **Clinical features** – early signs include irritability and confusion. Drowsiness and coma develop over hours to weeks. Reversible causes must be excluded (e.g. hypoglycaemia, sedatives). Tremor, liver 'flap' and sustained clonus may be elicited.

• **Diagnosis** is clinical, supported by elevated ammonia levels and specific EEG findings (e.g. high amplitude δ and triphasic waves), although most EEGs show non-specific diffuse slowing. HpE grades (Fig. d) are of limited value due to fluctuations in coma level.

Management

Management is mainly supportive but early involvement of a specialist liver unit is essential. (Figure c) lists appropriate investigations. In survivors, liver regeneration may be associated with complete recovery.

• **General:** glucose infusions (i.e. 10% dextrose) prevent hypoglycaemia. Potassium supplements may be required. Infection must be treated (e.g. broad-spectrum antibiotics, antifungals) promptly but prophylactic antibiotics are ineffective. Antacids prevent stress ulceration but H₂ blockers and PPI can cause CNS side-effects due to impaired drug metabolism.

• **Nutrition** – avoid high protein diets and limit sodium intake. Branched-chain amino acids in TPN minimize HpE. Supplemental vitamin K, thiamine and folate are required.

• **Cardiorespiratory support:** the circulation is often hyperdynamic, vasodilated and volume-depleted. Careful resuscitation (e.g. CVP monitored) maintains organ perfusion but avoids pulmonary and cerebral oedema due to excessive fluid. Hypoxaemia (e.g. V/Q mismatch), inadequate ventilation (e.g. ascitic diaphragmatic splinting) and HpE (e.g. aspiration risk) may require mechanical ventilation.

• **Ascites, oedema (± hypokalaemia)** require fluid restriction, a low salt diet and potassium-sparing diuretics (spironolactone).

• **Coagulopathy** – vitamin K, platelets and FFP are given for active bleeding and invasive procedures but not prophylactically.

• **Cerebral oedema** is transiently reduced by hyperventilation and mannitol therapy (Chapter 53) but survival is not improved.

• **Encephalopathy:** is prevented by avoiding sedation and correcting precipitating factors. Bacterial generation and bowel absorption of nitrogenous toxins is reduced with a low protein diet (<40 g/day), laxatives (e.g. lactulose) to reduce bowel transit time (e.g. GI bleeding) and non-absorbable antibiotics (e.g. neomycin) to sterilize the bowel. Convulsions are treated aggressively (Chapter 45).

• **Specific therapies:** are limited.

• **N-acetylcysteine** benefits most patients but is essential in paracetamol-induced ALF (Chapter 50).

• **Liver transplantation** is a last resort with 1-year survivals between 50% and 75%. It has a limited but definite role in paracetamol-induced ALF but is less successful in alcohol-related ALF (Appendix 5). Limited organ availability means that ~50% of candidates die awaiting a donor.

Prognosis

Overall ALF survival rates are 20–30%. Mortality depends on cause (i.e. hepatitis A ~33–55%; paracetamol-induced ~47–65%; hepatitis B ~61–76%; and non-A, non-B hepatitis >85%), age (i.e. worse if >40 years) and HpE grade. Other poor prognostic factors are bilirubin level (>300 μmol/L), metabolic acidosis (pH < 7.3), prothrombin time (>3.5) and organ failure (e.g. renal).

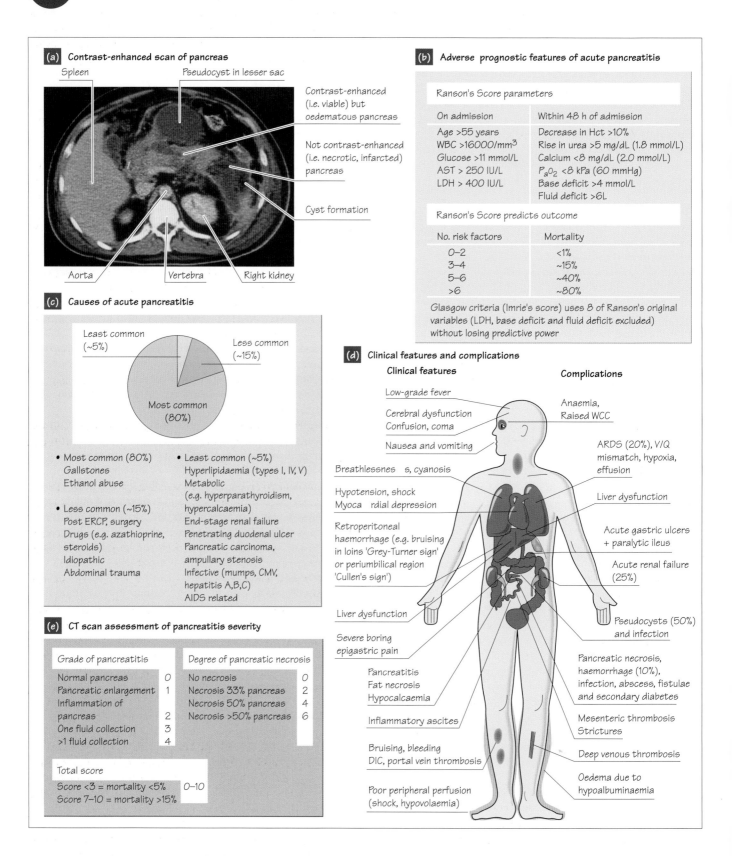

(a) Contrast-enhanced scan of pancreas

- Spleen
- Pseudocyst in lesser sac
- Contrast-enhanced (i.e. viable) but oedematous pancreas
- Not contrast-enhanced (i.e. necrotic, infarcted) pancreas
- Cyst formation
- Aorta
- Vertebra
- Right kidney

(b) Adverse prognostic features of acute pancreatitis

Ranson's Score parameters

On admission	Within 48 h of admission
Age >55 years	Decrease in Hct >10%
WBC >16000/mm^3	Rise in urea >5 mg/dL (1.8 mmol/L)
Glucose >11 mmol/L	Calcium <8 mg/dL (2.0 mmol/L)
AST > 250 IU/L	P_aO_2 <8 kPa (60 mmHg)
LDH > 400 IU/L	Base deficit >4 mmol/L
	Fluid deficit >6L

Ranson's Score predicts outcome

No. risk factors	Mortality
0–2	<1%
3–4	~15%
5–6	~40%
>6	~80%

Glasgow criteria (Imrie's score) uses 8 of Ranson's original variables (LDH, base deficit and fluid deficit excluded) without losing predictive power

(c) Causes of acute pancreatitis

- Least common (~5%)
- Less common (~15%)
- Most common (80%)

- **Most common (80%)**
  Gallstones
  Ethanol abuse

- **Less common (~15%)**
  Post ERCP, surgery
  Drugs (e.g. azathioprine, steroids)
  Idiopathic
  Abdominal trauma

- **Least common (~5%)**
  Hyperlipidaemia (types I, IV, V)
  Metabolic (e.g. hyperparathyroidism, hypercalcaemia)
  End-stage renal failure
  Penetrating duodenal ulcer
  Pancreatic carcinoma, ampullary stenosis
  Infective (mumps, CMV, hepatitis A,B,C)
  AIDS related

(d) Clinical features and complications

Clinical features
- Low-grade fever
- Cerebral dysfunction Confusion, coma
- Nausea and vomiting
- Breathlessness, cyanosis
- Hypotension, shock Myocardial depression
- Retroperitoneal haemorrhage (e.g. bruising in loins 'Grey-Turner sign' or periumbilical region 'Cullen's sign')
- Liver dysfunction
- Severe boring epigastric pain
- Pancreatitis Fat necrosis Hypocalcaemia
- Inflammatory ascites
- Bruising, bleeding DIC, portal vein thrombosis
- Poor peripheral perfusion (shock, hypovolaemia)

Complications
- Anaemia, Raised WCC
- ARDS (20%), V/Q mismatch, hypoxia, effusion
- Liver dysfunction
- Acute gastric ulcers + paralytic ileus
- Acute renal failure (25%)
- Pseudocysts (50%) and infection
- Pancreatic necrosis, haemorrhage (10%), infection, abscess, fistulae and secondary diabetes
- Mesenteric thrombosis Strictures
- Deep venous thrombosis
- Oedema due to hypoalbuminaemia

(e) CT scan assessment of pancreatitis severity

Grade of pancreatitis		Degree of pancreatic necrosis	
Normal pancreas	0	No necrosis	0
Pancreatic enlargement	1	Necrosis 33% pancreas	2
Inflammation of pancreas	2	Necrosis 50% pancreas	4
One fluid collection	3	Necrosis >50% pancreas	6
>1 fluid collection	4		

Total score	
Score <3 = mortality <5%	0–10
Score 7–10 = mortality >15%	

Acute pancreatitis may be clinically mild (75%) or severe (25%). Mild pancreatitis usually resolves with analgesia and fluid therapy alone. In severe pancreatitis, prompt identification and management of organ failure and local complications (e.g. necrosis, pseudocysts) improves outcome. However, mortality is still ~25%.

Aetiology

• *Causes* Gallstones and alcohol cause 80% of cases (Fig. c).
• *Pathogenesis* Ductal obstruction (e.g. gallstones) with biliary reflux into the pancreatic duct or cytotoxic injury (e.g. alcohol) initiates pancreatic auto-digestion by the enzymes trypsin, lipase and elastase.
• *Histology* Acute pancreatitis is classified as oedematous (~75%) or necrotizing (~25%). Necrotic tissue is identified as failure of contrast enhancement on CT scanning (Fig. a).

Clinical features (Fig. d)

Pancreatitis presents with severe, persistent 'boring' epigastric and/or back pain. Nausea, vomiting and low-grade fever are common. Pain and fluid loss cause tachycardia, hypotension and shock. Acute lung injury may cause respiratory distress (Chapter 35). Peritonitis is unusual because the pancreas is retroperitoneal but epigastric tenderness and abdominal distension due to ileus are often present. Bruising in the loins (Grey–Turner's sign) and around the umbilicus (Cullen's sign) are rare manifestations of retroperitoneal haemorrhage.
There are two clinical phases during severe pancreatitis:
1 **The early phase** (0–14 days) is due to inflammation (i.e. mediator release, SIRS) and large fluid shifts. It causes shock, ARDS, acute kidney injury, coagulopathy, fat necrosis and hypocalcaemia.
2 **The late phase** is associated with local complications including pancreatic necrosis, infection (±abscess), pseudocyst, fistula, ascites, strictures, ileus, portal vein thrombosis and diabetes.

Investigation

• **Laboratory:** raised WCC, uraemia, hypocalcaemia, hypoglycaemia and hypoalbuminaemia are common. Serum amylase levels three to five times normal strongly suggests pancreatitis, but may be raised in many abdominal emergencies and normal in 30% of confirmed pancreatitis. Consequently, amylase levels have little prognostic value. Raised serum lipase is more specific but not widely available.
• **Radiological:** abdominal X-rays may show localized ileus (e.g. 'sentinel loop', 'colon cut-off sign') or calcification in chronic pancreatitis. Abdominal USS detects gallstones, biliary duct dilation and pancreatic pseudocysts but pancreatic visualization is poor. CT scans best visualize the pancreas (e.g. oedema) and associated complications (e.g. necrosis) but only confirms the cause in ~25%.

Prognosis

Mortality is ~10% in sterile and ~35% in infected pancreatitis. **Early deaths** (0–14 days) are due to SIRS and MOF. **Late deaths** are usually due to infection, which develops in 40–60% of necrotizing pancreatitis. The risk of infection increases with the amount of necrosis and the time from onset.

Severity assessment several scoring systems assess severity and prognosis (e.g. APACHE II). Of the specific scoring systems, Ranson's criteria are most commonly used (Fig. b). Other prognostic factors include: (i) **Cause (i.e. cytotoxic vs gallstone):** death occurs early in alcohol-induced (i.e. inflammation related) and later in gallstone-induced (i.e. sepsis-related) pancreatitis. Mortality is ~50% if gallstones are not removed. Pancreatic haemorrhage carries the worst prognosis. (ii) **Histology (i.e. oedematous vs necrotic):** necrosis is associated with increased mortality (Fig. e). (iii) **Pancreatic infection:** CT-guided fine needle aspiration reliably assesses development of infection in necrotic pancreatic tissue. (iv) **Multiorgan failure (MOF):** number of organ failures correlates with mortality.

Management

Uncomplicated, oedematous pancreatitis Management includes:
1 **Fluid resuscitation and electrolyte replacement** to correct hypovolaemia due to 'third space' and GI (e.g. ileus, vomiting) losses. Inotropic support may be needed in severe pancreatitis.
2 **Nutrition:** oral feeding is initially withheld (i.e. to reduce pancreatic enzyme release) and nasogastric tube drainage initiated (although benefit has not been established). In uncomplicated pancreatitis, nutritional support is of limited value. However, in severe pancreatitis, early enteric feeding through a naso-jejunal tube is well tolerated and reduces infectious complications. Parenteral nutrition is only justified if enteral feeding fails.
3 **Pain control** can be difficult. Theoretical concerns that morphine may evoke ampullary spasm are probably not justified.
4 **Prophylactic antibiotics** are given in gallstone-induced pancreatitis (i.e. high incidence of biliary tract infection) and all cases with shock; but not in uncomplicated cases.
5 **Stress-ulcer prophylaxis** (e.g. omeprazole) reduces upper GI bleeding but pancreatitis is unaffected.
6 **Early gallstone extraction** reduces mortality, infective complications and severity of pancreatitis. ERCP is as successful as surgery if accomplished within 48 hours.
7 **Non-specific sepsis measures** include glucose control, activated protein C and steroids for relative adrenocortical insufficiency (Chapter 22).

Severe necrotizing pancreatitis is treated as above; but since the development of infected necrosis substantially increases mortality, prevention and treatment of infection are essential.
1 **Antibiotic therapy** reduces infection and late mortality in necrotizing pancreatitis. High-dose cefuroxime or meropenem is started when necrosis is confirmed and continued for 10–14 days.
2 **Radiological percutaneous drainage** of infected collections may avoid the need for surgery.
3 **Surgery.** Infected necrotizing pancreatitis may be fatal without surgical debridement (necrosectomy). Endoscopic irrigation techniques are currently being assessed. In early sterile necrotizing pancreatitis surgery does not reduce mortality but may be considered later in the disease for patients who remain systemically unwell (e.g. fever, weight loss).
4 **Somatostatin and octreotide** are frequently used to reduce pancreatic secretions but have not been shown to improve outcome.

Complications and long-term sequelae

Complications of acute pancreatitis are illustrated in Fig. (d). **Pseudocysts** are collections of pancreatic secretions and occur in ~20% of cases. Indications for drainage are pain, size >6cm, gastric outlet obstruction and secondary infection or haemorrhage.

Chronic pancreatitis follows recurrent pancreatitis and causes chronic pain, pancreatic calcification and impaired endocrine and exocrine pancreatic function (e.g. diabetes, malabsorption).

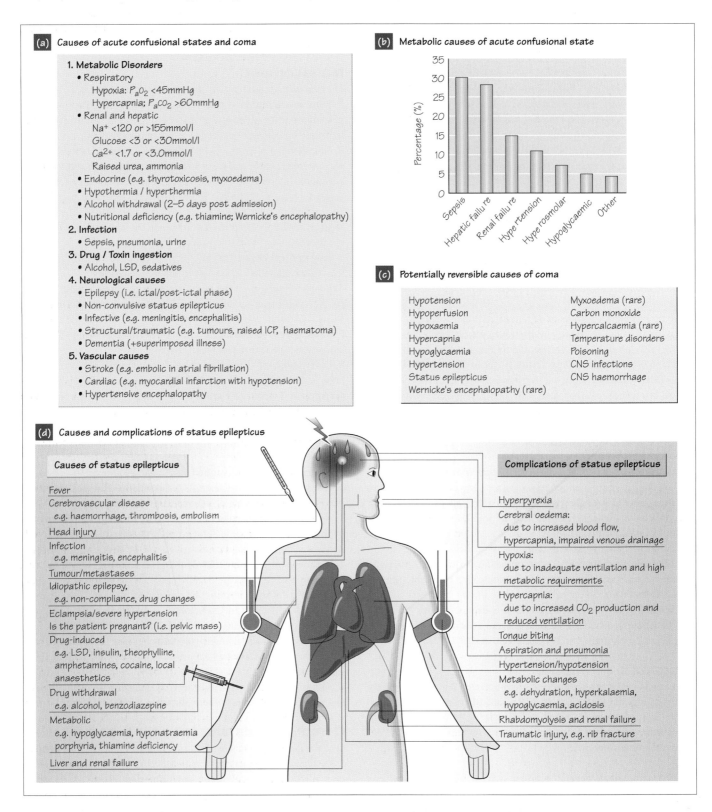

(a) Causes of acute confusional states and coma

1. **Metabolic Disorders**
   - Respiratory
     - Hypoxia: P_aO_2 <45mmHg
     - Hypercapnia; P_aCO_2 >60mmHg
   - Renal and hepatic
     - Na^+ <120 or >155mmol/l
     - Glucose <3 or <30mmol/l
     - Ca^{2+} <1.7 or <3.0mmol/l
     - Raised urea, ammonia
   - Endocrine (e.g. thyrotoxicosis, myxoedema)
   - Hypothermia / hyperthermia
   - Alcohol withdrawal (2–5 days post admission)
   - Nutritional deficiency (e.g. thiamine; Wernicke's encephalopathy)
2. **Infection**
   - Sepsis, pneumonia, urine
3. **Drug / Toxin ingestion**
   - Alcohol, LSD, sedatives
4. **Neurological causes**
   - Epilepsy (i.e. ictal/post-ictal phase)
   - Non-convulsive status epilepticus
   - Infective (e.g. meningitis, encephalitis)
   - Structural/traumatic (e.g. tumours, raised ICP, haematoma)
   - Dementia (+superimposed illness)
5. **Vascular causes**
   - Stroke (e.g. embolic in atrial fibrillation)
   - Cardiac (e.g. myocardial infarction with hypotension)
   - Hypertensive encephalopathy

(b) Metabolic causes of acute confusional state

Bar chart: Percentage (%) on y-axis (0 to 35). Categories on x-axis: Sepsis (~31), Hepatic failure (~28), Renal failure (~15), Hypertension (~11), Hyperosmolar (~7), Hypoglycaemic (~5), Other (~4).

(c) Potentially reversible causes of coma

Hypotension	Myxoedema (rare)
Hypoperfusion	Carbon monoxide
Hypoxaemia	Hypercalcaemia (rare)
Hypercapnia	Temperature disorders
Hypoglycaemia	Poisoning
Hypertension	CNS infections
Status epilepticus	CNS haemorrhage
Wernicke's encephalopathy (rare)	

(d) Causes and complications of status epilepticus

Causes of status epilepticus

Fever
Cerebrovascular disease
  e.g. haemorrhage, thrombosis, embolism
Head injury
Infection
  e.g. meningitis, encephalitis
Tumour/metastases
Idiopathic epilepsy,
  e.g. non-compliance, drug changes
Eclampsia/severe hypertension
Is the patient pregnant? (i.e. pelvic mass)
Drug-induced
  e.g. LSD, insulin, theophylline,
  amphetamines, cocaine, local
  anaesthetics
Drug withdrawal
  e.g. alcohol, benzodiazepine
Metabolic
  e.g. hypoglycaemia, hyponatraemia
  porphyria, thiamine deficiency
Liver and renal failure

Complications of status epilepticus

Hyperpyrexia
Cerebral oedema:
  due to increased blood flow,
  hypercapnia, impaired venous drainage
Hypoxia:
  due to inadequate ventilation and high
  metabolic requirements
Hypercapnia:
  due to increased CO_2 production and
  reduced ventilation
Tongue biting
Aspiration and pneumonia
Hypertension/hypotension
Metabolic changes
  e.g. dehydration, hyperkalaemia,
  hypoglycaemia, acidosis
Rhabdomyolysis and renal failure
Traumatic injury, e.g. rib fracture

Acute confusional state (ACS)

ACS is common, especially in the elderly. It affects ~10–15% of medical and surgical ward patients, increasing mortality unless due to sedation. Characteristic features are impaired consciousness usually worse at night, disorientation in time and place, abnormal behaviour, altered perception particularly visual hallucinations, emotional lability (e.g. fear, anxiety) and memory loss. Figures (a) and (b) show common causes. Patients are nursed in quiet, gently lit rooms, with reassurance, orientation and constant observation. The cause must be treated (e.g. infection) but cautious use (i.e. slowly titrate dose) of haloperidol and/or benzodiazepines may be required (Chapter 19).

Coma

Definition Coma is a state of unconsciousness from which the patient cannot be aroused. It is often defined as a Glasgow Coma Score (GCS; Chapter 53) of ≤8. ACS or gradual loss of consciousness may precede coma. **Cause** may be metabolic, infective, traumatic or neurological (Fig. a).

Immediate management

Assess airway, breathing and circulation. Give oxygen, support the circulation, treat seizures and protect (± stabilize) the cervical spine as required. Consider intubation if the GCS is < 8 to protect the airway or to aid investigation (e.g. CT scan). Check the blood glucose (e.g. BM stix) and give intravenous dextrose if hypoglycaemia is suspected. Correct reversible causes of coma (Fig. c). Naloxone and flumazenil temporarily reverse opiate- and benzodiazepine-induced coma respectively (Chapter 19). Give thiamine if alcohol abuse or Wernicke's encephalopathy is suspected. Subsequent management including antibiotics, anticoagulants, anticonvulsants and ICP reduction depends on differentiation of medical and neurological causes of coma (Chapters 46, 47, 53).

Assessment

1 Brief history (i.e. from family, witnesses): often establishes the cause (e.g. trauma, overdose). An abrupt onset suggests a seizure or vascular event whereas a slower onset suggests a metabolic cause, tumour or extradural haematoma. Recent symptoms (e.g. headache, fever), previous illness (e.g. diabetes, sinusitis, AF), travel and drug therapy direct subsequent investigation.

2 Examination: vital signs (e.g. BP, temperature) aid diagnosis (Fig. a). Exclude trauma (e.g. haematoma, 'panda eyes') and immobilize the cervical spine if suspicious. Smell the breath (i.e. alcohol, ketones, hepatic foetor). Examine for stigmata of systemic disease (e.g. cirrhosis, uraemia, alcoholism, diabetes), focal infection (e.g. pneumonia, endocarditis), venepuncture marks (i.e. illicit drug use) and neurological disease (e.g. stroke, meningitis). Incontinence and tongue lacerations indicate seizure. Neurological examination (mnemonic: SPERM) should include:

- **State of consciousness** (i.e. alert, lethargic (i.e. responds to command), stuporous (i.e. arousal to pain) or comatose (i.e. unrousable)). Record the GCS.
- **Pupillary reactions**. Bilateral unreactive and pinpoint pupils suggest a brainstem lesion although many drugs affect pupillary response (e.g. morphine causes pin-point pupils). Normal pupillary reactions during coma suggest a metabolic cause or a structural lesion above the midbrain.
- **Eye movements** are altered by frontal lobe, cortical or brainstem lesions. Loss of oculocephalic and oculovestibular reflexes (Chapter 24) suggests pontomedullary-midbrain damage.
- **Respiratory pattern.** Tachypnoea is non-specific (e.g. acidosis) whereas ataxic breathing indicates severe brainstem dysfunction.
- **Motor function.** The best response is noted (e.g. spontaneously moves all limbs, no response to pain). Pontine damage causes decerebrate (i.e. extensor) posturing, whereas lesions above the pons cause decorticate (i.e. flexor) posturing.

Full neurological examination (+ fundoscopy) localizes focal signs and differentiates between structural and metabolic causes.

3 Investigations: depend on the cause but include biochemistry, glucose, CRP, toxicology (± alcohol level), microbiology (± malaria), blood gases, carboxyhaemoglobin level, CXR, CT scan, EEG and lumbar puncture (if ICP normal).

Prognosis deteriorates with duration of coma. It can be assessed from posture, pupillary and oculovestibular reflexes but only after drug, metabolic, cranial nerve and tympanic membrane defects have been excluded (Chapters 24, 53). Outcome can also be determined reproducibly from the GCS (Chapter 53). Patients with >3 days postanoxic coma (i.e. cardiac arrest) rarely survive without severe disability. Poor prognostic features include decerebrate posturing and rigidity for >24 hours in non-trauma and >2 weeks in trauma patients, absent pupillary reflexes for >24 hours in post-anoxic brain injury or >3 days in other patients, and absent oculovestibular reflexes for >24 hours.

Status epilepticus (SEp)

Definition Seizures lasting >30 minutes or repeated seizures without intervening consciousness. Prolonged seizures cause permanent brain damage due to hypoxia, hypotension, cerebral oedema and neuronal injury. Damage is proportional to seizure duration with mortality rates of 15–30%.

Causes (Fig. d) Patients with epilepsy and metabolic disturbances have a good prognosis, whereas those with global hypoxia, structural damage or infective lesions have a poor prognosis.

Clinical features and complications (Fig. d) Severe lactic acidosis (i.e. pH < 7.0), metabolic imbalance, high fever, cerebral oedema and raised ICP may occur during SEp.

Investigations Immediately exclude (or treat) hypoglycaemia (i.e. bedside BM stix). The following are checked after treatment has started: routine blood tests, toxicology, ECG and anticonvulsant levels in known epileptics. In patients with new-onset seizures, CT imaging detects structural lesions (>50%) and EEG differentiates primary and secondary (focal) generalized seizures. In undiagnosed coma the EEG occasionally reveals non-convulsive SEp.

Management

- **General:** open and maintain the airway (i.e. prevent aspiration, recovery position). Give oxygen (>60%) and thiamine if malnourished (i.e. alcoholics). Support the circulation but avoid hypotonic fluids which increase cerebral oedema. Correct pyrexia and electrolyte disturbances. Continuous EEG monitoring is indicated in severe SEp.
- **Anticonvulsants:** rapid control of seizures is often achieved with slow i.v. bolus or rectal benzodiazepines (e.g. diazepam). If fitting continues a phenytoin or diazepam infusion may be required. In resistant SEp alternative therapies include sodium valproate, vigabatrin, barbiturates and i.v. anaesthetic agents (e.g. propofol).
- **Other therapies:** include hyperventilation (± osmotic diuretics) for cerebral oedema, dexamethasone for tumours or vasculitis, and surgery for space-occupying lesions (e.g. haemorrhage).

46

(a) Clinical features of stroke

Feature	Thrombotic	Embolic	Haemorrhagic
Time course	Slow, stuttering onset	Sudden, maximal defect	Abrupt, rapid onset
Location	Cortical infarcts	Cortical infarcts	Internal capsule, cortical, basal ganglia
Preceding history	TIA ± amaurosis fugax, Retinal artery occlusion	Recent MI, Arrhythmias (e.g. AF)	Anticoagulation, Recent thrombolysis
Predisposing factors	DM, smoking, HT, hyperlipidaemia, heart disease	Endocarditis, ASD + PE, LV aneurysm and thrombus, air embolism, AF	HT, vascular malformation, herald bleeds and headache, cardiac catheterization
Treatment	Endarterectomy, Aspirin (± thrombolysis?)	Aspirin, anticoagulation	Surgical evacuation, Correct coagulopathy

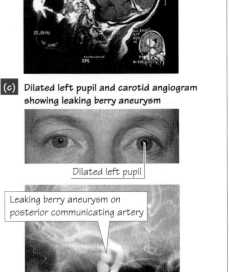

(b) Haemorrhagic stroke on CT scan showing 'bright white' blood

Haemorrhagic stroke

(c) Dilated left pupil and carotid angiogram showing leaking berry aneurysm

Dilated left pupil

Leaking berry aneurysm on posterior communicating artery

Carotid artery

A 44-year-old woman presents with severe headache and dilated left pupil due to the pressure of a posterior communicating aneurysm on the pupillary parasympathetic 'constrictor' fibres lying on the surface of the left third cranial nerve

Strokes

Strokes result from localized areas of intracerebral haemorrhage (ICH; ~20%) or thromboembolic infarction (TE; ~80%), usually manifest as abrupt or gradually progressive focal neurological deficits lasting >24 hours. They may present as confusion or seizures. Incidence is 1/100/ year after 75 years of age. Figure (a) summarizes features of:
• **Thrombotic strokes:** follow atherothrombosis, vasculitis or coagulopathy. In hypertension (HT), small internal capsule infarcts cause large functional deficits. CT scans reveal hypodense areas. Haemorrhage occurs in large infarcts.
• **Embolic strokes:** are less common. Arterial procedures, arrhythmias (e.g. AF), endocarditis and surgery increase the risk.
• **Haemorrhagic strokes:** occur in the basal ganglia (~50%) and pons (~5%) due to HT or in the cortex (Fig. b) and cerebellum (~45%) due to arteriovenous malformations (AVM). Other risk factors are drug abuse, anticoagulation and thrombolysis. Mortality is ~50%.
• *Clinical features* Cortical (50%) and basal ganglia (25%) strokes cause hemiplegia. Brainstem cerebrovascular accidents (CVA; 25%) cause quadraparesis, pinpoint pupils, coma, locked-in syndrome and gaze palsies. Cerebellar lesions cause ataxia and vomiting.
• *Management* Arrange an early CT scan (<12–24 hours), treat hypoxia, arrhythmias and seizures and avoid rapid BP reductions, as even a 20% fall may be harmful (Chapter 29). Aspirin (300 mg p.o.) improves outcome in TE strokes. Thrombolysis using TPA (alteplase) within 3 hours of stroke onset may reduce neurological sequelae but there is small risk of ICH. Anticoagulation is contraindicated in ICH, HT or large strokes. Patients at risk of emboli are anticoagulated after 48 hours, if repeat CT scans exclude haemorrhage. Surgical evacuation improves outcome in cerebellar haemorrhage. Admission to a stroke unit improves care and reduces mortality by ~25%. Prophylactic measures prevent DVT, peptic ulcers, pressure sores and aspiration.

Subarachnoid haemorrhage (SAH)

SAH is spontaneous bleeding from intracranial aneurysms (~85%; Fig. c) or AVM (~15%). Risk factors include family history of SAH, connective tissue disease, polycystic disease and HT.
• *Clinical features* SAH usually presents as a sudden headache, like 'a kick to the back of the head', with nausea, vomiting, confusion or coma. The headache is not always severe. Neck stiffness, subhyaloid

haemorrhage (~25%) and focal neurological signs, due to vasospasm or mass effect, develop later. Complications include arrhythmias, pulmonary oedema and hydrocephalus. Grading systems utilize symptom severity, GCS and motor deficit.
• *Investigation* CT imaging (± lumbar puncture) detects >95% of SAH within 24 hours. Angiography (Fig. c) locates the aneurysm (~80% anterior cerebral circulation).
• *Treatment* requires resuscitation, analgesia and anticonvulsants. Nimodipine, a calcium channel blocker, prevents cerebral artery vasospasm. Aneurysms may be surgically clipped or embolized with 'Guglielmi coils' during radiological endovascular procedures.
• *Prognosis* Initial mortality is ~40%, and ~25% have repeat bleeds. Severe neurological deficits affect ~30% of survivors.

Extradural haematoma is due to middle meningeal artery rupture after head injury. A lucid period precedes rapid GCS deterioration. Prognosis is good following early surgical drainage if the initial GCS was high.

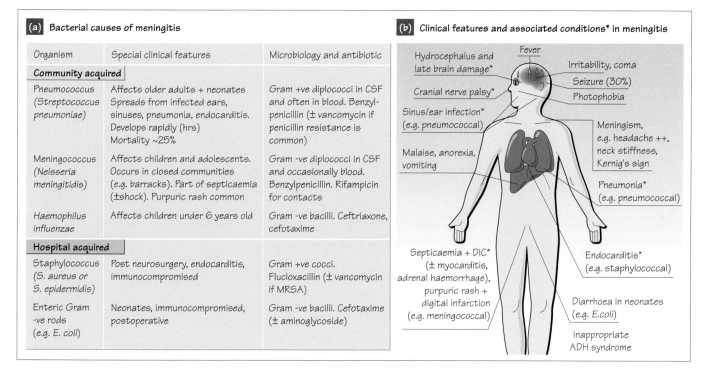

(a) Bacterial causes of meningitis

Organism	Special clinical features	Microbiology and antibiotic
Community acquired		
Pneumococcus (Streptococcus pneumoniae)	Affects older adults + neonates. Spreads from infected ears, sinuses, pneumonia, endocarditis. Develops rapidly (hrs) Mortality ~25%	Gram +ve diplococci in CSF and often in blood. Benzyl-penicillin (± vancomycin if penicillin resistance is common)
Meningococcus (Neisseria meningitidis)	Affects children and adolescents. Occurs in closed communities (e.g. barracks). Part of septicaemia (±shock). Purpuric rash common	Gram -ve diplococci in CSF and occasionally blood. Benzylpenicillin. Rifampicin for contacts
Haemophilus influenzae	Affects children under 6 years old	Gram -ve bacilli. Ceftriaxone, cefotaxime
Hospital acquired		
Staphylococcus (S. aureus or S. epidermidis)	Post neurosurgery, endocarditis, immunocompromised	Gram +ve cocci. Flucloxacillin (± vancomycin if MRSA)
Enteric Gram -ve rods (e.g. E. coli)	Neonates, immunocompromised, postoperative	Gram -ve bacilli. Cefotaxime (± aminoglycoside)

(b) Clinical features and associated conditions* in meningitis

Meningitis

Bacterial meningitis presents with fever, headache, neck stiffness and photophobia but should be suspected in any patient with fever and confusion, as meningism is not always present. It is often associated with rapidly progressive, life-threatening sepsis. Early recognition and treatment is life-saving. Viral meningitis is rarely severe.

Causes Bacteria are listed in Fig. (a). Viruses (e.g. enterococcus), *Mycobacterium tuberculosis* (TB) and leptospirosis (Weil's disease) present less acutely. *Listeria monocytogenes* and *Cryptococcus neoformans* meningitis affect immunocompromised patients (e.g. AIDS).

Clinical features (e.g. septicaemia, meningism) are illustrated in Fig. (b). Precipitating causes must be excluded (e.g. pneumococcal meningitis is often secondary to chest, ear or sinus infection). Chronic TB meningitis is easily missed. SAH, malignancy and abscess may present with meningism. **Complications** (Fig. b) include seizures, digital infarctions, cerebral oedema and obstructive hydrocephalus.

Investigation A CT scan is performed before lumbar puncture if there is a CNS deficit, papilloedema, trauma or suspected mass lesion. Cerebrospinal fluid (CSF) in bacterial infections reveals raised polymorphs ($>500\,mm^3$) and increased protein (0.5–3 g/L), low CSF : blood sugar ratio (CSF/BS < 40%) and bacteria on stain or culture. Blood cultures may be positive. In viral meningitis CSF finds raised lymphocytes ($<500\,mm^3$) and protein (0.5–1 g/L), but normal CSF/BS ratio (~60%). Viral culture and immunology of CSF, throat swabs or faeces are diagnostic. In TB meningitis CSF shows raised lymphocytes ($<500\,mm^3$), protein (1–5 g/L) and a low CSF/BS ratio (<40%). Detection of acid-fast bacilli confirms TB. India ink stains detect *Cryptococcus*.

Treatment (Fig. a) Benzylpenicillin is effective against most pneumococcal and meningococcal meningitis. Cefotaxime or ceftriaxone treats *H. influenzae*. Until an organism has been isolated treat with empirical cefotaxime (±penicillin) and await cultures. Aminoglycosides and antistaphylococcal agents are required in hospital-acquired meningitis. TB meningitis is treated with standard quadruple therapy. Steroids improve outcome and reduce complications in bacterial and tuberculous meningitis. Rifampicin is given to close contacts of meningococcal and *H. influenzae* meningitis.

Encephalitis

This is an acute, usually viral, brain infection (e.g. herpes simplex). It is a rare complication of common viral diseases (e.g. mumps). Immunocompromised patients are at greatest risk. Initial features include drowsiness, irritability, fever, meningism and occasionally focal neurological signs. Severe cases progress to seizures, coma and death. CSF reveals lymphocytosis and raised protein. Viral serology may identify the cause. Management is supportive but aciclovir treats herpes simplex and ganciclovir, CMV infections. Prognosis varies but mortality is high with some viruses (e.g. Japanese B).

Other neurological infections

• **Tetanus:** a toxin-mediated disease caused by *Clostridium tetani* infection of necrotic wounds. Generalized muscle rigidity, spasms and respiratory failure require heavy sedation, paralysis and mechanical ventilation. Cardiovascular instability is controlled with magnesium infusions. Antibiotics, surgical debridement and immune globulin treat the infection and toxin.

• **Poliomyelitis, botulism and rabies:** cause paralytic infections.

• **Others:** cerebral abscesses, cerebral malaria, prion disease.

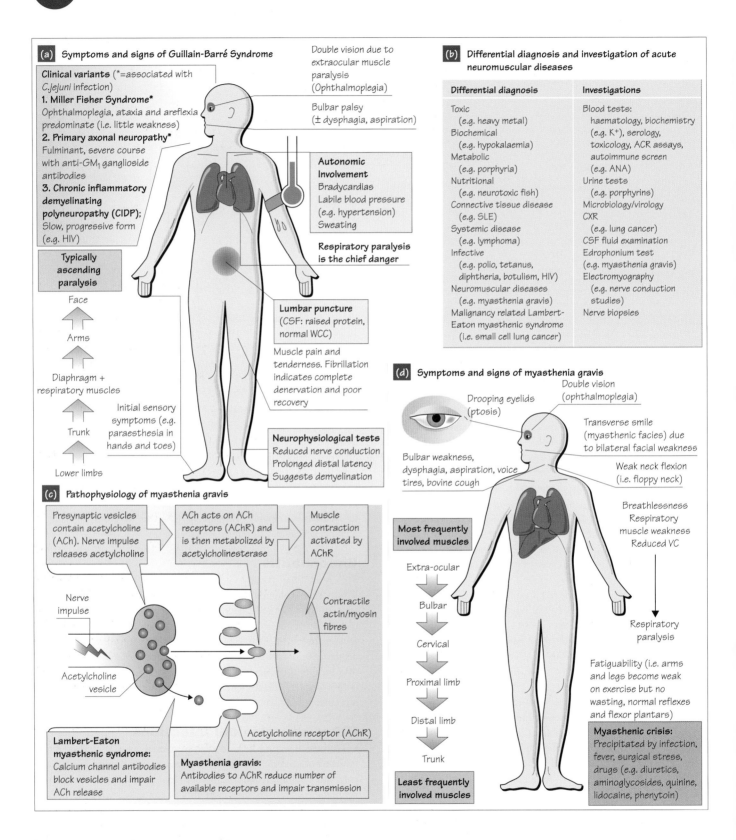

(a) Symptoms and signs of Guillain-Barré Syndrome

Clinical variants (*=associated with C.jejuni infection)
1. Miller Fisher Syndrome*
Ophthalmoplegia, ataxia and areflexia predominate (i.e. little weakness)
2. Primary axonal neuropathy*
Fulminant, severe course with anti-GM₁ ganglioside antibodies
3. Chronic inflammatory demyelinating polyneuropathy (CIDP);
Slow, progressive form (e.g. HIV)

Double vision due to extraocular muscle paralysis (Ophthalmoplegia)

Bulbar palsy (± dysphagia, aspiration)

Autonomic Involvement
Bradycardias
Labile blood pressure (e.g. hypertension)
Sweating

Respiratory paralysis is the chief danger

Typically ascending paralysis

Face → Arms → Diaphragm + respiratory muscles → Trunk → Lower limbs

Initial sensory symptoms (e.g. paraesthesia in hands and toes)

Lumbar puncture (CSF: raised protein, normal WCC)

Muscle pain and tenderness. Fibrillation indicates complete denervation and poor recovery

Neurophysiological tests
Reduced nerve conduction
Prolonged distal latency
Suggests demyelination

(b) Differential diagnosis and investigation of acute neuromuscular diseases

Differential diagnosis	Investigations
Toxic (e.g. heavy metal)	Blood tests: haematology, biochemistry (e.g. K⁺), serology, toxicology, ACR assays, autoimmune screen (e.g. ANA)
Biochemical (e.g. hypokalaemia)	
Metabolic (e.g. porphyria)	
Nutritional (e.g. neurotoxic fish)	Urine tests (e.g. porphyrins)
Connective tissue disease (e.g. SLE)	Microbiology/virology
Systemic disease (e.g. lymphoma)	CXR (e.g. lung cancer)
Infective (e.g. polio, tetanus, diphtheria, botulism, HIV)	CSF fluid examination
	Edrophonium test (e.g. myasthenia gravis)
Neuromuscular diseases (e.g. myasthenia gravis)	Electromyography (e.g. nerve conduction studies)
Malignancy related Lambert-Eaton myasthenic syndrome (i.e. small cell lung cancer)	Nerve biopsies

(c) Pathophysiology of myasthenia gravis

Presynaptic vesicles contain acetylcholine (ACh). Nerve impulse releases acetylcholine

ACh acts on ACh receptors (AChR) and is then metabolized by acetylcholinesterase

Muscle contraction activated by AChR

Nerve impulse

Acetylcholine vesicle

Contractile actin/myosin fibres

Acetylcholine receptor (AChR)

Lambert-Eaton myasthenic syndrome:
Calcium channel antibodies block vesicles and impair ACh release

Myasthenia gravis:
Antibodies to AChR reduce number of available receptors and impair transmission

(d) Symptoms and signs of myasthenia gravis

Drooping eyelids (ptosis)

Double vision (ophthalmoplegia)

Transverse smile (myasthenic facies) due to bilateral facial weakness

Bulbar weakness, dysphagia, aspiration, voice tires, bovine cough

Weak neck flexion (i.e. floppy neck)

Breathlessness
Respiratory muscle weakness
Reduced VC

Most frequently involved muscles

Extra-ocular → Bulbar → Cervical → Proximal limb → Distal limb → Trunk

Least frequently involved muscles

Respiratory paralysis

Fatiguability (i.e. arms and legs become weak on exercise but no wasting, normal reflexes and flexor plantars)

Myasthenic crisis:
Precipitated by infection, fever, surgical stress, drugs (e.g. diuretics, aminoglycosides, quinine, lidocaine, phenytoin)

Guillain–Barré Syndrome (GBS)

Incidence The commonest cause of acute generalized flaccid paralysis affecting ~1.7/10^5/population/yr.

Pathophysiology An acute, inflammatory, demyelinating polyradiculoneuropathy, often occurring a few weeks after surgery, flu vaccination or minor respiratory (45%) or gastrointestinal (20%) infections. Implicated organisms include *Campylobacter jejuni* (20–45%), CMV (10–20%), Epstein–Barr virus and mycoplasma. Cross-reactivity between the immune response to an organism and peripheral nerves is the likely mechanism. Figure (b) lists other acute neuropathies.

Clinical features (Fig. a) Initial symptoms are often sensory (e.g. distal paraesthesia 50–75%). Subsequent ascending weakness (i.e. lower limbs to face), areflexia and paralysis can be surprisingly rapid. In severe cases bulbar (e.g. ophthalmoplegia) and autonomic involvement (e.g. bradycardia) occur. Respiratory paralysis is the chief danger. **Clinical variants** (Fig. a) include: (i) **Miller Fisher Syndrome:** mainly ophthalmoplegia, ataxia and areflexia; (ii) **primary axonal neuropathy:** fulminant, severe illness with poor prognosis; and (iii) **chronic inflammatory demyelinating polyneuropathy** (CIDP): slow, stepwise deterioration and prolonged course.

Prognosis Flaccid quadriparesis and respiratory paralysis can occur within 24–72 hours. About 30% require mechanical ventilation (MV) for a few days to >1 year. Neurological deficit usually peaks at ~14–21 days, followed by gradual recovery over weeks or months. Mortality is <10% but ~10% of survivors have residual neurological deficits. Outcome is worse in the elderly and those with rapid onset or axonal damage.

Investigation (Fig. b) excludes other causes of weakness (e.g. hypokalaemia). **Electrophysiology** may suggest demyelination (i.e. ↓ nerve conduction velocity, ↑ distal latency). **CSF analysis** reveals raised protein (>0.5 g/L) and a normal white cell count.

Management Monitor respiratory reserve (i.e. vital capacity (VC)) every 4 hours as respiratory distress and arterial blood gas (ABG) deterioration are late features of respiratory failure (RF). Intubation is indicated if VC is <15 ml/kg (~1 L) or pharyngeal paralysis impairs secretion clearance. Respiratory function usually recovers within 2–3 weeks but consider a tracheostomy if paralysis persists. Chest physiotherapy and microbiological monitoring reduce respiratory infections. Monitor autonomic dysfunction (e.g. hypotension, arrhythmia, ileus) and minimize with fluid resuscitation and sedation. Profound bradycardia occasionally requires temporary pacemaker insertion. **General measures** include skin care, nutrition, analgesia (e.g. neuropathic pain), thromboembolic prophylaxis and physiotherapy to prevent joint contractures. **Specific measures** include high-dose (i.v.) immunoglobulin therapy and plasma exchange (plasmapheresis). Both speed recovery if used early (<7 days). Steroids are of no benefit except for radicular (root) pain and in CIDP.

Myasthenia gravis (MG)

An autoimmune disorder characterized by skeletal muscle fatigability and weakness. Antibodies to postsynaptic, acetylcholine receptors (AChR) are detected in 90%. AChR loss reduces transmission across the neuromuscular junction (Fig. c). It affects 5/10^5 population (1 : 2 M : F ratio). Women are affected earlier (<50 years) and men later (>50 years) in life. The thymus gland is abnormal in 75%; mainly thymic hyperplasia in young women and benign thymoma (~10%) in elderly males. MG is associated with autoimmune disorders (e.g. hyperthyroidism, SLE), drugs (e.g. penicillamine) and thymic tumours.

Clinical features (Fig. d) MG usually develops insidiously over weeks. Typically muscle weakness increases with repetitive use and recovers with rest. Extraocular muscles are most frequently involved, trunk muscles least (Fig. d). Ptosis and diplopia are the commonest presenting features. MG is confined to the extraocular muscles in 20%. Bulbar muscle involvement causes dysphagia, aspiration and a snarling smile (myaesthenic facies). **Myaesthenic crisis** describes a life-threatening deterioration precipitated by infection, fever, surgical stress or drugs (e.g. aminoglycosides). Rapid RF requires intubation and MV.

Investigations include blood for AChR antibodies. CXR and CT scans exclude thymoma. **Electromyography** shows declining muscle action potentials on repetitive stimulation. The **edrophonium (Tensilon) test** is diagnostic. Edrophonium prevents breakdown of acetylcholine (ACh) by acetylcholinesterase. Increased ACh temporarily restores neuromuscular transmission, abolishing weakness, ptosis and diplopia. However, AChR stimulation may cause autonomic side-effects (e.g. sweating, bradycardia) requiring treatment with atropine. A test dose of edrophonium (2 mg) is injected, followed by a further 8 mg if side-effects are not excessive. Improved strength within 1 minute, lasting several minutes, supports the diagnosis. Facilities for intubation must be available because excess ACh inhibits neuromuscular transmission and may precipitate a **cholinergic crisis** (e.g. apnoea, paralysis, bulbar palsy, excessive secretions, colic).

Management Monitor respiratory function in patients with dyspnoea or difficulty swallowing. Consider intubation if VC is <15 ml/kg (~1 L) or secretion clearance is inadequate. MV is required in ~10%. Assess swallowing in dysphagic patients and start thromboembolic prophylaxis.

Specific treatments include: (i) **Anticholinesterase drugs** (e.g. pyridostigmine). Slowly increase the dose to achieve optimal symptomatic relief. Excessive therapy, in an attempt to abolish all weakness, may result in cholinergic crisis. Anticholinergics are used to control muscarinic side-effects (e.g. salivation, colic, diarrhoea). (ii) **Immunosuppressive therapy.** Steroids may benefit patients with isolated ocular MG or a poor response to anticholinesterases. Improvement after several weeks follows initial deterioration. Azathioprine is required in severe MG. (iii) **Plasma exchange** produces short lived (~4 weeks) but marked improvements during myaesthenic crisis or ventilator weaning. (iv) **Thymectomy** improves ~80% of MG, hastening remission induction and reducing mortality compared to medical therapy alone.

Other neuromuscular disorders

Many neuromuscular diseases (e.g. muscular dystrophy, poliomyelitis) require ventilatory support following RF or surgical intervention. Weaning from MV can be difficult.

Critical illness polyneuropathy occurs after sepsis, MOF or high dose steroids particularly if combined with prolonged paralysis. Axonal degeneration of the motor (±sensory) peripheral nerves leads to weakness, wasting, weaning failure and loss of reflexes. Nerve conduction studies confirm axonal loss. Treatment is symptomatic and recovery may take many months.

49 Coagulation disorders and transfusion

(a) Initial (previous extrinsic pathway) and amplification (previous intrinsic pathway) phases of the clotting cascade and causes of prolonged PT (vitamin K dependent factors) and APPT (measures amplification phase)

(i) Initial phase produces relatively little thrombin but activates the amplification phase (thrombin activates ($\rightarrow$) factors V, VIII, XI)

(ii) Amplification phase produces >90% of thrombin produced (measured by APPT)

*As IXa, Xa only work when tethered to AP via PL, clotting is confined to the platelet plug

TF=tissue factor (thromboplastin)
PL=phospholipid, AP=activated platelets
PT= prothrombin time, APPT= activated partial thromboplastin time
INR=international normalized ratio
DIC=disseminated intravascular coagulation

PT prolonged by:
Liver disease + DIC
Warfarin
Vitamin K deficiency
Salicylate poisoning
Circulating anticoagulants
Excessive heparin
Circulating anticoagulants
PT is expressed as the INR, the ratio of the PT to a standardized reference sample. INR is normally 1

APPT prolonged by:
Haemophilia
Heparin
Von Willebrand's Disease
Under-filled blood bottle (e.g. spurious result)
Delay in assay performance
Circulating anticoagulants

(b) Causes of thrombocytopenia

Decreased Platelet Production
- Leukaemias, marrow depression
- Infiltration by malignancy
- Drugs e.g. chlorpropamide, thiazides, gold, penicillin, methyldopa, quinine, TB therapy, chloroquine, chloramphenicol

Increased Platelet Consumption
- Sepsis (most important)
- Shock
- Disseminated intravascular coagulation
- Splenomegaly with hypersplenism
- Idiopathic thrombocytopenic purpura (ITP) due to anti-platelet IgG autoantibodies
- Thrombotic thrombocytopenic purpura (TTP)
- Haemolytic uraemic syndrome (HUS)
- Heparin-induced thrombocytopenia (HIT)

Extracorporeal Platelet Loss
- Cardiopulmonary bypass
- Renal replacement therapy

(c) Factors contributing to coagulation failure in acute illness

- Vessel trauma e.g. surgical, traumatic
- Acquired factor deficiencies e.g. trauma, transfusion, liver failure, DIC, extracorporeal circuits
- Anticoagulants e.g. heparin, thrombolytics
- Thrombocytopenia e.g. heparin-induced, idiopathic thrombocytopenic purpura (ITP), sepsis
- Hereditary factors e.g. haemophilia
- Hypothermia

(d) Conditions predisposing to disseminated intravascular coagulation (DIC)

- Sepsis e.g. E. coli, malaria, viral
- Surgery e.g. cardiac bypass
- Liver failure
- Malignancy e.g. promyelocytic leukaemia
- Incompatible transfusions
- Intravascular haemolysis
- Shock e.g. burns, trauma
- Poisoning e.g. snake venom
- Autoimmune disease
- Pregnancy-related e.g. eclampsia, puerperal sepsis, amniotic fluid embolism etc.

(e) Management of bleeding, transfusion reactions and effects of massive transfusion

RESUSCITATE | CORRECT COAGULATION

Immediate i.v. fluid to prevent hypovolaemia chapter 6

Give blood to maintain haemoglobin level >8g/dl

Give fresh frozen plasma to replace coagulation factors

Give platelets to maintain count >50x10^9/L when bleeding

Give cryoprecipitate to replace fibrinogen

GIVE OXYGEN to prevent hypoxaemia

* Platelets may be needed with normal platelet count if aspirin or NSAID taken recently

TAKE BLOOD SAMPLES for coagulation studies + platelets

STOP THE BLEEDING !!
1. Pressure on bleeding site
2. Non-surgical haemostasis (e.g. embolization)
3. Surgical haemostasis

Give clotting factors as required (e.g. VIII in haemophilia)

Give Vitamin K in liver failure + to reverse warfarin (effect<12h)

Give protamine to reverse heparin effects

Consider (i) Aprotinin (ii) factor VIIa therapy which may help control massive haemorrhage

RISKS OF TRANSFUSION
1. **Acute haemolytic reactions**
   - due to incompatible blood group
   - 50% due to administrative error
   - urticaria, rigors, shock, asthma, etc
2. **Non-haemolytic reactions (~3%)**
   - reaction to donor white cells
   - fever, chills, urticaria
3. **Infection**
   - viral hepatitis risk ~1% per unit even after testing
4. **Acute lung Injury**
5. **Delayed immune reactions**

ADVERSE EFFECTS OF MASSIVE TRANSFUSION
1. Coagulopathy e.g. dilutional, DIC
2. Biochemical e.g. $\uparrow K^+$, $\downarrow pH$, $\downarrow Ca^{2+}$
3. Hypothermia
4. Volume overload
5. ARDS
6. Infection (hepatitis)

Blood and blood components

Blood is expensive and because it is antigenic requires cross-matching. Screening for HIV, hepatitis, HTLV1, syphilis and CMV reduces infection risk. Donated **whole blood** is collected into CPD-A (citrate, phosphate, dextrose-adenine) anticoagulant; 1 unit is ~430 ml. Subdivision of blood (i.e. red cells, platelets) aids storage (i.e. shelf-life) and targets use at specific needs. Centrifugation separates red cells which are resuspended in SAG-M (sodium chloride, adenine, glucose; mannitol prevents haemolysis). These **packed red cells** have a haemocrit of ~0.65 and a shelf-life of ~42 days. The platelet-rich plasma fraction (~250 ml) is divided into platelets and plasma. **Platelets** have a short shelf-life of ~7 days and 1 unit increases the platelet count by ~4–9 × 10^9/L. **Fresh frozen plasma** (FFP) contains all the clotting factors but ≥4 units are required for clinically useful increases in serum levels. Storage time is ~12 months. FFP can be further separated into **cryoprecipitate** (factor VIII, fibrinogen) and supernatant (albumin). **Fresh whole blood** is rich in clotting factors and platelets but transfusion reactions are common. It is only used to reduce clotting factor dilution during massive transfusions. **Stored blood** is metabolically active; pH, 2,3-DPG, ATP, platelets and clotting factors decrease, K^+ increases (cell rupture) and microaggregates form.

Coagulation disorders

Coagulation disorders occur when the normal haemostatic balance between **vascular endothelium**, **platelets** and the **clotting–fibrinolytic system** is disrupted. In severe illness the cause is often multifactorial (Fig. c), whereas hereditary disorders stem from a single soluble factor deficiency. **Bleeding disorders** are rapidly identified, as clinical abnormalities are obvious and laboratory monitoring widely available. By contrast, **hypercoagulability** and microvascular thrombosis is less easily recognized.

Coagulation tests

Figure (a) illustrates the clotting cascade. **Prothrombin time** (PT) is the time to clot formation following addition of thromboplastin (TF) and Ca^{2+}; normally 12–14 seconds. It measures vitamin K dependent clotting factor (II, VII, X) activity (e.g. warfarin control). Causes of prolonged PT are listed in Fig. (a). **Activated partial thromboplastin time** (APPT) is time to clot formation after adding kaolin (surface activator), phospholipid and Ca^{2+} to plasma; normally ~40 seconds. It measures the amplification phase factor activities (but not factor VII). Figure (a) lists causes of prolonged APPT. **Platelet counts** <20 × 10^9/L (<50 × 10^9/L with co-existing platelet dysfunction) increase the risk of spontaneous bleeding. **Bleeding time** tests platelet function primarily. Following a standard skin incision, bleeding should stop within 9 minutes. **Activated clotting time**, a bedside test of heparin action, examines clotting in whole blood but is prolonged by thrombocytopenia, hypothermia and fibrinolysis. **Factor assays** (e.g. fibrinogen, VII) are available. **Fibrinogen degradation products** (FDPs) and **d-dimers** are products of fibrinolysis and increase during DIC, sepsis, trauma and VTE. FDP assays are widely available. D-dimers are sensitive but not specific for VTE; a negative result reliably excludes VTE (Chapter 30). **PT, APPT and platelet count** detect most acquired bleeding disorders following a detailed history (i.e. previous haemorrhage) and medication review (e.g. aspirin).

Bleeding disorders

• **Genetic coagulopathies:** the haemophilias are sex-linked, recessive diseases causing spontaneous bleeding in affected males. **Haemophilia A** is due to factor VIII deficiency. **Haemophilia B** (Christmas disease) is less common and due to factor IX deficiency. Treatment is with factors VIII and IX respectively. **Von Willebrand's disease**, an autosomal dominant trait, is the commonest hereditary coagulation disorder. It decreases factor VIII activity and reduces platelet adherence to vascular injury sites. Treatment with DDAVP augments factor VIII and reduces haemorrhagic risk in mild cases. Cryoprecipitate and FFP also correct the deficit.

• **Liver disease, malnutrition and antibiotic therapy:** cause vitamin K-dependent coagulation factor deficiency. Rapid correction follows vitamin K therapy except in severe hepatocellular damage.

• **Anticoagulation agents:** oral anticoagulants deplete vitamin K-dependent clotting factors. FFP transiently reverses and vitamin K therapy corrects warfarin-induced anticoagulation. **Heparin** potentiates antithrombin III, which blocks the action of thrombin (± factors IX, X), inhibiting coagulation and prolonging APPT. It is reversed by protamine sulphate. Antibodies to heparin can cross-react with platelet antigens causing heparin-induced thrombocytopenia (HIT; ~10%) and thrombosis. **Antiplatelet agents** (e.g. aspirin) irreversibly inhibit platelet function for ~10 days. **Thrombolysis** may cause haemorrhage (e.g. GI tract). Intracranial bleeding occurs in <0.5–2%. FFP and platelets stop bleeding. **Circulating anticoagulants** develop with some drugs (e.g. penicillin) and diseases (e.g. AIDS, SLE).

• **Disseminated intravascular coagulation (DIC):** follows extensive activation of coagulation and fibrinolysis (e.g. sepsis) with simultaneous bleeding, often the presenting feature, and thrombosis. Platelets and fibrinogen fall and PT, APPT and FDP increase. Red cell fragmentation may occur. Figure (d) lists causes of DIC. Treat the cause, supplement clotting factors (± platelets) and start low-dose heparin.

• **Thrombocytopenia:** is due to decreased production, increased consumption or extracorporeal loss of platelets (Fig. b). Treat the cause (e.g. steroids and immune globulin in immune thrombocytopaenia (ITP), FFP and plasma exchange in thrombotic thrombocytopaenia (TTP)).

Transfusion and management of bleeding

Full cross-matching takes ~45 minutes but ABO type can be determined in ≤10 minutes. O-negative blood (universal donor) is given when blood is needed immediately, but may provoke minor transfusion reactions. Type specific (ABO-, rhesus-compatible) blood is preferred if time permits. After ~5 units of blood, dilutional clotting disorders and biochemical abnormalities (e.g. hypocalcaemia) develop and may require correction. Blood filters are recommended during large transfusions. Management of bleeding and the consequences of transfusions are illustrated in Fig. (e).

Hypercoagulable disorders

Thromboembolism (Chapter 30) involves a predisposing genetic disorder in ~20% of cases (e.g. antithrombin III deficiency, protein C and S deficiency, lupus anticoagulant). A family history of thrombosis, repeated thrombosis, unusual sites (e.g. arms) and recurrent spontaneous abortions are suggestive.

50 Drug overdose and poisoning

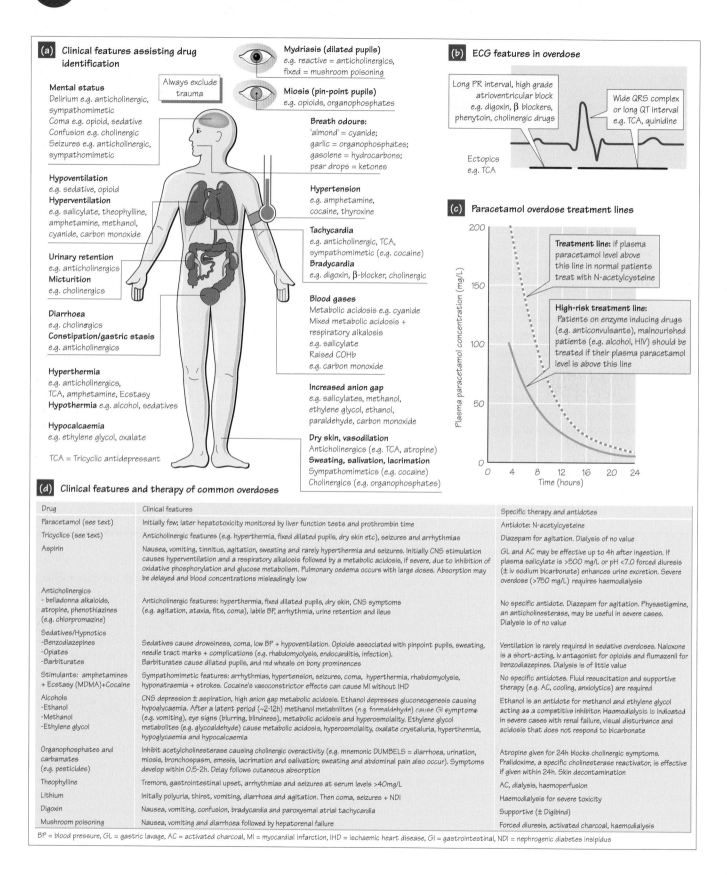

(a) Clinical features assisting drug identification

Always exclude trauma

Mental status
Delirium e.g. anticholinergic, sympathomimetic
Coma e.g. opioid, sedative
Confusion e.g. cholinergic
Seizures e.g. anticholinergic, sympathomimetic

Hypoventilation
e.g. sedative, opioid
Hyperventilation
e.g. salicylate, theophylline, amphetamine, methanol, cyanide, carbon monoxide

Urinary retention
e.g. anticholinergics
Micturition
e.g. cholinergics

Diarrhoea
e.g. cholinergics
Constipation/gastric stasis
e.g. anticholinergics

Hyperthermia
e.g. anticholinergics, TCA, amphetamine, Ecstasy
Hypothermia e.g. alcohol, sedatives

Hypocalcaemia
e.g. ethylene glycol, oxalate

TCA = Tricyclic antidepressant

Mydriasis (dilated pupils)
e.g. reactive = anticholinergics, fixed = mushroom poisoning

Miosis (pin-point pupils)
e.g. opioids, organophosphates

Breath odours:
'almond' = cyanide;
garlic = organophosphates;
gasolene = hydrocarbons;
pear drops = ketones

Hypertension
e.g. amphetamine, cocaine, thyroxine

Tachycardia
e.g. anticholinergic, TCA, sympathomimetic (e.g. cocaine)
Bradycardia
e.g. digoxin, β-blocker, cholinergic

Blood gases
Metabolic acidosis e.g. cyanide
Mixed metabolic acidosis + respiratory alkalosis
e.g. salicylate
Raised COHb
e.g. carbon monoxide

Increased anion gap
e.g. salicylates, methanol, ethylene glycol, ethanol, paraldehyde, carbon monoxide

Dry skin, vasodilation
Anticholinergics (e.g. TCA, atropine)
Sweating, salivation, lacrimation
Sympathomimetics (e.g. cocaine)
Cholinergics (e.g. organophosphates)

(b) ECG features in overdose

Long PR interval, high grade atrioventricular block e.g. digoxin, β blockers, phenytoin, cholinergic drugs

Wide QRS complex or long QT interval e.g. TCA, quinidine

Ectopics e.g. TCA

(c) Paracetamol overdose treatment lines

Treatment line: if plasma paracetamol level above this line in normal patients treat with N-acetylcysteine

High-risk treatment line: Patients on enzyme inducing drugs (e.g. anticonvulsants), malnourished patients (e.g. alcohol, HIV) should be treated if their plasma paracetamol level is above this line

(Plasma paracetamol concentration (mg/L) vs Time (hours))

(d) Clinical features and therapy of common overdoses

Drug	Clinical features	Specific therapy and antidotes
Paracetamol (see text)	Initially few; later hepatotoxicity monitored by liver function tests and prothrombin time	Antidote: N-acetylcysteine
Tricyclics (see text)	Anticholinergic features (e.g. hyperthermia, fixed dilated pupils, dry skin etc), seizures and arrhythmias	Diazepam for agitation. Dialysis of no value
Aspirin	Nausea, vomiting, tinnitus, agitation, sweating and rarely hyperthermia and seizures. Initially CNS stimulation causes hyperventilation and a respiratory alkalosis followed by a metabolic acidosis, if severe, due to inhibition of oxidative phosphorylation and glucose metabolism. Pulmonary oedema occurs with large doses. Absorption may be delayed and blood concentrations misleadingly low	GL and AC may be effective up to 4h after ingestion. If plasma salicylate is >500 mg/L or pH <7.0 forced diuresis (± iv sodium bicarbonate) enhances urine excretion. Severe overdose (>750 mg/L) requires haemodialysis
Anticholinergics - belladonna alkaloids, atropine, phenothiazines (e.g. chlorpromazine)	Anticholinergic features: hyperthermia, fixed dilated pupils, dry skin, CNS symptoms (e.g. agitation, ataxia, fits, coma), labile BP, arrhythmia, urine retention and ileus	No specific antidote. Diazepam for agitation. Physastigmine, an anticholinesterase, may be useful in severe cases. Dialysis is of no value
Sedatives/Hypnotics -Benzodiazepines -Opiates -Barbiturates	Sedatives cause drowsiness, coma, low BP + hypoventilation. Opioids associated with pinpoint pupils, sweating, needle tract marks + complications (e.g. rhabdomyolysis, endocarditis, infection). Barbiturates cause dilated pupils, and red weals on bony prominences	Ventilation is rarely required in sedative overdoses. Naloxone is a short-acting, iv antagonist for opioids and flumazenil for benzodiazepines. Dialysis is of little value
Stimulants: amphetamines + Ecstasy (MDMA)+Cocaine	Sympathomimetic features: arrhythmias, hypertension, seizures, coma, hyperthermia, rhabdomyolysis, hyponatraemia + strokes. Cocaine's vasoconstrictor effects can cause MI without IHD	No specific antidotes. Fluid resuscitation and supportive therapy (e.g. AC, cooling, anxiolytics) are required
Alcohols -Ethanol -Methanol -Ethylene glycol	CNS depression ± aspiration, high anion gap metabolic acidosis. Ethanol depresses gluconeogenesis causing hypoglycaemia. After a latent period (~2-12h) methanol metabolites (e.g. formaldehyde) cause GI symptoms (e.g. vomiting), eye signs (blurring, blindness), metabolic acidosis and hyperosmolality. Ethylene glycol metabolites (e.g. glycoaldehyde) cause metabolic acidosis, hyperosmolarity, oxalate crystaluria, hyperthermia, hypoglycaemia and hypocalcaemia	Ethanol is an antidote for methanol and ethylene glycol acting as a competitive inhibitor. Haemodialysis is indicated in severe cases with renal failure, visual disturbance and acidosis that does not respond to bicarbonate
Organophosphates and carbamates (e.g. pesticides)	Inhibit acetylcholinesterase causing cholinergic overactivity (e.g. mnemonic DUMBELS = diarrhoea, urination, miosis, bronchospasm, emesis, lacrimation and salivation; sweating and abdominal pain also occur). Symptoms develop within 0.5-2h. Delay follows cutaneous absorption	Atropine given for 24h blocks cholinergic symptoms. Pralidoxime, a specific cholinesterase reactivator, is effective if given within 24h. Skin decontamination
Theophylline	Tremors, gastrointestinal upset, arrhythmias and seizures at serum levels >40mg/L	AC, dialysis, haemoperfusion
Lithium	Initally polyuria, thirst, vomiting, diarrhoea and agitation. Then coma, seizures + NDI	Haemodialysis for severe toxicity
Digoxin	Nausea, vomiting, confusion, bradycardia and paroxysmal atrial tachycardia	Supportive (± Digibind)
Mushroom poisoning	Nausea, vomiting and diarrhoea followed by hepatorenal failure	Forced diuresis, activated charcoal, haemodialysis

BP = blood pressure, GL = gastric lavage, AC = activated charcoal, MI = myocardial infarction, IHD = ischaemic heart disease, GI = gastrointestinal, NDI = nephrogenic diabetes insipidus

Overdoses (OD) and poisonings cause ~10% of hospital admissions. In-hospital mortality is <1% as most deaths occur before admission due to arrhythmia or respiratory arrest. A few drugs (e.g. paracetamol, tricyclic antidepressants) account for ~90–95% of self-administered OD. Most episodes are 'a cry for help' rather than genuine suicide attempts and occur in young people (<35 years old; M : F 1 : 1.5) with a history of similar episodes. Fatal overdoses are more likely in patients >45 years old with serious suicidal intent. In children, poisoning is usually accidental due to ingestion of a single agent.

In general, supportive care and prevention of absorption are more important than active measures to hasten drug elimination. Be guided by the poisons information services. A practical approach to overdose management entails:

1 **Resuscitation:** including airways protection, respiratory support, fluid replacement and acid–base balance. Prolonged unconsciousness is often associated with hypothermia, aspiration of gastric contents, rhabdomyolysis and compartment syndrome. Drug-induced hyperthermia (e.g. salicylates, anticholinergics) is uncommon (Chapter 21).

2 **Substance identification:** although **history** is unreliable, important information includes: *drugs taken* (± time taken, dosage, route); *past history* (i.e. previous OD); *circumstances* (e.g. witnesses, empty containers, syringes) and *associated trauma*.

  • **Examination** (Fig. a) provides important diagnostic clues.
  • **Investigations** (Figs a, b) include: drug identification (e.g. blood, urine, gastric aspirates); paracetamol, aspirin and alcohol levels; routine blood tests including liver function tests, coagulation and serum osmolality (e.g. methanol, ethylene glycol); blood gases and anion gap (Chapter 18); CXR (e.g. pulmonary oedema with salicylates); and ECG (e.g. myocardial ischaemia with cocaine).

3 **Prevention of absorption:** is best achieved with:

  • **Activated charcoal (AC)** – an effective adsorbent that promotes drug elimination (e.g. salicylates) and is first line therapy for most poisonings. It is best given within 1 hour of drug ingestion (later if drug delays gastric emptying), after gastric lavage (GL) and at 4-hourly intervals with specific drugs (e.g. theophylline). AC does not bind iron, lithium, alcohols, acids, alkalis, cyanide or pesticides. It causes constipation and may be given with a cathartic (e.g. sorbitol) as an aqueous slurry.
  • **Gastric lavage (GL)** – ineffective unless performed within 1 hour of drug ingestion. Occasionally, late GL may recover drugs which form concretions (e.g. theophylline) or impair gastric emptying (e.g. anticholinergics). GL is harmful after caustic or petroleum product ingestion and ineffective following alcohol OD. Lavage is performed in the left lateral position using a large bore (~ 38 Fr) orogastric tube to facilitate removal of pill fragments. Consider intubation in obtunded patients as gastric aspiration is the main risk. Oropharyngeal trauma and oesophageal perforation also occur.
  • **Additional measures** include: (i) **cathartics** which promote diarrhoea and reduce drug absorption but risk fluid and electrolyte loss; (ii) **skin decontamination** for transdermally absorbed toxins (e.g. organophosphates); and occasionally (iii) **endoscopy/surgery** (e.g. iron overdose, body packers). Induced vomiting is not recommended as it is ineffective, limits AC use and risks aspiration (± oesophageal tears).

4 **Enhanced drug elimination:** only indicated in life-threatening poisoning as some techniques have associated risks.

  • **Gut dialysis** uses repeated doses of AC to bind drugs with an enterohepatic circulation which are excreted in bile (e.g. theophylline, digoxin, carbamazepine).
  • **Forced diuresis** – enhances drug excretion by increasing urine production to 2–5 ml/kg/h with intravenous fluid (± diuretic) but risks fluid overload. Alkalinization with sodium bicarbonate promotes salicylate, tricyclic antidepressant and barbiturate excretion but is only used in severe cases.
  • **Haemodialysis** – removes low molecular weight, water soluble molecules, with a small volume of distribution and low protein binding (e.g. salicylates, methanol, theophylline).
  • **Haemoperfusion** – using charcoal or resin columns is useful for lipid soluble drugs (e.g. theophylline, barbiturates) but may cause hypocalcaemia and coagulopathy.

Specific management

Figure (d) summarizes the clinical features and management of OD and poisonings. Paracetamol and tricyclic antidepressants are most common, often in combination with alcohol.

• **Paracetamol overdose (POD):** depletes hepatic glutathione stores, causing accumulation of a hydroxylamine metabolite which causes liver and renal damage. Malnourished patients (e.g. alcoholics) and those taking anticonvulsants are at greatest risk of hepatotoxicity. In the UK, POD causes 200 deaths/yr and >12 g (150 mg/kg) can be lethal. Initially there are few symptoms apart from nausea, vomiting and abdominal pain. Signs and biochemical evidence of hepatocellular necrosis present after 24 hours and peak at 3–4 days. The recovery phase lasts ~8 days. Management during the initial 4 hours includes GL and AC. If paracetamol levels at 4 hours are above the treatment line (Fig. c) or if >10 g has been ingested, treatment with intravenous *N*-acetylcysteine (NAC) raises glutathione levels, reduces toxicity and improves outcome. It is most effective within 12 hours. Rapid administration can cause bronchospasm, urticaria and anaphylaxis. Methionine is an oral alternative to NAC. Early referral to a liver unit is required if liver failure develops. Liver transplantation may be indicated in established liver failure.

• **Tricyclic antidepressants (TCA):** cause most overdose fatalities (~300 deaths/yr in the UK) but in-hospital mortality is still <1%. Toxicity is due to anticholinergic effects which cause fixed dilated pupils, dry red skin, hyperthermia, tachycardia, urine retention and CNS hyperreactivity (e.g. psychosis, hallucinations, seizures). Severely intoxicated patients are accurately described as 'hot as a hare, blind as a bat, dry as a bone and mad as a hatter'. There is no specific antidote. GL and AC are essential due to associated ileus, delayed gastric emptying and enterohepatic circulation. The ECG signals cardiac and CNS toxicity when the QRS complex is >0.12 seconds. Potentially life-threatening arrhythmias and hypotension respond to correction of hypoxia, acidosis and cardioversion but can be very resistant to antiarrhythmic agents. Lidocaine (lignocaine) or phenytoin are the most beneficial antiarrhythmics. Type 1a drugs (e.g. quinidine) further impair conduction and should be avoided. Recovery occurs in ~24 hours due to rapid metabolism.

(a) Clinical features of AIDS and causes of critical illness

Clinical features and diseases that are indicators of AIDS

Cerebral
HIV encephalopathy, dementia
Cerebral toxoplasmosis
Cryptococcus neoformans
Primary brain lymphoma

General
Weight loss, fatigue
Lymphadenopathy
CMV retinitis

Respiratory
Pneumocystis carinii
  pneumonia
Mycobacterium avium
  intracellulare
Mycobacterium tuberculosis
Pneumonia
(e.g. S.pneumoniae)

Gastrointestinal
Diarrhoea
Cytomegalovirus colitis
Oral and oesophageal candida
Small bowel lymphoma

Skin
Herpes simplex
Kaposi's sarcoma
Dermatitis

Malignancy
Non-Hodgkin's lymphoma
Burkitt's lymphoma

Blood
Lymphopenia
Bacteraemia

Causes of critical illness *commonest

Neurological emergencies*
Seizures
Meningitis
Encephalitis
Infection

Upper airways obstruction

Hypotension*
Sepsis (e.g. candida)
Adrenal insufficiency
Cardiac arrhythmias

Respiratory failure*
Pneumocystis carinii
  pneumonia
Tuberculosis
Interstial pneumonitis

Gastrointestinal
GI bleeding

Malignancy
Side effects of therapy
Secondary infection
Drug toxicity

Other
Drug toxicity
Self harm

(b) Cerebral CT scan illustrating cerebral toxoplasmosis with ring enhancement following contrast

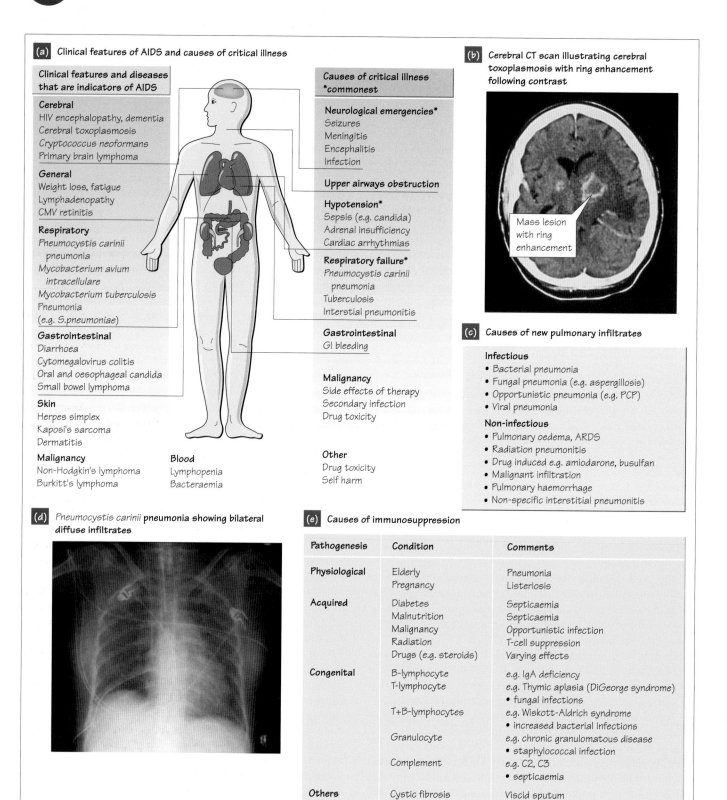

Mass lesion with ring enhancement

(c) Causes of new pulmonary infiltrates

Infectious
• Bacterial pneumonia
• Fungal pneumonia (e.g. aspergillosis)
• Opportunistic pneumonia (e.g. PCP)
• Viral pneumonia

Non-infectious
• Pulmonary oedema, ARDS
• Radiation pneumonitis
• Drug induced e.g. amiodarone, busulfan
• Malignant infiltration
• Pulmonary haemorrhage
• Non-specific interstitial pneumonitis

(d) *Pneumocystis carinii* **pneumonia showing bilateral diffuse infiltrates**

(e) Causes of immunosuppression

Pathogenesis	Condition	Comments
Physiological	Elderly	Pneumonia
	Pregnancy	Listeriosis
Acquired	Diabetes	Septicaemia
	Malnutrition	Septicaemia
	Malignancy	Opportunistic infection
	Radiation	T-cell suppression
	Drugs (e.g. steroids)	Varying effects
Congenital	B-lymphocyte	e.g. IgA deficiency
	T-lymphocyte	e.g. Thymic aplasia (DiGeorge syndrome)
		• fungal infections
	T+B-lymphocytes	e.g. Wiskott-Aldrich syndrome
		• increased bacterial infections
	Granulocyte	e.g. chronic granulomatous disease
		• staphylococcal infection
	Complement	e.g. C2, C3
		• septicaemia
Others	Cystic fibrosis	Viscid sputum
		• pneumonia

General factors

Malnutrition, disease (e.g. diabetes, AIDS) and medical interventions (e.g. chemotherapy) impair the immune system and risk critical illness due to **infection** and **non-infectious** (e.g. neoplasia, drug reactions, graft vs. host disease) causes (Figs a, e). Primary failure of **T-lymphocyte** (cell-mediated) function predisposes to viral and fungal infections or neoplasia. **B-lymphocyte** (antibody-mediated; 'humoral') disorders and **granulocytopenia** are associated with bacterial infections. Fever in profoundly neutropenic (<1000 granulocytes/mm^3) patients is an emergency, particularly when due to infection, and survival depends on rapid diagnosis and treatment. Unfortunately, infection with commensal organisms (e.g. *Pneumocystis*, *Aspergillus*) and lack of localized inflammation often make diagnosis difficult. Primary bacteraemia and soft tissue (e.g. mucosal) infections are characteristic although any site can be infected. **Pulmonary infiltrates** do not always indicate infection, as there are many non-infective causes (Fig. c). Establishing the diagnosis may require invasive techniques (e.g. bronchoscopy, biopsy) with associated risks (e.g. haemorrhage).

General management

Survival of febrile neutropenic patients depends on **early empirical antibiotic (± antifungal) therapy** effective against potential infecting organisms including gram-negative rods (e.g. *Pseudomonas*), staphylococci and fungi (e.g. *Aspergillus*). Impaired cell-mediated immunity predisposes to *Pneumocystis* and *Candida* infection. **Cultures** of blood, urine, sputum and skin lesions must be obtained before starting **broad-spectrum antibiotics** including extended-spectrum penicillins, third generation cephalosporins, aminoglycosides and in some cases cover against methicillin-resistant *Staphylococcus aureus* (MRSA) infections. Many centres advocate the addition of **antifungal therapy** (e.g. amphotericin) if fever persists for >72 hours after starting antibiotics.

Specific causes

Acquired immunodeficiency syndrome (AIDS)

AIDS is caused by human immunodeficiency virus (HIV) which infects, replicates within, impairs and eventually depletes CD4 T-lymphocytes. HIV is transmitted by sexual contact, in blood products, during pregnancy from mother to child and through breast milk. Over 40 million people are infected worldwide. AIDS is defined by the presence of indicator diseases (see below) in HIV-infected individuals with a blood CD4 count <200/ml (or a CD4 count <14% of all lymphocytes). Clinical features, diseases and critical illnesses which indicate AIDS (Fig. a) include:

- *Pneumocystis jirovecii (carinii)* pneumonia **(PCP)** with respiratory failure. Although common, incidence has decreased with prophylactic Septrin therapy.
  - **Clinical features** include fever, dry cough and dyspnoea. Pneumothorax occurs in ~2% cases.
  - **Investigations** demonstrate generalized alveolitis with impaired diffusion on lung function tests and exercise desaturation. Chest radiography typically shows bilateral interstitial infiltrates (Fig. d) but may be normal or focally consolidated. Giemsa, silver and immunofluorescent stains of sputum, particularly if induced with nebulized 3N saline, detects pneumocystis in >70% cases. Bronchoscopic washings detect >90% of cases but transbronchial lung biopsies are most reliable.

- **Treatment** is with oxygen (± CPAP) and high dose intravenous co-trimoxazole (Septrin), which can cause severe skin rashes (~30%), vomiting, colitis and hepatitis. Alternative therapy with pentamidine also causes side effects. High dose steroids reduce alveolitis, respiratory failure and mortality.
- **Other opportunistic infections** include pulmonary TB, toxoplasmosis (Fig. b), candidiasis, *Cryptococcus neoformans*, CMV and herpes simplex. HIV patients with undiagnosed respiratory illness should be isolated until TB has been excluded.

Hospital precautions Assume all patients are HIV-positive and take appropriate precautions (e.g. gloves, masks). The infection risk following HIV-contaminated needlestick injury is ~0.4%. After cleansing, seek expert advice and start prophylactic therapy.

Other specific causes

1 Malignant diseases: are increasingly associated with improved prognosis, especially haematological and lymphoproliferative disorders. Acute hospital admission for treatment of potentially reversible life-threatening effects of the tumour (e.g. hypercalcaemia) or associated therapy (e.g. chemotherapy) may be required. These patients are susceptible to infection due to the profound leucopenia that occurs 10–14 days after chemotherapy or bone marrow transplantation, disease-mediated immunosuppression and invasive procedures (e.g. line insertion). In general, mortality rates are high (>70%) when patients with malignant disease develop acute illness but prolonged, high quality, survival justifies aggressive management in selected cases.

2 Post splenectomy: infection may be fatal as loss of splenic phagocytic function allows rapid bacterial proliferation and spread. Infection is usually due to encapsulated bacteria (e.g. pneumococci, *Haemophilus*). Prophylactic antibiotics (e.g. penicillin) and vaccination against influenza, pneumococcus, *H. influenza* and meningococcus are recommended.

3 Systemic disease: can increase infection risk (e.g. diabetes). **Cirrhosis** impairs hepatic phagocytic function. **Connective tissue diseases** (e.g. SLE) can be immunosuppressive due to associated leucopenia and the effects of therapy (e.g. steroids). **Primary immunodeficiency disorders** (e.g. DiGeorge syndrome) occasionally cause infection.

4 Transplant surgery: requires postoperative immunosuppressive therapy (e.g. ciclosporin, steroids, azathioprine) to prevent graft vs. host organ rejection. Ciclosporin acts mainly on T-cells rather than B-cells, is less immunosuppressive and prevents rejection better than azathioprine. This has reduced infections and increased graft survival. Risk of rejection is greatest in the first 6–12 weeks post-transplant, after which the body develops a degree of tolerance to the graft and ciclosporin dose can be reduced. During this period of intense T-cell suppression, transplant recipients are prone to CMV, cryptococcus, PCP, herpes simplex and *Aspergillus* infections. The long-term risk of opportunistic infections, and to a lesser extent that of malignancy (e.g. lymphoma), is also increased.

5 Immunosuppressive therapy: is required for many common disorders (e.g. Crohn's disease, rheumatoid arthritis). These drugs (e.g. steroids, cyclophosphamide, azathioprine, methotrexate) and therapies (e.g. radiotherapy) are immunosuppressive and associated with an increased risk of infection.

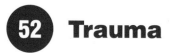

(a) Manual in-line cervical immobilization

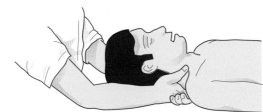

(c) Classification of haemorrhage severity

Class	Circulating volume loss	Approx volume loss (70kg man)	Clinical signs
Class 1	<15%	<750mL	Minimal signs
Class 2	15-30%	<1500mL	↑HR + ↓BP; sweating ↓pulse pressure
Class 3	30-40%	<2000mL	Agitated, sweating, oliguria, ↑HR (>120/min) ↓BP (systolic ~90mmHg)
Class 4	>40%	>2000mL	Preterminal, drowsy ↓BP (systolic <90mmHg)

(b) C2 hangman's fracture and C2 on C3 facet joint fracture dislocation (arrow) causing loss of alignment, bony contour and lordosis with interspinous opening

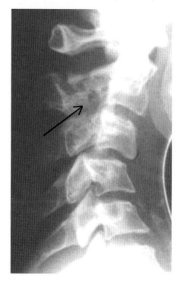

(d) Examining the cervical X-ray and examples of cervical fracture (#)

Cervical X-rays compromise 3 views AP, lateral and open mouth. The lateral must clearly visualize the occiput to the C7/T1 junction
Check the following on the 3 views to assess the presence of injury

1. Alignment (see figure)
The following indicate injury a. loss of lordosis b. ↑ anterior soft tissue shadows >4mm at C4, >15mm at C6 c. ↑ interspinous distance d. malaligned spinous processes e. cortical discontinuity

2. Bony abnormality

3. Contours (+ cartilages)
Check vertebral bodies and spinous processes. Look for avulsion, burst and wedge fractures (i.e. >3mm height difference between front and back of the body)

4. Disc spaces and soft tissues
e.g. distance from C3 to the back of the pharynx (>4mm = haematoma)

5. Odontoid peg
Open mouth and lateral views. Distance between the anterior arch of C1 and the peg should be <3mm

Normal alignment

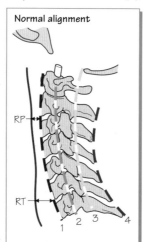

RP→

RT→

1 2 3 4

1. Anterior vertebral line
2. Posterior vertebral line
3. Spinolaminar line
4. Spinous process line
5. RP= retropharyngeal Soft tissue space C4 <4mm
6. RT=retrotracheal space C6 <15mm

Odontoid process fracture
a) AP view through mouth
b) Lateral view in extension. Usually an unstable injury, that requires stabilization. Rarely associated with cord injury, as injury to the cord at this level leads to sudden death

(a)   (b)

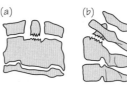

Burst fractures
A compression injury tends to be stable unless significant displacement of bony fragments posteriorly causes cord damage

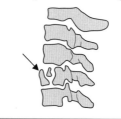

Extension injuries
These injuries occur commonly in the elderly, are associated with central cord neurological deficit and are usually stable and may be treated expectantly. The role for surgical decompression is equivocal

Fracture dislocations (distraction) injuries
Very unstable injuries with both anterior and posterior ligamentous and bony disruption with a high association of cord damage. Usually requires surgical correction and fixation to stabilize the spine

Trauma is the leading cause of death in young people (<40 years old). **The Advanced Trauma Life Support (ATLS) Programme** recommends a **structured approach** to the management of severe and multiple trauma, by a well organized **trauma team**. Assessment, diagnosis and therapy should be concurrent and lack of a definitive diagnosis must not delay appropriate therapy. Treat the greatest risk to life first; recognizing that **airways obstruction** is more rapidly fatal than **inadequate ventilation**, which is more serious than **loss of circulating volume,** followed by expanding **intracranial mass lesions** (i.e. ABC system)

Although early resuscitation reduces morbidity and mortality, **prehospital treatment** is limited to ensuring adequate oxygenation, ventilation and spinal immobilization. Fluid resuscitation should not delay transfer to hospital. The sequence of trauma management is:

Primary survey/initial resuscitation

Assess and treat:

1 Airway and cervical spine: ensure a patent upper airway (Chapters 12, 13) and start oxygen therapy. Immobilize the spine with manual in-line cervical stabilization (MILS; Fig. a) or a hard cervical collar, sandbags and tape. If the airway is at risk, intubate using rapid sequence induction with MILS and cricoid pressure (Chapter 15). Profound hypotension may occur during anaesthestic induction due to hypovolaemia.

2 Breathing: treat immediate life-threatening chest injuries (e.g. flail segment, haemothorax) and anticipate pneumothorax (±tension), especially during mechanical ventilation (MV). Consider prophylactic MV in head injured patients at risk of hypoxia, hypercapnia and BP fluctuations (Chapters 53, 54).

3 Circulation: control external haemorrhage with direct pressure, establish intravenous access (i.e. large bore peripheral (± central) cannulae), institute ECG monitoring and cross-match blood. Shock is usually hypovolaemic due to blood loss, but other causes include sepsis, tension pneumothorax, neurogenic shock and myocardial contusion or tamponade (secondary survey). Clinical signs indicate haemorrhage severity (Fig. c) but hypotension (± shock) may not be apparent until loss of >30% circulating volume in young patients. Early fluid replacement, guided by appropriate monitoring, prevents tissue ischaemia and subsequent organ dysfunction (Chapters 3, 4, 6). Fluid is warmed as hypothermia will increase bleeding. Blood is given if haemocrit is <0.3 or haemoglobin level <10 g/dl. **Immediate surgery** may be required to control bleeding.

4 Neurological status: record pupillary light responses and GCS (Chapters 45, 53). Record blood alcohol levels.

5 General management: undress the patient to aid examination but avoid hypothermia. Catheterize to monitor urine output after excluding urethral injury. In basal skull fractures, nasogastric tubes may cause meningeal infection. The oro-gastric route is preferred.

Secondary survey/definitive therapy

Detailed clinical examination and referral for specialist treatment follows resuscitation.

- **Head and face:** inspect for lacerations, haematomas, depressed fractures, eye and orbit injury and mobile mid-face or mandible segments. Clinical features of basal skull fracture include racoon eyes, bruising over the mastoids (Battle's sign), subhyaloid haemorrhage, haemotympanum and CSF rhinorrhoea or otorrhoea. Head injury is discussed in Chapter 53.

- **Chest:** life-threatening tracheobronchial injuries, pulmonary or cardiac contusions and aortic, oesophageal or diaphragmatic ruptures must be detected and treated (Chapter 54).

- **Abdomen:** concealed intra-abdominal bleeding or viscus perforation should be suspected if shock persists despite fluid replacement. Associated abdominal bruising, lacerations, tenderness and distention are frequently detected. Rectal examination reveals bleeding after bowel injury, a high prostate suggests urethral injury and reduced perianal sensation and sphincter tone occurs in spinal injury. Abdominal ultrasound, CT scan, diagnostic peritoneal lavage and rarely laparotomy may be required if examination is unreliable in unconscious, ventilated or persistently hypotensive patients.

- **Peripheral trauma:** long-bone fractures are associated with occult haemorrhage and neurovascular injuries which must be detected and treated. Crush injuries may cause compartment syndromes requiring decompressive fasciotomy. Associated rhabdomyolysis causes hypovolaemia, hyperkalaemia and renal failure unless preventative measures are instituted (Chapters 38, 39).

- **Spinal injury:** occurs in ~3% of major trauma victims (Fig. b). Most injuries occur in the cervical region (~50%). The commonest sites are $C_{5/6}$, $C_{6/7}$ and T_{12}/L_1.

Examination Carefully log-roll the patient to allow palpation of the spine for tenderness and 'step-off' deformity (Fig. d). Neurological assessment is vital, particularly motor and sensory function below suspected cord lesions, which has prognostic implications.

Investigations Cervical (i.e. lateral anteroposterior and open mouth views), thoracic and lumbar spine X-rays are essential although injury may occur *without radiographic abnormality*. CT scans assess injured regions not clearly visualized on X-ray. MRI scans detect ligament and cord damage.

Management Aims to prevent secondary cord damage by immobilization and spinal cord ischaemia with resuscitation.

- **Spinal stability** – disruption of the posterior ligamentous complex produces an unstable spine. Early referral for fixation is advocated by many specialist centres. Potentially unstable cervical fractures (Fig. d) may require stabilization with a halo frame.

- **Respiration** – cord lesions above C_4 inhibit diaphragmatic function and always require ventilatory support. Intercostal muscles are innervated by T_2–T_{12}. Patients with lesions above this level depend on diaphragmatic breathing with reduced tidal volumes and impaired cough.

- **Circulation** – following immediate hyperstimulation and hypertension, subsequent loss of sympathetic control in cord lesions above T_{1-6}, limits the cardiovascular stress response causing bradycardia, peripheral vasodilation, hypotension and neurogenic shock (Chapter 6). Unopposed vagal activity (e.g. after bronchial suctioning) can cause profound bradycardia.

- **Neurology** – spinal shock describes muscle flaccidity and areflexia following spinal injury. It lasts for 2–70 days and muscle contractures and spasms may follow resolution. Autonomic dysreflexia occurs with cord injuries above T_7 (~65%). Stimulation below the level of the lesion (e.g. bladder distention) causes a sympathetic reflex with flushing, sweating, hypertension and bradycardia that can precipitate seizures or strokes. **Early steroids** may improve neurological outcome.

- **General factors** include hypothermia due to vasodilation, thromboprophylaxis, paralytic ileus and bladder atony requiring catheterization. Meticulous nursing avoids pressure sores.

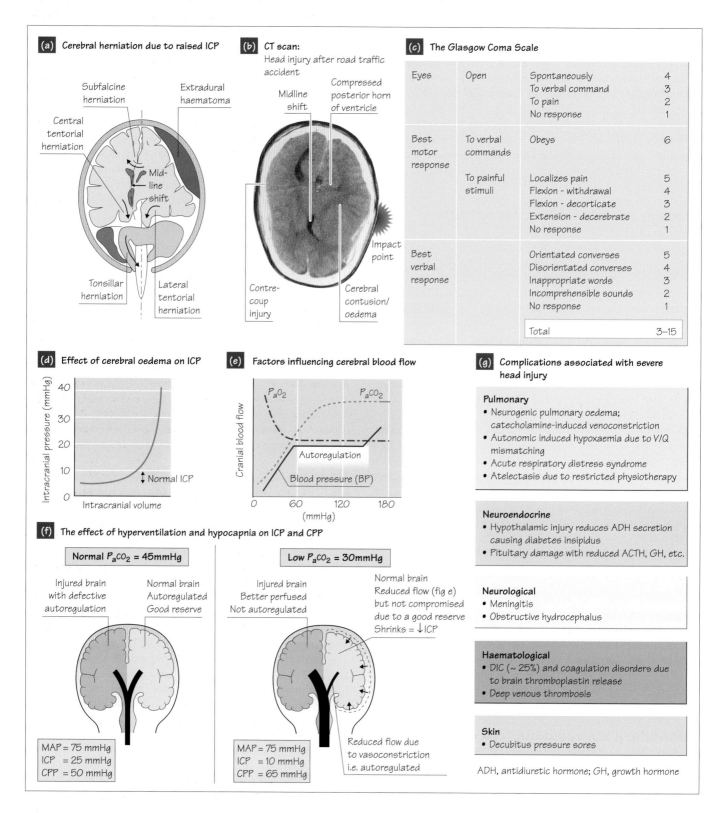

(a) Cerebral herniation due to raised ICP

- Subfalcine herniation
- Extradural haematoma
- Central tentorial herniation
- Mid-line shift
- Tonsillar herniation
- Lateral tentorial herniation

(b) CT scan: Head injury after road traffic accident

- Midline shift
- Compressed posterior horn of ventricle
- Contre-coup injury
- Cerebral contusion/oedema
- Impact point

(c) The Glasgow Coma Scale

Eyes	Open	Spontaneously	4
		To verbal command	3
		To pain	2
		No response	1
Best motor response	To verbal commands	Obeys	6
	To painful stimuli	Localizes pain	5
		Flexion - withdrawal	4
		Flexion - decorticate	3
		Extension - decerebrate	2
		No response	1
Best verbal response		Orientated converses	5
		Disorientated converses	4
		Inappropriate words	3
		Incomprehensible sounds	2
		No response	1
		Total	3–15

(d) Effect of cerebral oedema on ICP

Intracranial pressure (mmHg) vs Intracranial volume. Normal ICP indicated.

(e) Factors influencing cerebral blood flow

Cranial blood flow vs Blood pressure (BP) (mmHg). P_aO_2, P_aCO_2, Autoregulation.

(f) The effect of hyperventilation and hypocapnia on ICP and CPP

Normal P_aCO_2 = 45mmHg

- Injured brain with defective autoregulation
- Normal brain Autoregulated Good reserve

MAP = 75 mmHg
ICP = 25 mmHg
CPP = 50 mmHg

Low P_aCO_2 = 30mmHg

- Injured brain Better perfused Not autoregulated
- Normal brain Reduced flow (fig e) but not compromised due to a good reserve Shrinks = ↓ICP
- Reduced flow due to vasoconstriction i.e. autoregulated

MAP = 75 mmHg
ICP = 10 mmHg
CPP = 65 mmHg

(g) Complications associated with severe head injury

Pulmonary
- Neurogenic pulmonary oedema; catecholamine-induced venoconstriction
- Autonomic induced hypoxaemia due to V/Q mismatching
- Acute respiratory distress syndrome
- Atelectasis due to restricted physiotherapy

Neuroendocrine
- Hypothalamic injury reduces ADH secretion causing diabetes insipidus
- Pituitary damage with reduced ACTH, GH, etc.

Neurological
- Meningitis
- Obstructive hydrocephalus

Haematological
- DIC (~ 25%) and coagulation disorders due to brain thromboplastin release
- Deep venous thrombosis

Skin
- Decubitus pressure sores

ADH, antidiuretic hormone; GH, growth hormone

Head injury accounts for ~33% of trauma deaths. Road traffic accidents, falls, assaults and gunshot wounds account for most serious head injuries. Two mechanisms cause neural tissue damage:

1 Primary injury: sustained during trauma and includes brain lacerations, contusions and diffuse axonal injury due to shear forces during acceleration or deceleration. It is irreversible.

2 Secondary injury (Figs a, b): due to **raised intracranial pressure (ICP)** and **inadequate cerebral perfusion**. It accounts for ~50% of deaths. Preventive therapy may improve outcome. Causes are:

- **Intracranial** including cerebral oedema, hydrocephalus, space occupying lesions (SOL; e.g. extradural haemorrhage), cerebral ischaemia (e.g. vasospasm, seizures) and inflammatory mediators.
- **Systemic** including hypotension, hypoxia, anaemia, hyper-/hypoglycaemia, hyper-/hypocapnia and hyperthermia.

Pathophysiology

The skull is a fixed volume containing brain, blood and CSF. Initially cerebral oedema (±SOL) displaces blood and CSF with little effect on the ICP (~5–10 mmHg). Further swelling rapidly raises ICP (Fig. d). After trauma, ICP peaks at ~72 hours and may cause cerebral herniation (Fig. a). Increased ICP (e.g. >25 mmHg) reflects the severity of brain injury but reduced **cerebral perfusion pressure** (CPP), which is the difference between mean arterial pressure (MAP) and ICP, is more important, as this impairs cerebral blood flow (CBF) causing ischaemia. Therapy aims to maintain a normal CPP (>60 mmHg) as neuronal failure and death occur at <40 and <20 mmHg respectively.

Normally CBF is independent of BP (i.e. autoregulated) but is sensitive to P_aO_2 and P_aCO_2 (Fig. e). In injured brain autoregulation fails and perfusion directly parallels CPP.

- **Hypoxia or hypercapnia:** dilates normal vessels and diverts blood flow away from damaged cerebral tissue. The associated increase in cerebral blood volume (CBV) raises ICP, reduces CPP and CBF and further aggravates ischaemia in damaged brain tissue.
- **Hypocapnia** (Fig. f): constricts normal vessels, reducing CBV and ICP. This increases CPP and improves CBF. In addition, vasoconstriction in normal tissue and failure of autoregulation in damaged tissue divert blood flow to injured brain relieving ischaemia. Unfortunately, raised CPP eventually increases oedema and ICP in damaged brain and excess vasoconstriction may cause ischaemia in normal tissue. Consequently a low-normal P_aCO_2 (~35–40 mmHg) is currently recommended.

Immediate management

(i) **Prompt resuscitation.** Supplemental oxygen corrects hypoxaemia, ventilatory support prevents hypercapnia and fluid resuscitation and antiarrhythmics maintain BP, haemodynamic stability and CPP. (ii) **Spinal immobilization.** Assume all head-injured patients have spinal injuries. (iii) **Airways protection** in obtunded patients. Manual in-line cervical stabilization is required during intubation (Chapter 52). (iv) **Detect other injuries:** ~50% have potentially lethal thoracic or abdominal injuries. (v) **Sedation (±paralysis).** Prevents ICP elevation and spinal injury in agitated patients.

Assessment

The **Glasgow Coma Score** (GCS) is a prognostic, reproducible method of assessing patient responsiveness (Fig. c). Severe head injury is defined as a GCS ≤ 8; post-resuscitation GCS ≤ 8 within 48 hours of injury; or any intracranial contusion, haematoma or laceration.

- **Physical examination:** detects head wounds and spinal cord damage. Basilar skull fractures are recognized as CSF rhinorrhoea, blood behind the tympanic membrane, 'racoon eyes' or bruising behind the ears (Battle's sign). Papilloedema indicates raised ICP. Neurological examination is essential.
- **Radiographic evaluation:** includes skull radiographs and/or CT scan (Fig. b). Immediate CT scan is indicated during coma or for deteriorating consciousness, GCS ≤ 8, GCS 9–13 with skull fractures, or planned surgery. Intracranial haematoma is 10-fold more common following skull fractures.
- **Monitoring:** GCS is adequate in mild injuries. Severe head injury may require **ICP monitoring** using extradural, subarachnoid space or direct brain tissue (e.g. Camino bolt) pressure transducers. Infection risks and inaccuracy limit use. **Cerebral oxygen saturation** (S_jO_2) is measured using a jugular venous bulb fibreoptic catheter. $S_jO_2 < 55\%$ suggests inadequate CBF. **Blood sugar** (BS) is monitored and occasionally **EEG**.

Management

Management aims to prevent secondary cerebral damage.

- **General measures:** optimize CBF (i.e. MAP > 70 mmHg, ICP < 15–20 mmHg, CPP > 60 mmHg) and oxygenation (i.e. $P_aO_2 > 90\%$, $S_jO_2 > 55\%$).
- **Reduce ICP:** treatment options are: (i) **hyperventilation** (P_aO_2 25–30 mmHg) which rapidly (~30 seconds) reduces ICP (~25%) but is not recommended routinely (see above); (ii) **loop diuretics** (e.g. furosemide (frusemide)) **and osmotic agents** (e.g. mannitol) effectively but transiently (~6–8 hours) reduce ICP which may prevent cerebral herniation. Mannitol increases intravascular osmotic pressure and resulting fluid shifts reduce brain cell volume and ICP; (iii) **improved venous drainage.** Hard collars, neck flexion and tracheostomy ties can impede venous drainage and increase ICP. Drainage is optimum with midline head position and 15–30° elevation. Suctioning, physiotherapy and PEEP increase venous pressure; and (iv) **ventriculostomy drainage/decompressive surgery** is considered if other methods fail. CSF drainage is particularly useful in obstructive hydrocephalus. **Steroids** do not reduce ICP or improve outcome.
- **Reduce cerebral metabolism:** therapeutic strategies include: (i) **tight glycaemic control** (BS 4–7 mmol/L). Improves outcome by reducing cerebral lactate production associated with hyperglycaemia; (ii) **prophylactic anticonvulsants.** Prevent seizures that complicate ~10–40% of severe head injuries; (iii) **sedation and paralysis.** Decreases agitation and metabolism. Propofol may be neuroprotective. Barbiturates (e.g. thiopentone) reduce cerebral metabolic demand but cause haemodynamic instability. Benzodiazepines are a good alternative; and (iv) **antipyretics and cooling.** Prevent hyperthermia which damages injured brain. Moderate hypothermia (33–34 °C) may be neuro-protective.
- **Treat complications** associated with head injury (Fig. g). Avoid nasogastric tubes in basilar skull fractures and treat signs of meningitis with antibiotics.

Prognosis

Road safety measures (e.g. seat belts, helmets, drink-driving legislation) have reduced head injury related deaths. Nevertheless, in the USA, ~50,000 severely head injured patients (GCS ≤ 8) die before reaching hospital and ~50,000 after hospital admission. Of survivors with an initial GSC ≤ 8, ~33% never regain independent function, whereas ~66% are largely self-reliant.

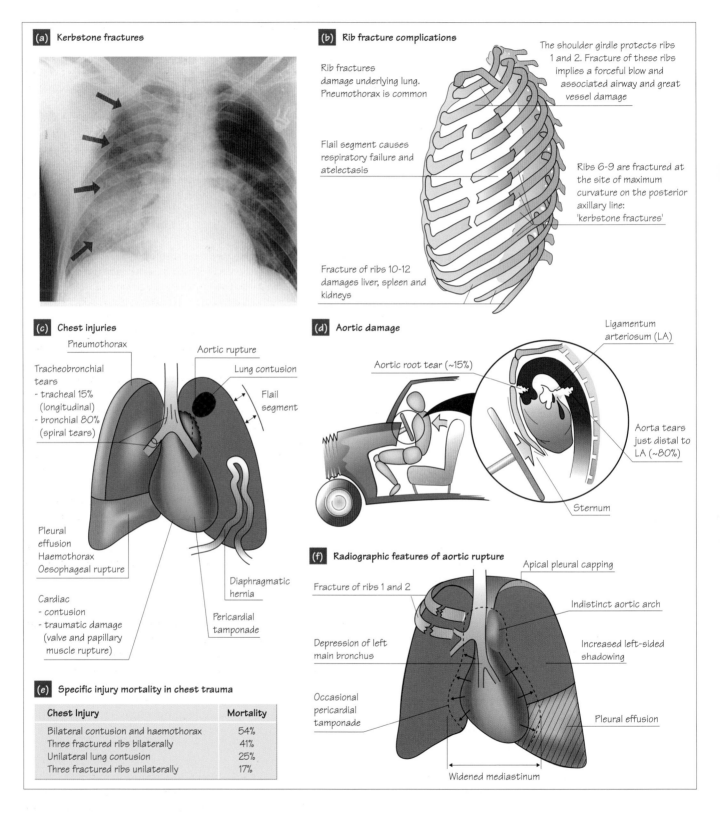

(a) Kerbstone fractures

(b) Rib fracture complications

Rib fractures damage underlying lung. Pneumothorax is common

The shoulder girdle protects ribs 1 and 2. Fracture of these ribs implies a forceful blow and associated airway and great vessel damage

Flail segment causes respiratory failure and atelectasis

Ribs 6-9 are fractured at the site of maximum curvature on the posterior axillary line: 'kerbstone fractures'

Fracture of ribs 10-12 damages liver, spleen and kidneys

(c) Chest injuries

Pneumothorax

Aortic rupture

Lung contusion

Tracheobronchial tears
- tracheal 15% (longitudinal)
- bronchial 80% (spiral tears)

Flail segment

Pleural effusion
Haemothorax
Oesophageal rupture

Diaphragmatic hernia

Cardiac
- contusion
- traumatic damage (valve and papillary muscle rupture)

Pericardial tamponade

(d) Aortic damage

Ligamentum arteriosum (LA)

Aortic root tear (~15%)

Aorta tears just distal to LA (~80%)

Sternum

(f) Radiographic features of aortic rupture

Apical pleural capping

Fracture of ribs 1 and 2

Indistinct aortic arch

Depression of left main bronchus

Increased left-sided shadowing

Occasional pericardial tamponade

Pleural effusion

Widened mediastinum

(e) Specific injury mortality in chest trauma

Chest Injury	Mortality
Bilateral contusion and haemothorax	54%
Three fractured ribs bilaterally	41%
Unilateral lung contusion	25%
Three fractured ribs unilaterally	17%

Chest trauma may be penetrating or blunt and is often associated with multiple trauma (Chapters 52, 53). Treatment of accompanying hypoxaemia, hypercapnia and hypotension prevents secondary organ damage (Chapters 6, 12). Ongoing management aims to anticipate complications and detect missed injuries.

Penetrating chest trauma

• **Stab (e.g. knife) and low velocity gunshot wounds:** cause haemopneumothorax. Simple chest drainage is effective therapy in most cases. Indications for thoracotomy include transmediastinal injury, cardiac tamponade and >1.5–2 L initial blood loss from the chest drains or >200–250 ml drainage/h indicating ongoing bleeding.

• **High velocity gunshot wounds:** cause extensive cavitation and tissue injury due to kinetic energy release. Early surgery is required to control haemorrhage or air leaks, evacuate blood clots and remove damaged lung. Air embolism may complicate any parenchymal lung damage but is more common in high velocity gunshot wounds and during mechanical ventilation (MV). It is suspected if neurological (e.g. CVA) or cardiac (e.g. arrhythmias) complications develop.

Blunt chest trauma

Non-penetrating blunt chest trauma is relatively common. There may be few external clinical signs apart from bruising. A high index of suspicion is required to avoid delayed diagnosis of serious internal injury (Fig. e).

Three mechanisms cause intrathoracic injury:

1 Rib fractures (Figs a and b): damage underlying structures (e.g. pneumothorax, haemothorax, lung contusion) and cause severe pain with splinting, hypoventilation and atelectasis. Older patients are most frequently affected. In young patients chest wall flexibility causes intrathoracic damage without rib fractures. Treatment involves chest drainage, physiotherapy, nerve blocks and potent opioid (± epidural) analgesia.

2 Increased intrathoracic pressure: abrupt elevation of intracavitary pressures may rupture air- or fluid-filled structures. Alveolar, oesophageal and diaphragmatic rupture cause pneumothorax, mediastinitis and herniation of abdominal structures into thoracic cavity respectively (Fig. c).

3 Shear stress: intrathoracic structures are tethered to adjacent tissues. The shear forces produced by differential organ motion cause visceral or vascular tears including aortic rupture (Fig. d), tracheobronchial disruption and pulmonary haematoma.

Specific injuries

Lung, tracheobronchial and diaphragmatic injuries

(Fig. e)

• **Pneumothorax/haemothorax:** are common and require drainage (Chapter 36).

• **Pulmonary contusions:** present as ill defined infiltrates at the site of trauma on CXR. Haemoptysis and hypoxaemia are due to localized bleeding, oedema and associated V/Q mismatch.

• **Flail chest:** occurs when multiple fractures, usually at two sites, result in a 'free' section of chest wall or sternum. 'Paradoxical' movement of the flail segment (i.e. moves in during inspiration and out during expiration) causes hypoventilation and atelectasis in the underlying lung. Discomfort also impedes ventilation, cough and secretion clearance and requires effective analgesia. Thoracic epidural is the most effective technique. If respiratory failure develops, MV (± tracheostomy) may be required for ~7–14 days to restore normal inspiratory/expiratory movement of the flail segment. External chest wall stabilization (e.g fixation, taping) is of no benefit.

• **Tracheobronchial tears:** must be suspected after fracture of the first and second ribs, with bilateral pneumothoraces, haemoptysis, mediastinal/subcutaneous emphysema and persistent air leaks. Typically longitudinal tears occur in the posterior membranous portion of the lower trachea (~15%) and spiral tears in the main bronchi (~80%). Bronchoscopy confirms the diagnosis and early surgical repair prevents atelectasis, infection and late development of bronchial stenosis (± bronchiectasis). Occasionally a main bronchus is completely severed. The 'drop' lung is easily recognized and surgical repair is associated with no long-term complications.

• **Diaphragmatic injuries:** occur in ~7%, mostly on the left (~80%) as the right diaphragm is protected by the liver. Mortality is high because of associated splenic or hepatic rupture.

• **Lung torsion** (i.e. rotation on the hilar axis): is rare.

Heart and great vessel injuries

• **Cardiac contusion:** causes local oedema and microvascular haemorrhage at the site of cardiac impact resulting in myocardial ischaemia, arrhythmias, heart block and ventricular failure. Cardiac enzymes, ECG, echocardiography and occasionally angiography or myocardial perfusion scans establish the diagnosis. Treatment is non-specific including management of arrhythmias and circulatory failure (Chapters 7, 27, 28).

• **Aortic tears and dissection:** due to shear stresses associated with abrupt deceleration accidents (Fig. d). Most cases are fatal at the scene of the accident. Clinically there may be no evidence of external trauma and rib fractures are not always present. Tears are most common just distal to *ligamentum arteriosum* (~80%). Aortic root tears (~15%) occasionally damage the valve or coronary arteries. Figure (f) illustrates CXR features of aortic rupture. Aortography or contrast CT scans confirm the diagnosis.

• **Pericardial tamponade:** may be due to aortic root disruption, coronary artery laceration or rupture of the free ventricular wall. It usually requires surgical drainage.

• **Traumatic damage:** may involve the heart, valves (aortic ~60%, mitral ~30%) or papillary muscles. Transmural rupture is rapidly fatal in >80% of cases. Early surgery is often required

Other injuries

• **Oesophageal rupture:** suspected when haematemesis or subcutaneous emphysema occurs with post-traumatic pleural effusion, pneumothorax or mediastinitis. Aspirated pleural fluid may reveal food particles and a raised amylase. A gastrografin swallow confirms the diagnosis whereas endoscopy and CT scans are often unhelpful. Mortality is high without immediate surgical repair.

• **Fat embolism syndrome:** occurs 1–72 hours after multiple longbone or pelvic fractures. Lipases liberate unsaturated fatty acids which cause lung toxicity and coagulopathy (e.g. DIC). Small fat emboli also pass through pulmonary capillaries to occlude retinal, skin and CNS vessels. The characteristic clinical triad includes **confusion, pulmonary dysfunction** (e.g. cough, dyspnoea, pleurisy, ARDS) and a **petechial skin rash** over the upper torso. Investigations reveal hypoxaemia, a normal early CXR and lipase and fat globules in urine and serum.

55 Acute abdominal emergencies

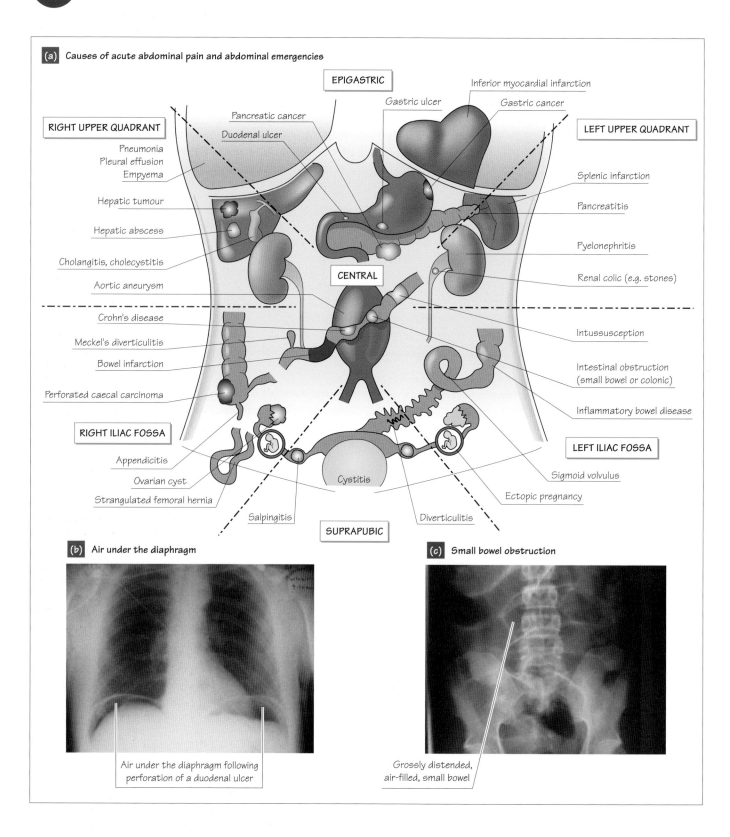

(a) Causes of acute abdominal pain and abdominal emergencies

EPIGASTRIC

Inferior myocardial infarction

Gastric ulcer

Gastric cancer

RIGHT UPPER QUADRANT

Pancreatic cancer

Duodenal ulcer

LEFT UPPER QUADRANT

Pneumonia
Pleural effusion
Empyema

Hepatic tumour

Hepatic abscess

Cholangitis, cholecystitis

Aortic aneurysm

Splenic infarction

Pancreatitis

Pyelonephritis

Renal colic (e.g. stones)

CENTRAL

Crohn's disease

Meckel's diverticulitis

Bowel infarction

Perforated caecal carcinoma

Intussusception

Intestinal obstruction
(small bowel or colonic)

Inflammatory bowel disease

RIGHT ILIAC FOSSA

Appendicitis

Ovarian cyst

Strangulated femoral hernia

LEFT ILIAC FOSSA

Sigmoid volvulus

Ectopic pregnancy

Cystitis

Salpingitis

Diverticulitis

SUPRAPUBIC

(b) Air under the diaphragm

Air under the diaphragm following
perforation of a duodenal ulcer

(c) Small bowel obstruction

Grossly distended,
air-filled, small bowel

Acute and Critical Care Medicine at a Glance, 2e. By R. Leach. Published 2009 by Blackwell Publishing. ISBN 978-1-4051-6139-8.

In the acute setting, abdominal emergencies (Fig. a) rarely present with typical symptoms and signs, as characteristic features (e.g. peritonitis) are masked by coma, spinal injury or drugs (e.g. analgesics). Relatively minor features including diarrhoea, vague discomfort or feeding intolerance may be the only indicators of pathology. Early diagnosis requires a high index of suspicion, vital sign monitoring (e.g. temperature, BP), repeated examination and timely investigation (e.g. amylase). CT scans provide the best images but USSs are portable and readily detect liver, renal and pelvic disease. If surgery is likely to be required, limit analgesia, withhold feeding and involve the surgeons early. Always exclude non-abdominal pathology (e.g. inferior MI causes epigastric pain). Peritonitis, bacteraemia and subsequent multiple organ failure complicate many abdominal emergencies (Chapter 22).

Peptic ulceration and perforation

Duodenal (5–10%) rather than gastric (<1%) ulcers are most likely to perforate and there may be no previous history of peptic ulcer disease. Perforation occurs at any age but is most common in 20- to 40-year-old patients. It usually presents with sudden, severe mid-abdominal pain. Patients appear ill, lie still and take shallow breaths to minimize pain. Examination reveals a rigid, 'board-like' abdomen and absent bowel sounds. Elderly or critically ill patients, and those on steroids or NSAIDs, may not exhibit peritonitis. An erect chest radiograph (Fig. b) or left lateral decubitus view of the abdomen detects free air in the abdominal cavity (~80%).

Management includes fluid resuscitation, antibiotics and naso-gastric (NG) tube drainage. In unstable patients duodenal ulcers are oversewn whereas resection and vagotomy is performed in stable patients. Whenever possible, gastric ulcers are resected because of associated cancer risk.

Small bowel obstruction (SBO)

SBO may be simple or associated with vascular compromise (e.g. volvulus). It presents with nausea, vomiting, cramping abdominal pain and distension. Initially, bowel sounds are high pitched ('tinkling') but become infrequent with prolonged obstruction. Adhesions from previous surgery cause ~75% of SBO; and incarcerated hernias, malignancy and volvulus ~25%. Intussusception, gallstones and inflammatory bowel disease (IBD) are less common. Upright or decubitus abdominal radiographs (AXR) demonstrate dilated small bowel (>3 cm) with or without air/fluid levels (Fig. c). It is often difficult to distinguish between prolonged post-surgical ileus and SBO.

Management involves fluid/electrolyte resuscitation and gastric decompression with NG tube suction. **Surgery** is indicated if symptoms persist or the clinical condition fails to improve after 24–48 hours.

Large bowel obstruction

Colonic obstruction (± perforation) usually affects the elderly. It presents with acute abdominal pain, vomiting (~50%), constipation (~50%) and distension. Colonic cancer, diverticular disease, sigmoid volvulus and faecal impaction are common causes. Electrolyte imbalance, myxoedema, anticholinergic drugs and medical debility cause pseudo-obstruction (i.e. ileus rather than a mechanical barrier) with colonic dilation (± caecal perforation). Toxic megacolon (± perforation) occurs in severe ulcerative colitis. Plain AXRs showing colonic distension, volvulus and sub-diaphragmatic air are often diagnostic. A caecal diameter >9 cm suggests imminent perforation.

Management includes stopping sedative or narcotic drugs, fluid/electrolyte correction and colonic decompression by rectal tube or colonoscopy. **Surgery:** imminent caecal perforation requires decompressive caecostomy. A limited right hemicolectomy, ileostomy and mucous fistula are recommended after perforation.

Acute bowel ischaemia (ABI)

Mesenteric ischaemia affects the elderly with heart and vascular disease. Mortality is ~70%. Superior mesenteric artery (SMA) occlusion causes ~50% of ABI. It presents with severe abdominal pain, leucocytosis but few physical signs. Inferior mesenteric artery (IMA) thrombosis causes ~25% of ABI and presentation may be subtle. Proximal SMA or IMA occlusion is usually due to atherosclerosis and presentation may be acute or gradual (i.e. with pain after meals). Embolic occlusion occurs with atrial fibrillation or post-MI mural thrombosis. Less common causes of occlusive ischaemia include vasculitis and mesenteric venous thrombosis. Non-occlusive ABI due to hypotension, cardiac failure or vasopressor drugs is increasingly recognized. Initially, ABI produces mucosal injury with bleeding and/or bloody diarrhoea (~50%). Mucosal sloughing, bowel necrosis, perforation, peritonitis, sepsis, shock and death follow. Refractory metabolic (lactic) acidosis with hyperkalaemia is characteristic.

Management includes fluid resuscitation, electrolyte correction and antibiotics. In selected cases angiography confirms the diagnosis, allows vasodilator infusion (e.g. nitroglycerin) and may aid surgical revascularisation. **Surgery** initially resects gangrenous bowel. Re-exploration at 24–36 hours allows demarcation and further resection of non-viable tissue. Unfortunately, delayed diagnosis or extensive infarction often renders the situation hopeless.

Cholecystitis and cholangitis

Gallstone obstruction of the cystic duct causes ~90% of cholecystitis and cholangitis. Acalculous cholecystitis is common in seriously ill patients due to cholestasis or biliary reflux but is often unrecognized as the cause of associated sepsis. The classical triad of fever, rigors and right upper quadrant (RUQ) pain occurs in ~70%. Vomiting, RUQ mass (~20%) and elevated WCC (~70%), bilirubin, alkaline phosphatase and amylase (without pancreatitis) are also typical. Ultrasonography and CT scans demonstrate biliary tract dilation due to gallstones. A distended gallbladder (>5 cm), thickened wall (>3 mm), sediment and pericholecystic fluid collections suggest acalculous cholecystitis. Common infective organisms are *E. coli*, *Klebsiella*, *Streptococcus faecalis* and anaerobes.

Management: includes resuscitation, analgesics, broad-spectrum antibiotics and, until the patient is stable, T-tube drainage of the biliary tract. Cholecystectomy may be required later. Percutaneous drainage is an option in high risk patients but can cause potentially lethal bile peritonitis.

Other acute abdominal emergencies

Pancreatitis (Chapter 44), ruptured or leaking aortic aneurysms, pelvic disease in females (e.g. pelvic inflammatory disease, ectopic pregnancy, ovarian torsion), appendicitis, retroperitoneal haematoma (e.g. renal trauma) and renal calculi may all present as acute abdominal emergencies.

(a) Causes of maternal deaths

Medical condition	Rate/million pregnancies	Deaths/year in UK
Thromboembolism	21.8	~48
Intracranial bleeding (e.g. SAH)	10.9	~25
Pregnancy-induced hypertension	9.1	~20
Amniotic fluid embolism	7.7	~17
Obstetric haemorrhage (e.g. APH)	5.5	~12
Eclampsia/HELLP syndrome	0.1	~1

(b) Features used to define pre-eclampsia and severe pre-eclampsia (American College of Obstetricians and Gynecologists)

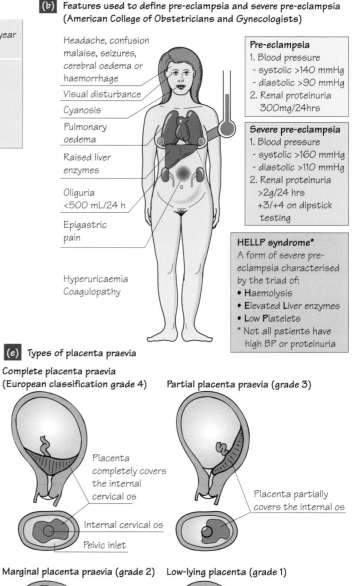

Headache, confusion malaise, seizures, cerebral oedema or haemorrhage

Visual disturbance

Cyanosis

Pulmonary oedema

Raised liver enzymes

Oliguria <500 mL/24 h

Epigastric pain

Hyperuricaemia
Coagulopathy

Pre-eclampsia
1. Blood pressure
   - systolic >140 mmHg
   - diastolic >90 mmHg
2. Renal proteinuria 300mg/24hrs

Severe pre-eclampsia
1. Blood pressure
   - systolic >160 mmHg
   - diastolic >110 mmHg
2. Renal proteinuria >2g/24 hrs +3/+4 on dipstick testing

HELLP syndrome*
A form of severe pre-eclampsia characterised by the triad of:
• Haemolysis
• Elevated Liver enzymes
• Low Platelets
* Not all patients have high BP or proteinuria

(c) Amniotic fluid embolism

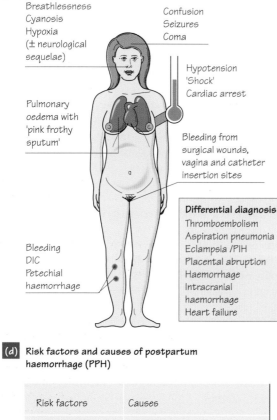

Breathlessness
Cyanosis
Hypoxia
(± neurological sequelae)

Confusion
Seizures
Coma

Hypotension
'Shock'
Cardiac arrest

Pulmonary oedema with 'pink frothy sputum'

Bleeding from surgical wounds, vagina and catheter insertion sites

Bleeding
DIC
Petechial haemorrhage

Differential diagnosis
Thromboembolism
Aspiration pneumonia
Eclampsia /PIH
Placental abruption
Haemorrhage
Intracranial haemorrhage
Heart failure

(e) Types of placenta praevia

Complete placenta praevia (European classification grade 4)

Placenta completely covers the internal cervical os

Internal cervical os

Pelvic inlet

Partial placenta praevia (grade 3)

Placenta partially covers the internal os

Marginal placenta praevia (grade 2)

Placental edge reaches but does not cross the internal os

Low-lying placenta (grade 1)

Lower edge of placenta reaches into the lower uterine segment and within 2 cm of internal os but does not cover it

2 cm range from internal cervical os

(d) Risk factors and causes of postpartum haemorrhage (PPH)

Risk factors	Causes
Placenta praevia	Retained products of conception
Placental abruption	Uterine atony
Pre-eclampsia	Trauma
HELLP syndrome	Uterine rupture
Operative delivery	Bi rth canal lacerations
Caesarian section	DIC
Previous PPH	Bleeding diathesis
Obesity	
Chorioamnionitis	

Life-threatening obstetric emergencies occur antepartum and postpartum. In the developed world, maternal and foetal mortality has decreased but avoidable deaths continue to occur. Figure (a) reports the main causes and associated death rates.

Pre-eclampsia or pregnancy-induced hypertension (PIH)

PIH is defined as 'gestational hypertension with proteinuria developing during pregnancy or labour'. It affects ~2–10% of pregnancies, usually at 32–38 weeks' gestation and resolves 2–3 days after delivery. Figure (b) illustrates the features that define pre-eclampsia and severe PIH. Eclampsia is diagnosed if grand mal convulsions occur. The main causes of maternal death are cerebral or pulmonary oedema, intracranial haemorrhage and liver damage.

Management aims to control BP, prevent seizures (± end-organ damage) and maintain uterine perfusion (i.e. nurse in a semi-lateral position); but only delivery is curative. Monitor urine output, proteinuria, liver function, platelet count and urate.
- **Antihypertensive therapy** (e.g. nifedipine, labetalol): aims to reduce BP without impairing uterine perfusion.
- **Fluid balance:** difficult as pulmonary oedema is a risk despite intravascular depletion and CVP is unreliable. Initially give crystalloid at ~75–100 ml/h. Consider invasive monitoring if oliguria persists.
- **Magnesium sulphate:** the drug of choice to prevent (± treat) convulsions in PIH due to its CNS depressant, cerebral vasodilator and mild antihypertensive actions. In overdose it causes muscle weakness, respiratory paralysis and heart block but can be inhibited by calcium gluconate.
- **Early foetal delivery:** may be required. If the pregnancy is <34 weeks, dexamethasone aids foetal lung maturation with best results if delivery can be delayed for 48 hours.

Amniotic fluid embolism (AFE)

AFE causes 5–10% of maternal deaths and affects 1 in 20–80 000 pregnancies. It occurs when amniotic fluid (±foetal matter, meconium) enters the maternal circulation. Figure (c) illustrates the clinical features. Classically AFE presents with severe dyspnoea, cyanosis and hypotension (±cardiac arrest) in older, multiparous mothers with large babies during oxytocin driven labour. However it can occur throughout pregnancy (e.g. amniocentesis, termination, membrane rupture). Initial survivors develop seizures (~20%), DIC with bleeding (~40%) and pulmonary oedema (~75%). Management is symptomatic (e.g. oxygen) and supportive (e.g. ventilation). Mortality can be >80% with ~50% dying within the first hour.

Severe obstetric haemorrhage (SOH)

Peripartum haemorrhage causes 15% (25% if ectopic pregnancies included) of maternal deaths. Blood loss >40% is life-threatening and requires prompt resuscitation with fluids, blood and clotting factors (Chapters 6, 8, 49). Compression of the aorta against the vertebral column (pressure above the umbilicus) allows time to institute therapy. Obstetric intervention depends on the cause.

Antepartum haemorrhage (APH)

Bleeding from the birth canal after >20 weeks of pregnancy puts the foetus at risk. The main causes are placental abruption (~25%), placenta praevia (~20%), uterine rupture and placental abnormalities (e.g. vasa praevia). Ultrasound scan determines the cause.
- **Placental abruption (PA)** occurs when a normally implanted placenta separates from the uterine wall. Precipitating factors include hypertension, trauma or sudden changes in uterine size but usually there is no obvious cause. It affects ~1.5% of pregnancies and is more common in smokers and older, multiparous women. Perinatal mortality is high (~50%). Bleeding may be concealed or revealed and with increasing placental separation there is abdominal pain and tenderness. Retroplacental bleeding >500 ml can cause foetal death and >1 L results in serious maternal sequelae with shock and DIC.
- **Placenta praevia (PP)** affects ~1% of pregnancies. It is due to placental encroachment on the lower uterine segment (LUS); the more severe, the higher maternal mortality (Fig e). The LUS endometrium is less-well developed and placental attachment to underlying muscle (PP accreta) impairs separation during third stage delivery. It classically presents with painless vaginal bleeding in late pregnancy. Significant APH may require hospitalization in later pregnancy but management is conservative to allow foetal maturation. Delivery by caesarian section (CS) is usually required.

Primary postpartum haemorrhage (PPH)

This refers to >500 ml blood loss within 24 hours of delivery. It is severe if >1 L/24 h. Risk factors and causes are listed in Fig. (d).
- **Retained products of conception (RPC)** complicate 4% of deliveries and require uterine evacuation. Severe haemorrhage may entail embolization, iliac artery ligation or hysterectomy.
- **Uterine rupture** affects multiparous women with foetal malpresentations, operative trauma, breech delivery, PP accreta or oxytocic use.
- **Uterine atony** may be due to drugs (e.g. beta-blockers), uterine sepsis, bladder distension, multiparity or long labour but is uncommon since the advent of oxytocic drugs. Treatments include uterine massage, bimanual compression, oxytocin, uterine packing or intramyometrial prostaglandin.
- **Coagulation defects** follow PA, PIH, AFE, intrauterine death or sepsis.

Secondary PPH

Secondary PPH describes severe bleeding >24 hours post-partum until the end of the puerperium. It is often due to infected RPC and treated with antibiotics.

Sheehan's syndrome is panhypopituitarism following pituitary hypoperfusion during SOH. Failure of lactation and amenorrhoea are early features. Adrenal and thyroid gland failure follow (Chapter 41).

Medical emergencies in pregnancy

Cardiac arrest affects 1 in 30 000 pregnancies. Advanced life support (ALS) guidelines are followed (Chapter 5). Early intubation prevents hypoxaemia due to diaphragmatic splinting and increased oxygen consumption. Chest compressions are performed with a wedge below the right hip or manual uterine displacement to prevent caval compression which impairs venous return. Immediate foetal delivery by CS is required if resuscitation is unsuccessful. ALS is continued until after delivery. Gastric compression makes aspiration a risk.

Pulmonary thromboembolism (PE; Chapter 30) causes ~20% of maternal deaths and affects ~1 in 2000 pregnancies. Caval compression by the gravid uterus and pregnancy-induced hypercoagulability predispose to antepartum lower limb and pelvic vein thrombosis. Mobilization after delivery may precipitate PE. LMWH is the treatment and prophylaxis of choice.

Intracranial bleeds cause ~10% of maternal deaths and are primary or due to subarachnoid haemorrhage.

57 Burns, toxic inhalation and electrical injuries

(a) Classification of burns

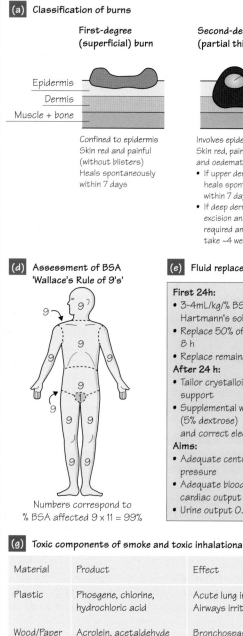

First-degree (superficial) burn

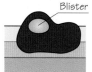

Epidermis
Dermis
Muscle + bone

Confined to epidermis
Skin red and painful (without blisters)
Heals spontaneously within 7 days

Second-degree (partial thickness) burn

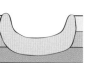

Blister

Involves epidermis + dermis
Skin red, painful, blistered and oedematous
- If upper dermis involved heals spontaneously within 7 days
- If deep dermis affected, excision and grafting required and healing may take ~4 weeks

Third-degree (full thickness) burn

Destroys all layers of skin + some underlying tissue (Fourth-degree burn involves muscle and bone)

Burn is white (or charred), painless (anaesthetic), indurated and firm.

Even after skin grafting there is functional limitation and scarring

(b) Criteria for hospital admission

Second-degree burn (SDB) >20-25% BSA
Third-degree burn (TDB) >5-10% BSA
Any SDB or TDB if >60 or <5 years old
Hand, feet, face, eye or perineal burns
Burns affecting major joints
Circumferential burns
Inhalational or airways burn injury
Chemical or electrical burns

(c) Symptoms in carbon monoxide poisoning

CO-Hb level	Symptoms
<15%	None
15-20%	Headache, confusion
20-40%	Disorientation, nausea, visual impairment
40-60%	Hallucinations, coma, shock
>60%	Death

(d) Assessment of BSA 'Wallace's Rule of 9's'

Numbers correspond to % BSA affected 9 x 11 = 99%

(e) Fluid replacement

First 24h:
- 3-4mL/kg/% BSA burn of Hartmann's solution
- Replace 50% of deficit in first 8 h
- Replace remainder over 16 h

After 24 h:
- Tailor crystalloid / colloid support
- Supplemental water (5% dextrose) and correct electrolytes

Aims:
- Adequate central venous pressure
- Adequate blood pressure + cardiac output
- Urine output 0.5-1.0mL/kg/h

(f) Burns complications and treatment

Complications

Fever + hypermetabolism
Corneal burns
Laryngeal oedema + airways obstruction
Bronchospasm
Toxic inhalation
Pneumonitis
Pneumonia/sepsis
ARDS
Pancreatitis
Acute gastric ulcers ± bleeding
Paralytic ileus
Acute renal failure
Perineal burns
Circumferential burns
Albumin-rich fluid loss
Bruising, bleeding, DIC

Treatment

Aggressive nutritional support
Protective tarsorrhaphy
Chloramphenicol ointment
100% oxygen
Nebulized adrenaline
Early intubation
Bronchodilators
Oxygen ± IPPV
Antibiotics
Histamine antagonists
Sucralfate
Nasogastric tube
i.v. fluids
Renal replacement therapy
Catheterization
Escharotomy to prevent limb ischaemia/ restricted ventilation
Colloid fluid replacement after 24 h
Correction of coagulation LMW heparin

ARDS = acute respiratory distress syndrome;
IPPV = intermittent positive pressure ventilation;
LMW = low molecular weight

(g) Toxic components of smoke and toxic inhalational injury

Material	Product	Effect
Plastic	Phosgene, chlorine, hydrochloric acid	Acute lung injury Airways irritation
Wood/Paper	Acrolein, acetaldehyde Formaldehyde, acetic acid	Bronchospasm, airways irritation, mucosal sloughing
Synthetic materials (e.g. nylon)	Nitrogen oxides (e.g. NO_2) Hydrogen cyanide	Cyanide poisoning, tissue hypoxia, pulmonary oedema
All the above	Carbon monoxide	Tissue hypoxia (see Fig. c)

 Acute and Critical Care Medicine at a Glance, 2e. By R. Leach. Published 2009 by Blackwell Publishing. ISBN 978-1-4051-6139-8.

In the UK, serious burns account for ~10 000 admissions/yr and ~500 die. Mortality is decreasing, largely due to management in specialized units, and patients may survive burns to >80% of body surface area (BSA). Burns are classified (Fig. a) by the skin layers affected, appearance and healing, as **first degree** (superficial), **second degree** (partial thickness) or **third degree** (full thickness) burns.

Assessment of burns

- **Depth:** determines healing time, scarring and appropriate therapy (e.g. grafting). The important decision is whether a burn is full or partial thickness (Fig. a). It is difficult even when experienced.
- **Size:** estimated from the 'rule of nines' in adults (Fig. d). It aids assessment of fluid loss and inflammatory response.
- **Cause:** may be dry (e.g. flame), moist (e.g. hot liquids), blast, electrical or chemical.
- **Time:** replace fluid from the time of the burn, not admission.
- **Site affected:** face (e.g. eyelids), perineum, hands, feet and circumferential burns require specialist attention.
- **Smoke inhalation** (e.g. in enclosed spaces): increases mortality.

Management of major burns

Figure (b) indicates the criteria for hospital admission and/or referral to specialist burns centres. Figure (f) illustrates complications of burns injury.

1 Resuscitation: burns activate the inflammatory cascade causing vasodilation and increased vascular permeability. Fluid shifts (i.e. intravascular to extravascular) and exudative loss from burns causes hypovolaemia (±shock). Burns >15% BSA (>10% with smoke inhalation) require immediate fluid replacement to maintain organ function and preserve viable skin tissue by restoring perfusion.

- **First 24 hours** – crystalloid-only regimes are usually used. Neither colloid nor hypertonic solutions improve outcome. The Parkland formula recommends 4 ml/kg/%BSA burn/day, of Hartmann's solution, with 50% given in the first 8 hours (Fig. e). However, formulae are only guidelines and fluid replacement should also be guided by clinical response (e.g. urine output). Excessive fluid can be harmful; but only specialists should use hypertonic solutions to reduce tissue oedema.
- **After 24 hours** – sodium requirements and vessel permeability decrease. Low sodium solutions and colloids are used to maintain circulating volume and electrolyte balance.
- **Vasoactive agents** – may be required (e.g. sepsis), but avoid α-adrenergic agonists (e.g. norepinephrine (noradrenaline)) which decrease blood flow to injured skin.

2 Airway complications: often cause early death. Facial or neck burns, oropharyngeal swelling, cough, carbonaceous sputum, respiratory distress or stridor suggest smoke inhalation and upper airways damage. Hyperventilation and hypercapnia due to increased metabolism may also cause respiratory failure.

- **Airways obstruction** – hot gases (e.g. steam) and toxic chemicals in smoke cause rapid upper airways obstruction. Early intubation is recommended with second or third degree facial burns, as it may be impossible later due to oedema. If intubation is not required, monitor pulmonary function tests and give humidified oxygen and nebulized bronchodilators (± ephedrine). Steroids do not reduce oedema and increase infection risks.
- **Toxic inhalational injury (TII)** – highly soluble gases (e.g. SO_2, Cl) dissolve in upper airway secretions forming potent acids which cause mucosal inflammation, ulceration and bronchospasm (Fig. g). Low solubility toxins (e.g. NO_2, phosgene) penetrate to the lower respiratory tract causing alveolar damage, pulmonary oedema and V/Q mismatch. In severe TII, mucosa sloughs at ~72 hours and requires 7–14 days to regenerate. Secondary infection and pneumonitis are common.
- **Carbon monoxide (CO) poisoning** causes 75% of fire deaths. Affinity of CO for Hb is ~250 times that of oxygen. Low CO concentrations (e.g. 0.1%) readily displace oxygen to produce non-functional carboxyhaemoglobin (CO-Hb). Symptoms of CO poisoning are those of tissue hypoxia and correlate with CO-Hb levels (Fig. c). Co-oximeters with multiwavelength spectroscopy differentiate between CO-Hb and oxyhaemoglobin; pulse oximeters cannot do this and record inappropriately high saturations. Treatment with 100% oxygen decreases Hb-CO half-life from 240 to 40 minutes and is continued until the CO-Hb is <10%. Hyperbaric oxygen therapy reduces neuropsychiatric sequelae if CO-Hb levels are >30% but practical issues usually outweigh benefits.
- **Cyanide (CN) poisoning** causes histotoxic hypoxia. In smoke inhalation, lactic acid levels correlate with CN levels. Mild poisoning is treated with oxygen and inhaled amyl nitrite, more severe poisoning with sodium thiosulphite (i.e. speeds metabolism) or hydroxycobalamin (i.e. forms inactive complexes).

3 Metabolism and nutrition: increased basal metabolic rate, reflected by fever (~38.5 °C) and hypercapnia, peaks at ~7 days and is proportional to burn size and associated infection. High environmental temperatures (e.g. ~32 °C ± high humidity) reduce heat and water loss and calorie expenditure. Start early enteral feeding and calculate the high calorie requirements from burn size. Prophylaxis (e.g. ranitidine) reduces stress ulceration.

4 Burn wound care and skin grafts: initially cover burns with saline gauze (± clingfilm). Partial thickness burns are protected with biological or synthetic (e.g. Duoderm) dressing. Early excision and split-skin grafting of full thickness burns improves survival and decreases infection, pain and healing time. Transplant or biosynthetic skins can be used for burns >60% BSA. Topical antibiotics (e.g. silver sulphadiazine) reduce early staphylococcal and later pseudomonal colonization.

5 Infection: the commonest cause of death following severe burns due to skin barrier loss, reduced immunity or pulmonary sepsis after TII. Isolation, microbiological surveillance, early sepsis detection and judicious antibiotic use improve outcome.

6 Analgesia: initially intravenous opioids (e.g. morphine) are required. Ketamine provides good analgesia for dressing changes when combined with a benzodiazepine. Drug levels are monitored due to altered renal and hepatic clearance.

7 Complications (Fig. f): circumferential contraction of neck, chest or limb burns can cause life-threatening ventilatory impairment or distal limb ischaemia requiring immediate escharotomies.

Chemical and electrical burns

- **Chemical burns:** copiously irrigate with water and then treat like thermal burns. In acid or alkali burns avoid neutralizing solutions as exothermic reactions may cause further thermal damage.
- **Electrical burns** (e.g. lightning, high voltage): produce extensive internal tissue damage and rhabdomyolysis with little external evidence of injury. Exit wounds (e.g. hands, feet) are often overlooked. Monitor for arrhythmias and myocardial injury.

Case studies and questions

Case 1

A 68-year-old woman with a history of type II diabetes mellitus, nephropathy and mild renal impairment (creatinine ~130 μmol/L) and recurrent urinary tract infections is admitted to the accident and emergency (A+E) department as an emergency. She has a 24-hour history of fever, dysuria and urinary frequency and her husband reports that she has become progressively more confused during the hours prior to hospital admission. At admission she is obtunded, flushed, febrile (38.5 °C), tachycardic (heart rate 140/min), tachypnoeic (respiratory rate 30/min) and hypotensive with a BP of 90/50 mmHg and a dilated, hyperdynamic (bounding) circulation. She is tender suprapubically but examination is otherwise unremarkable. A central line is inserted and a 250-ml fluid challenge is given. The central venous pressure (CVP) response is measured (Fig. a).

1 *What initial investigations would you perform?*
2 *How would you resuscitate this patient and what is the relevance of the fluid challenges in Fig. (a) and the later response in Fig. (b)?*
3 *When would you start antibiotic therapy?*

Case 1

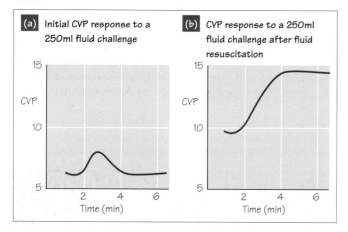

This patient is given 4 L of normal saline during her 2 hours in the A+E department which partially restores her BP to 105/60 mmHg, however following transfer to HDU her blood pressure falls to 80/40 mmHg and urine output falls to <20 ml/h. Further investigation reveals a haemoglobin of 100 g/L, P_aO_2 13 kPa, S_aO_2 98%, $S_{cv}O_2$ 65%, lactate 4 mmol/l and creatinine 190 μmol/L. Her cardiac output by thermodilution measurement is 8.5 L/min and she has a dilated circulation with a low systemic vascular resistance. Despite a further 2 L of gelofusin the BP remains low but a repeat 250-ml fluid challenge produces the response in Fig. (b).

4 *How would you maintain the blood pressure in this patient and what other therapies would you consider?*
5 *What is the oxygen delivery in this patient at the time of admission to HDU and why is the lactate raised?*
6 *The patient is found to have a persisting acidosis and a low urine output despite restoration of normal BP following recovery. How can this be explained?*

Case 2

Four men have been admitted to the HDU with progressive breathlessness and all four have an initial arterial P_aO_2 of 6.6 kPa when breathing air. The first patient is grossly obese and is complaining of a sore throat and an upper respiratory tract infection but has a normal CXR. Investigation has excluded pulmonary embolism. The second patient with non-specific interstitial pneumonitis has a reduced gas transfer (i.e. mainly diffusion defect), is *on* treatment with steroids and has developed a mild lower respiratory tract infection. The third patient has a true right to left shunt due to a longstanding atrial septal defect and apart from a slightly enlarged heart has a normal CXR. The fourth patient, a welder who inhaled NO_2 whilst at work, has developed acute lung injury with widespread alveolar shadowing on CXR. Each patient is to be treated with oxygen. You are the attending physician.

1 *Why is each patient hypoxaemic and what will happen when the F_iO_2 is raised to 1.0 (i.e. 100% oxygen therapy)? Precise answers cannot be calculated but assume reasonable values for unknown data.*
2 *How will you ensure improved oxygenation in each patient?*

Case 3

A 55-year-old man who is normally healthy but slightly overweight, smokes 15 cigarettes a day and has untreated borderline hypertension presents to the accident and emergency (A+E) department with severe epigastric and lower chest pain, nausea, vomiting and profuse sweating. He is currently breathless and reports dizziness. He has been having recurrent indigestion over the last 2 weeks, usually whilst walking to work but lasting for increasingly long periods before settling spontaneously. Over the last 2 days he has experienced similar but increasingly severe pain at rest. He takes regular oral antacids with no relief of the pain. The past medical history and review of systems were unremarkable. In particular, he had no history of peptic ulceration, cholecystitis, pancreatitis or diarrhoea. His father had a myocardial infarction (MI) at 65 years old and his brother suffers with angina. On examination he was in pain, pale and sweaty. He has a heart rate of 55/min and a blood pressure of 95/55 mmHg. The heart sounds were normal. The chest was normal with no crepitations. There was no chest wall tenderness or evidence of calf DVT. Abdominal examination was unremarkable, in particular there was minimal epigastric tenderness, normal bowel sounds and no melaena on rectal examination.

1 *What is the most likely diagnosis and what is your differential diagnosis?*
2 *What will you do immediately?*
3 *Is pain always a feature of this condition?*
4 *What investigations would you perform to establish the diagnosis in this case?*

The initial electrocardiogram (ECG) demonstrates sinus rhythm with Q-waves, T-wave inversion and ST-elevation in leads II, III and aVF. Subsequent ECGs show intermittent Mobitz I second degree heart block (Wenckebach phenomenon). The CXR was normal. Troponin T and cardiac enzymes are raised. An echocardiogram shows inferior left ventricular hypokinesia with a reduced ejection fraction.

5 *How would you treat this patient?*

6 *What are the complications of this condition, does this patient have any and how would you manage them? What is the significance of the hypotension?*

7 *Following recovery from the acute condition, what advice and follow-up management is required?*

Case 4

A 65-year-old man presents with severe wheeze and breathlessness following a minor upper respiratory tract infection. He is a longstanding smoker of 20 cigarettes a day and is known to have moderate COPD (FEV_1 1.2 L, FVC 2.7 L) treated with salbutamol and ipratropium bromide inhalers. In the past he has had a myocardial infarction and has echocardiographic evidence of left ventricular impairment with an ejection fraction of 35–40% requiring treatment with cardioselective beta-blockers, ACE inhibitors and a small dose of diuretic. He has mild ankle oedema and occasional orthopnoea but the review of systems was otherwise unremarkable. He can normally climb two flights of stairs and is a recently retired porter. On examination he is afebrile, breathless, cyanosed and sweaty. His respiratory rate is 28/min. He has a heart rate of 120/min and a blood pressure of 135/90 mmHg. The JVP is slightly raised at 2–3 cm, the heart sounds were inaudible due to wheeze and there was mild ankle oedema. The chest examination reveals poor air entry bilaterally with widespread wheeze and coarse basal crepitations. His haemoglobin was 160 g/L, white cell count 12×10^{-9}/L, urea 8 mmol/L and creatinine 135 µmol/L. Electrolytes, liver function tests, troponin T and d-dimers are all normal. The ECG show changes of an old anterior MI. Arterial blood gases on air are pH 7.29, P_aO_2 7.5 kPa, P_aCO_2 8.5 kPa and HCO_3 34 mmol/L. The chest radiograph shows hyperinflation, a large heart, enlarged hila with infiltrative changes in both lower lobes.

1 *What are the two most likely diagnoses and how would you differentiate between them?*

2 *What is the A–a gradient in this patient and what is its relevance?*

3 *How would you manage this case? In particular discuss oxygen dose, target saturation, ABG frequency, respiratory support and indications for intubation.*

4 *What factors are associated with success or failure of non-invasive ventilation (NIV) and when should NIV be considered to have failed?*

5 *How would you adjust NIV if the P_aCO_2 remained elevated, the P_aO_2 was persistently low or patient ventilator synchronization was poor?*

6 *When would you consider use of continuous positive airways pressure (CPAP) ventilation?*

Case 5

A 58-year-old lady was referred to casualty with a suspected chest infection. Following her return from a holiday in New Zealand 3 weeks previously she had developed a flu-like illness associated with fever, sore throat and cough that had lasted for a week. Initially she appeared to recover but 3 days ago the fever and cough recurred. Over the last 48 hours she had developed increasing breathlessness and deteriorated despite starting antibiotics 24 hours ago. She had no significant past medical history. On arrival in casualty she was unwell and breathless with a temperature of 37.9 °C, heart rate 120 beats/min, BP 110/65 mmHg, respiratory rate 31/min and S_aO_2 85% on air. Chest examination revealed left-sided upper and lower lobe and occasional right-sided basal coarse crepitations but there was no wheeze. The white cell count was elevated at 15×10^{-9}/L, urea 7.5 mmol/L, creatinine 124 µmol/L and the C-reactive protein (CRP) 94 mg/L at admission rising to 235 mg/L the following day. The P_aO_2 was 6.6 kPa and P_aCO_2 3.2 kPa on air. An ECG was normal and serology for atypical pneumonias (legionella, mycoplasma) was negative. The CXR at admission (Fig. ai) and after 24 hours (Fig. aii) are illustrated. You are the admitting SHO for the HDU and are reviewing the patient in casualty.

Case 5(a) CXR at admission (i) and after 24 hours (ii)

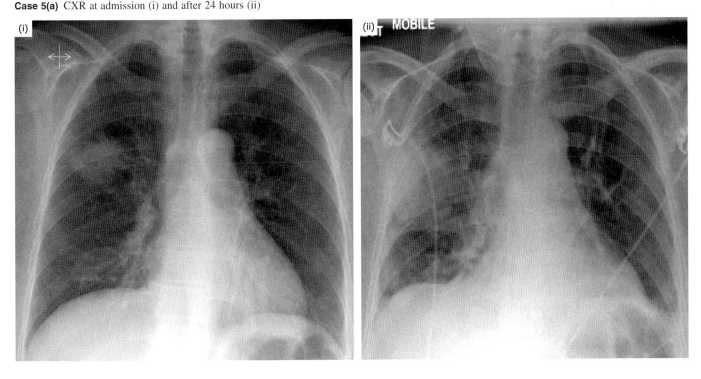

1 *What is the most likely diagnosis and would you admit this patient to HDU?*

2 *What was the admission A–a gradient in this patient?*

3 *How would you manage this patient and what immediate treatment would you recommend?*

On arrival in HDU the S_aO_2 is 95% on 60% oxygen therapy but desaturates to 75% when the mask is removed. Overnight she has episodes of confusion and the on-call doctor diagnoses an acute confusional state secondary to pneumonia and treats her with small doses of haloperidol. Overnight the confusion resolves and the patient appears to recover. Over the next 48 hours the patient deteriorates with persisting breathlessness, tachycardia, 'grumbling' fever and hypoxaemia. The nurses report further episodes of confusion and difficulty maintaining S_aO_2 > 90% and P_aO_2 > 8 kPa despite high dose oxygen.

4 *Is this patient's severe hypoxaemia consistent with pneumonia and how could this be explained?*

5 *What investigations will help establish the diagnosis?*

6 *In what other ways can this condition present?*

7 *What immediate treatment would you recommend?*

Case 5(b) CT scan

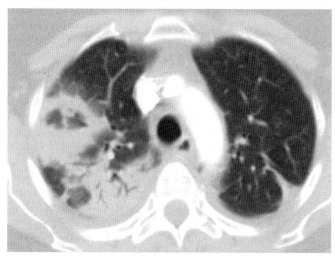

Immediately after her CT scan (Fig. b) the patient deteriorates. She is cold, clammy, cyanosed and confused. The pulse is 'thready', she is hypotensive (BP 90/40 mmHg) and the jugular venous pressure is raised. She is intubated and transferred to ICU. After initial stabilisation, her S_aO_2 is 95% on 100% oxygen, $S_{cv}O_2$ is 65% (right atrial blood sample) and her haemoglobin is 100 g/L. On air the S_aO_2 is 70% and her S_vO_2 40%. Shortly after admission to ICU she suddenly arrests.

8 *What is the degree of venous admixture (V/Q mismatch) and true shunt in this patient following ICU admission?*

9 *What is the likely cause of the arrest and what immediate management would you institute whilst awaiting the arrest team?*

10 *Would you consider thrombolytic therapy in this patient?*

Case 6

Two young boys (~16 years old) are found collapsed outside a night club at 3.00am in the morning. Both have lacerations to their foreheads, have been drinking alcohol and are confused, agitated and unresponsive except to painful stimuli. On arrival in accident and emergency both are tachycardic (120 beats/min), have blood pressures of 95/50 mmHg and are breathing through unobstructed airways. The first has a respiratory rate of 15 breaths/min, the second 35 breaths/min. Neither has any means of identification.

1 *What test would you perform immediately in both patients?*

2 *In the first patient the result of this test is low. How would you treat him?*

3 *In the second patient the result of this test is high. Why is he hyperventilating and what additional tests would you perform to confirm the diagnosis?*

4 *Having established the diagnosis how would you treat the second patient and in particular what 'pitfalls of management' would you be sure to avoid?*

5 *What are the likely precipitating causes in both patients and what additional tests might you perform?*

6 *What other causes of unconsciousness should be considered in these boys?*

Case studies answers

Case 1: Sepsis with shock

1 Investigation aims to identify the source and cause of the infection (Chapter 22). Routine blood tests, C-reactive protein, coagulation profile, arterial blood gases (ABG), dipstick urinalysis, ECG and CXR should all be performed at admission. Tests that the **sepsis guidelines** recommend but which are often forgotten include plasma lactate and central venous (superior vena cava/right atrial) S_aO_2 ($S_{cv}O_2$, e.g. from an internal jugular vein central line), which are measures of global oxygen delivery (Chapter 4). Appropriate cultures including blood, sputum, urine, CSF and wound pus *must* be taken before starting antibiotics providing this does not delay therapy. At least two blood cultures (≥1 drawn percutaneously and one through each vascular access device >48 hours old) are required. Specific investigations including lumbar puncture, ultrasonography and CT scans depend on the likely cause and the patient's condition. In this case urine dipstick testing revealed haematuria and an elevated nitrite level and a mid-stream urine examination confirmed an *E. coli* infection.

2 Fluid resuscitation is started *immediately* in patients with hypoperfusion (i.e. lactate >4 mmol/L, raised $S_{cv}O_2$) or hypotension. At the time of admission to HDU, the small unstained CVP response to the fluid challenge (Fig. a, p. 122) confirms that the patient is still hypovolaemic (Chapter 4). The sepsis guidelines (Chapter 22) recommend crystalloid (1 L) or colloid (0.5 L) fluid challenges aiming to achieve a CVP ≥ 8 mmHg (≥12 if ventilated); MAP ≥ 65 mmHg; urine output ≥0.5 ml/kg/h; and $S_{cv}O_2 \geq 70\%$. If the target $S_{cv}O_2$ is not achieved, consider packed red cell transfusion to a haemocrit $\geq30\%$ or a dobutamine infusion (max 20 µg/kg/min) to increase oxygen delivery and hence $S_{cv}O_2$. Reduce fluid administration if CVP increases without haemodynamic improvement. In this case the sustained increase in the CVP to a fluid challenge in Fig. (b) (p. 122) suggests that the heart is operating at optimal (or even hypervolaemic) filling pressures and is unlikely to benefit from further fluid administration.

3 Antibiotic therapy is started as early as possible in severe sepsis and always within the first hour. It is initially *empiric* using broad-spectrum agents active against the most likely causative pathogens and depends on the clinical features, whether community- or hospital-acquired, the site of primary infection and local antibiotic resistance patterns. Combination therapy is recommended in neutropenic patients and those infected with *Pseudomonas*. Ongoing therapy is modified according to microbiology results and unnecessary antibiotics stopped.

4 In early sepsis widespread vasodilation (i.e. low SVR) causes hypotension and relative hypovolaemia that may respond to fluid administration alone. However, once optimal cardiac filling pressures have been achieved (Fig. b) further fluid resuscitation risks pulmonary oedema. At this stage norepinephrine (noradrenaline), a vasopressor agent with α-receptor agonist properties, increases SVR and BP. In late sepsis, as toxic myocarditis impairs cardiac contractility, an inotropic agent like dobutamine, often used in combination with norepinephrine, increases both cardiac output and BP (Chapter 10). If hypotension is refractory to fluid and vasopressor support, the possibility of relative adrenocortical insufficiency should be considered. In these patients low dose steroid therapy (i.e. hydrocortisone 8 mg/h) can be beneficial. In septic shock activated protein C may improve outcome by modifying microcirculatory thrombosis and preventing organ ischaemia.

5 Oxygen delivery (DO_2; Chapter 4) is calculated from:

(i) $DO_2 = QT \times C_aO_2 = \text{normally} \sim 1000\,\text{ml/min}$

where: QT = cardiac output; C_aO_2 = arterial oxygen content.

(ii) $C_aO_2 = [\text{Hb} \times S_aO_2 \times k + (P_aO_2 \times 0.023)] = \text{normally} \sim 200\,\text{mlO}_2/\text{L}$

where: Hb = haemoglobin (g/L); k = coefficient of Hb oxygen binding capacity (1.36 ml O_2/g Hb); $P_aO_2 \times 0.023$ = oxygen dissolved in plasma.

In this case

(i) $C_aO_2 = 100 \times 0.98 \times 1.36 + (13 \times 0.023) = 133.5\,\text{ml O}_2/\text{L}$

(ii) $DO_2 = 8.5 \times 133.5 = 1135\,\text{ml/min}$

Although the DO_2 is greater than normal in this patient at 1135 ml/min, the hypotension, relative hypovolaemia and associated inappropriate distribution of cardiac output can cause regional (i.e. splanchnic, renal, skeletal) ischaemia resulting in raised lactate and in some cases low $S_{cv}O_2$. Inadequate hepatic lactate clearance in liver dysfunction or failure of oxygen utilization due to mitochondrial dysfunction in sepsis are also causes of a raised lactate.

6 This patient was initially resuscitated with large volumes of normal saline to correct sepsis-induced hypotension. She has previous chronic renal impairment due to diabetic nephropathy and a degree of 'hypotension-induced pre-renal' acute kidney injury (Chapter 38) indicated by the reduced urine output and the increasing creatinine (190 µmol/L) on this occasion. A litre of normal saline contains 154 mmol NaCl or 308 (154 mmol Na^+ + 154 mmol Cl^-) mosmol of solute; so 4 L of normal saline will contain 1232 mosmol of solute. Normal kidneys can achieve a maximum urine concentration of 1000 mosmol/L but much less in renal impairment (i.e. 500 mosmol/L). Consequently this large solute load (e.g. sodium, chloride) would be difficult to excrete (Chapters 8, 9), particularly with the reduced urine production. This causes hyperchloraemic acidosis (HCA) due to the high chloride (Cl^-) level and may have explained the persisting acidosis in this case. In this situation, the preferred fluid is a physiologically balanced solution (PBS) with low Cl^- content like Hartmann's. This is inexpensive and compared with normal saline causes less HCA and associated nausea, confusion and oliguria.

Case 2: Oxygenation and oxygen therapy Patient 1

1 This patient has a mild upper respiratory tract infection and no significant low respiratory tract pathology. However he is probably hypoventilating due to gross obesity restricting normal respiratory movement. Assuming his gas transfer and V/Q matching are normal, his P_aCO_2 can be calculated from the alveolar gas equation (Chapter 11):

$P_AO_2 = P_IO_2 - (1.25 \times P_aCO_2)$

where: $P_IO_2 = F_IO_2 \times$ (barometric − water vapour pressure) = $P_IO_2 = 0.21 \times (101 - 6.2) = 19.9$ kPa breathing air

Note: $1.25 \times P_aCO_2$ is a simplified expression of P_aCO_2/R where R is the respiratory quotient ($V_{CO2}/V_{O2} = \sim0.75$)

In this case P_aCO_2 must be 10.6 kPa if P_aO_2 is 6.6 kPa on air (and thus P_AO_2 6.6 kPa):

i.e. $P_AO_2 = 6.6 = 19.9 - (P_aCO_2 \times 1.25)$ thus $P_aCO_2 = 10.6$ kPa.

Therefore this patient has Type 2 respiratory failure with a raised P_aCO_2 (Chapter 12).

On 100% O_2 (F_iO_2 1.0):

$P_iO_2 = F_iO_2 \times$ (barometric pressure – water vapour pressure)
$\qquad = 1 \times (101 - 6.2)$
$\qquad = 95\,kPa.$

$P_AO_2 = P_iO_2 - (1.25 \times P_aCO_2)$
$P_AO_2 = 95 - (1.25 \times 10.6) = 95 - 13 = 82\,kPa$

Thus P_aO_2 will be about 81 kPa.

2 This patient has Type 2 respiratory failure (i.e. hypoxaemia drives ventilation not P_aCO_2). As P_aO_2 rises with increasing oxygen therapy, the drive to breath decreases and P_aCO_2 increases causing progressive respiratory acidosis, confusion, coma and death. Consequently this patient should be managed with low dose (24–28%) oxygen therapy aiming for a saturation of 88–92% and regular measurement of arterial blood gases (Chapters 12, 34). The optimal treatment to improve both oxygenation and to reduce hypercarbia in this patient would be non-invasive ventilation which would improve ventilation and alveolar gas exchange (Chapter 14).

Patient 2

1 This patient has a diffusion defect due to the interstitial lung disease (ILD) although usually there is a significant contribution of ventilation/perfusion (V/Q) mismatch to the hypoxaemia in these patients. The substantial increase in alveolar partial pressure ($P_AO_2 = P_iO_2 - (1.25 \times P_aCO_2)$; $P_AO_2 = 95 - (1.25 \times 4) = 90\,kPa$) when this patient is given 100% oxygen (F_iO_2 1.0) will more than overcome the partial diffusion defect associated with the ILD, and if this were a pure diffusion defect the P_aO_2 would approach 90 kPa. Even allowing for a wider than normal range of V/Q ratios in this patient, there would still be a substantial increase in P_aO_2 on 100% oxygen.

2 In this patient simply increasing the inspired oxygen concentration (F_iO_2 ~0.4–0.6) will correct the hypoxaemia. This patient probably has Type 1 respiratory failure because carbon dioxide (CO_2) diffuses twenty times better than oxygen and consequently the diffusion defect does not impair CO_2 clearance. The hypoxaemia will cause hyperventilation and the associated increase in minute ventilation ensures a low P_aCO_2 ($P_aCO_2 \propto 1$/alveolar ventilation). Consequently there is little risk of hypercapnia during use of high oxygen concentrations in this patient.

Patient 3

1 This patient is hypoxaemic due true right to left shunting causing admixture of venous blood to systemic blood. As in the second case the P_AO_2 will be 90 kPa with an F_iO_2 1.0. However the saturation is already 100% in oxygenated blood passing through the lungs and oxygen content will not be substantially increased by the high P_AO_2 apart from the small quantity of oxygen dissolved in blood (90×0.023 ml). The blood shunted from right to left through the atrial septal defect remains unaffected by the increased P_AO_2 and acts as venous admixture lowering oxygenation in the systemic circulation. Consequently, an F_iO_2 of 1.0 only fractionally increases systemic P_aO_2 perhaps to ~7.5 kPa in this case.

2 Only patient 3 will not show a substantial increase in P_aO_2 when given 100% O_2. In this case oxygenation will only be improved by decreasing the shunt fraction and reducing left-sided venous admixture. Figure (a) illustrates the effect of true shunt on the response to increasing F_iO_2.

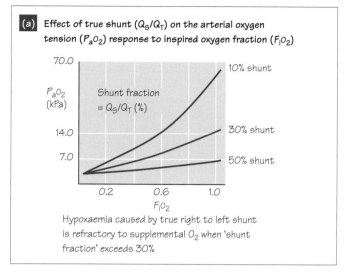

(a) Effect of true shunt (Q_S/Q_T) on the arterial oxygen tension (P_aO_2) response to inspired oxygen fraction (F_iO_2)

Hypoxaemia caused by true right to left shunt is refractory to supplemental O_2 when 'shunt fraction' exceeds 30%

Patient 4

1 This patient has acute lung injury with alveolar oedema due to alveolar epithelial damage and atelectasis due to loss of surfactant. A wider than normal range of V/Q ratios will be present throughout the lungs and the resulting V/Q mismatch causes hypoxaemia. Nevertheless the F_iO_2 of 1.0 will ensure a sufficiently high P_AO_2 even in low V/Q units to substantially increase P_aO_2. However, true shunt and units with a very low V/Q ratio cause hypoxaemia that is resistant to correction with increased F_iO_2.

2 In this patient an increase in inspired oxygen concentration (F_iO_2 ~0.4–0.6) will improve arterial oxygenation. However, there are a number of other strategies that may improve oxygenation in this case. Firstly, non-invasive ventilation with continuous positive airways pressure (CPAP; Chapter 14) will reinflate collapsed (atelectatic) alveoli, reducing V/Q mismatch which improves oxygenation. Secondly, reducing alveolar oedema by avoiding excessive fluid administration (± gentle diuresis, ± lowering pulmonary circulation hydrostatic pressure) will improve alveolar ventilation, reduce V/Q match and increase arterial oxygenation. Thirdly, prone positioning may improve oxygenation in severe acute lung injury because oedema and perfusion are greatest in dependent lung. Turning the patient prone ensures perfusion of ventilated non-dependent lung which is now dependent (Chapter 35). Finally inhaled nitric oxide dilates capillaries supplying ventilated alveoli (but not unventilated alveoli), tending to improve V/Q matching. However although nitric oxide improves oxygenation in the short term it can form toxic oxygen radicals which may eventually cause further damage to alveolar epithelium with increasing alveolar oedema. There is no evidence that nitric oxide improves outcome in severe acute lung injury (Chapter 35).

Case 3: Inferior myocardial infarction (MI)

1 The sudden onset of severe pain, nausea, bradycardia, reduced cardiac output (i.e. pale, sweaty and hypotensive) and absence of melaena and abdominal tenderness suggests that the most likely cause of this patient's symptoms is cardiac. Although the pain is epigastric (i.e. referred abdominal discomfort), this is often the case with inferior myocardial ischaemia and may be misinterpreted as abdominal pathology. The patient is a smoker with borderline hypertension and a family history of ischaemic heart disease (IHD) and the most likely diagnosis is myocardial ischaemia or MI. However, other causes of chest or epigastric pain that mimic myocardial ischaemia include reflux oesophagitis, peptic ulceration, oesophageal spasm, cholecystitis, costochondritis, anterior pleurisy, pericarditis and pulmonary embolism. A careful history and examination will often, but not always, differentiate the potential causes and further investigation may be required. In this case, a bleeding peptic ulcer with hypovolaemia and shock should have been considered, although a tachycardia would have been expected. Bradycardia (heart rate 55/min) is a common feature of inferior myocardial ischaemia as the atrioventricular node is usually supplied by the right coronary artery.

2 If a diagnosis of myocardial ischaemia or MI is suspected the patient should be given aspirin 300 mg immediately. Within 15 minutes of chewing a non-enteric aspirin tablet, irreversible cyclo-oxygenase inhibition prevents platelet aggregation, and in unstable angina reduces deaths from MI by 50%. Antiplatelet agents which inhibit glycoprotein IIb/IIIa are useful in patients with aspirin allergy but the onset of action is slow. Ideally the aspirin should be given prior to transfer to hospital.

3 Myocardial ischaemia normally causes 'crushing' or heavy substernal chest pain radiating to the neck and medial aspect of the left arm. However, pain associated with myocardial ischaemia may be atypical (i.e. burning), localized (i.e. jaw, left arm or epigastric only) or completely absent in ~20% of patients (e.g. diabetics). MI is characterized by an abrupt onset of severe, prolonged pain, autonomic symptoms, dyspnoea and anxiety. Angina (i.e. reversible myocardial ischaemia) is usually precipitated by exercise or anxiety, is short-lived and relieved by rest or sublingual nitrates. In this case the indigestion whilst walking to work was suggestive of angina. This was followed by unstable angina which refers to anginal pain occurring at rest, more frequently and for longer periods (>15 minutes). It is characterized by 'altered angina pattern' (i.e. with less exercise), 'a change in the character of previous anginal pain', autonomic manifestations (e.g. nausea, sweating) and radiation to new sites (e.g. jaw, arm). However unstable angina only precedes myocardial infarction in ~25% of cases (Chapters 25, 26).

4 Serial electrocardiograms (ECG) and cardiac enzymes usually establish the diagnosis of myocardial ischaemia. A raised cardiac troponin T (CTT) is particularly useful and confirms MI after surgery or when the ECG is non-specific (i.e. >40% of MI are non-Q wave). In non-MI acute coronary syndromes (e.g. unstable angina) a raised CTT indicates an increased risk of subsequent MI (Chapter 26). A chest radiograph will exclude other causes of chest pain and detect pulmonary oedema due to left ventricular failure following a MI. Echocardiography, although not often required immediately, establishes the degree of cardiac muscle impairment (i.e. ejection fraction) and excludes potential complications (e.g. papillary muscle rupture). The need for immediate angiography and percutaneous coronary angioplasty is discussed below.

5 This patient has had an inferior MI as confirmed by the raised troponin T and the ECG findings in leads II, III and aVF. The development of Mobitz type I, second degree heart block suggests atrioventricular node (AVN) ischaemia.

Immediate management aims to reperfuse ischaemic tissue and minimize MI size, which reduces hospital mortality from 13% to <10%. Initial management includes bed rest, pain relief, cardiac monitoring (~48 hours) and >60% oxygen. Aspirin prevents further platelet aggregation. Opiates (e.g. diamorphine) relieve anxiety and chest pain. They also improve cardiac output and reduce or prevent pulmonary oedema by reducing preload. Sublingual nitrates reduce chest pain and preload but often aggravate hypotension. Early beta-blockade (e.g. bisoprolol) limit infarct size, arrhythmias and mortality but contraindications include asthma, heart failure and bradycardia.

Revascularization with reperfusion of ischaemic myocardium, limits tissue damage and reduces future complications (e.g. heart failure, arrhythmias).

(i) *Percutaneous coronary intervention* (PCI) within ≤90 minutes of presentation is the preferred method of revascularization following MI if the facilities are available. Primary PCI within 6 hours reopens >90% of occluded coronary arteries with few complications and has the best outcomes. Rescue PCI is considered if TT fails but has a relatively high mortality (~40%) if unsuccessful.

(ii) Thrombolytic therapy (TT) clears coronary artery clot and reduces mortality by more than 25% if therapy occurs within 12 hours but is more effective within 3 hours. Reperfusion occurs in 50–75% of cases. TT accelerates conversion of plasminogen to plasmin, an enzyme that attacks fibrin. Consequently it increases the risk of haemorrhage and contraindications (e.g. peptic ulceration/stroke) prevent use in many cases. The thrombolytic agent streptokinase is allergenic and can only be used once. About 2% of patients have reactions (e.g. hypotension, pruritus) with the first use. Tissue plasminogen activator (TPA) is more expensive but only activates plasminogen bound to fibrin (i.e. better targeted at thrombus). If given within 3 hours, it is more effective than streptokinase but surprisingly causes more strokes. TPA is given if streptokinase has been used previously. Intravenous heparin is required for 48–72 hours after TPA because of its short half-life and fibrin specificity.

Angiotensin converting enzyme (ACE) inhibitors, orally, should be started 24 hours after admission and reduce heart failure in high risk patients. Unless contraindicated, prophylactic subcutaneous heparin prevents thromboembolic complications. Prophylactic antiarrhythmic therapy is not recommended but arrhythmias must be treated as required (see heart block below). Inotropic support may be required in patients with cardiogenic shock.

6 Complications after MI include arrhythmias (e.g. atrial fibrillation, ventricular tachycardia), papillary muscle or free wall rupture, pericarditis, cardiac aneurysms and ventricular septal defects. Heart failure can occur when >20% of the left ventricle is damaged and is characterized by breathlessness and pulmonary oedema on CXR. Cardiac auscultation often reveals a fourth heart sound and gallop rhythm. Hypotension (systolic BP < 90 mmHg), particularly with anterior ischaemia, suggests a large MI (i.e. >40% left ventricular damage) and heralds cardiogenic shock and the need for resuscitation (± inotropic support). Prophylactic anticoagulation is required in immobile patients who are at risk of DVT and in patients with large infarcts who are at risk of developing intracardiac thrombus and embolic sequela (e.g. stroke) in areas of akinetic cardiac muscle.

Bradycardia (± heart block) is more frequent after inferior MI. This is because the right coronary artery supplies the AVN and surrounding conducting tissue, as well as the inferior part of the heart. Although bradycardia and heart block are common after inferior MI, they are usually transient and rarely require intervention. By contrast, tachycardia usually accompanies anterior MI, and heart block in these patients suggests a large infarct and requires early pacemaker insertion. In this case, second degree heart block followed the MI. This occurs when some atrial beats are not conducted to the ventricles. *Mobitz 1 AVN block* (Wenkebach) causes progressive p–r interval lengthening, culminating in failure of transmission of an atrial impulse. This sequence is repetitive. Treatment is rarely required. *Mobitz II block* originates below the AVN in the His-Purkinje system. Every second or third atrial impulse initiates ventricular contraction ($2:1$; $3:1$ block). In this situation pacemaker insertion may be required (e.g. following an anterior MI) as symptoms or complete heart block may follow.

7 Risk factors must be reduced following recovery from the initial MI. Hypertension, hypercholesterolaemia and diabetes mellitus are treated and smoking cessation is strongly encouraged. The family history of IHD in this patient suggests the possibility of familial hypercholesterolaemia and cholesterol levels should be checked and followed up in other family members. Patients with IHD should be treated with lipid lowering drugs (e.g. statins) to lower the risk of future ischaemic episodes. Patients with unstable angina or at high risk for MI on exercise testing should be referred for angiography and early revascularization procedures (e.g. angioplasty, surgical coronary artery bypass grafting). Warfarin is administered for 3 months after a large usually anterior MI to prevent mural clot forming on akinetic heart wall and embolizing into the systemic circulation causing strokes or ischaemic legs or bowel. Aspirin should be continued indefinitely but beta-blockers and ACE inhibitors may be discontinued after 6–52 weeks in low risk patients (Chapter 26).

Case 4: COPD and Type 2 respiratory failure

1 Clinically the history and examination suggest an infective exacerbation of COPD with Type 2 respiratory failure. The raised bicarbonate on ABG analysis suggests an acute on chronic increase in P_aCO_2. Peak expiratory flow rate and lung function testing will aid the diagnosis of COPD. However, this patient also has a previous history of left ventricular failure and the clinical features of pulmonary oedema can be surprisingly difficult to differentiate from COPD (Chapter 28). **B-type natriuretic peptide (BNP)** has been particularly useful in detecting heart failure in patients with lung disease particularly when combined with echocardiography (Chapter 28). Most BNP is released from the ventricular myocardium. The serum BNP level, and its breakdown product NT-BNP, increase during myocardial wall stress and major studies demonstrate a high sensitivity (73–99%) and specificity (60–97%) for heart failure. Occasionally, invasive measurements of pulmonary artery wedge pressure and cardiac output may be required to confirm the diagnosis of heart failure (Chapters 3). Alternatively, a trial of therapy (e.g. diuretic) is less invasive and often the most effective means to establish or exclude the presence of pulmonary oedema.

2 The A–a gradient is calculated from the difference between the alveolar oxygen partial pressure and the arterial blood oxygen partial pressure (Chapter 11).

Alveolar oxygen tension (P_AO_2) is calculated from the simplified alveolar gas equation:

$$P_AO_2 = P_IO_2 - (1.25 \times P_aCO_2)$$

where P_IO_2 is the inspired oxygen partial pressure corrected for barometric pressure and water vapour pressure:

$$P_IO_2 = F_IO_2 \times (\text{barometric pressure(kPa)} - \text{water vapour pressure(kPa)})$$

Thus: breathing air:

$$P_IO_2 = 0.21 \times (101 - 6.2) = 19.9\,\text{kPa}$$

Thus:

$$P_AO_2 \,(\textbf{breathing air}) = 19.9 - (1.25 \times 8.5) = 19.9 - 10.63 = 9.3\,\textbf{kPa}$$

The alveolar – arterial oxygen tension difference is

$$P_{(A-a)}O_2 = P_AO_2 - P_aO_2 = 9.3 - 7.5 = 1.8\,\text{kPa}$$

The A–a gradient determines efficiency of gas exchange. By incorporating P_ACO_2 into the alveolar gas equation it is possible to determine when hypoventilation or hypercapnia are the cause of hypoxaemia (i.e.

a high P_ACO_2 lowers P_AO_2). Shunts, V/Q mismatch and diffusion impairment increase the A–a gradient. The normal A–a gradient is ~0.2–0.4 kPa but increases with age and F_IO_2. In this case, although the P_aO_2 is 7.5 kPa, the A–a gradient is only 1.8 kPa, indicating that a large component of the hypoxaemia is due to hypercapnia or hypoventilation rather than V/Q mismatch or shunt and suggests that improving alveolar ventilation (i.e. bronchodilation, use of non-invasive ventilation) is important.

3 In patients with Type 2 respiratory failure, low dose oxygen therapy should be delivered through fixed performance, Venturi masks aiming for a target saturation of 88–92% (Chapters 11, 12). A higher S_aO_2 has no advantages but in chronically hypoxaemic patients dependent on hypoxic ventilatory drive it can instigate hypoventilation, further hypercapnia and respiratory acidosis. Recheck ABG at 1 hour after starting oxygen therapy and at regular intervals whilst on oxygen particularly after oxygen dose changes. In the absence of an air compressor, nebulizers are driven with oxygen but only for 6 minutes to limit the risk of further hypercapnic respiratory failure. Non-invasive ventilation (NIV) should be considered in hypercapnic ($P_aCO_2 > 6\,\text{kPa}$) patients with acidosis (pH < 7.35), especially if the acidosis has persisted for over 30 minutes despite appropriate treatment (Chapter 14). Venturi masks can be changed to nasal cannulae at low flow rates 1–2 L/min when the patient is stable. High dose, aerosolized beta-agonists and anticholinergic bronchodilators and short courses of oral corticosteroids (i.e. 30 mg/day for 10 days) improve symptoms, gas exchange, lung function and aid recovery. Antibiotic therapy is directed at likely organisms (e.g. *H. influenzae*) and adjusted according to microbiological results (Chapter 34). Indications for intubation include a RR > 35/min, $P_IO_2 < 8\,\text{kPa}$ on >50% F_IO_2; $P_aCO_2 > 7.5\,\text{kPa}$, pH < 7.25, decreased conscious level (GCS < 8), inadequate secretion clearance, exhaustion and failure to improve within 1–4 hours with NIV (Chapters 11, 14).

4 Factors associated with successful NIV include a high P_aCO_2, pH 7.3–7.35, improvement in pH, low A–a gradient, reducing P_aCO_2 and respiratory rate within 1 hour of NIV and good conscious level. Factors associated with failure of NIV include pneumonia on CXR, pH < 7.25–7.3, poor nutritional status, impaired consciousness, copious secretions and poor mask fit. Benefit from NIV is usually evident at 1 hour and certainly after 4–6 hours of NIV. The point at which treatment is considered to have failed and should be withdrawn, depends on severity of respiratory failure, patient wishes and whether other factors (e.g. secretions) could be better managed following intubation (Chapter 14).

5 If the P_aCO_2 remains elevated on NIV, the inspiratory positive airways pressure (IPAP) should be increased or expiratory positive airways pressure (EPAP) decreased (Chapter 34), both of which will raise inspiratory pressure support, increasing tidal volume and alveolar minute ventilation with improved CO_2 clearance ($P_aCO_2 \propto 1/\text{alveolar ventilation}$). A persistently low P_aO_2 on NIV can be corrected by raising F_IO_2 or by increasing either IPAP or EPAP, both of which will encourage alveolar recruitment and improve ventilation (Chapter 34). Patient–ventilator synchronization can be optimized by ensuring a good mask fit, adjusting the trigger sensitivity and setting EPAP to overcome auto-PEEP, thus reducing the effort of triggering the ventilator (Chapter 34; Fig d(iii)).

6 CPAP primarily encourages alveolar recruitment, reduces V/Q mismatch and improves oxygenation. Consequently it is most effective in those conditions associated with alveolar atelectasis or oedema including cardiogenic pulmonary oedema and acute lung injury (Chapter 14).

CPAP does not assist inspiration (i.e. ventilation), although by preventing alveolar collapse and by increasing the functional residual capacity it may reduce the work of breathing by making the lungs easier to inflate (i.e. the steep upstroke of the lung pressure–volume relationship). In obstructive sleep apnoea it can prevents upper airways collapse.

Case 5: Community acquired pneumonia and pulmonary embolism

1 On the basis of the past history of an upper respiratory tract infection with subsequent fever, cough, crepitations on chest examination, raised white cell count and CRP and consolidation on the CXR, the most likely diagnosis appears to be community acquired pneumonia (CAP). The relatively normal CXR in comparison to the clinical findings at admission is sometimes seen with atypical pneumonias but this was subsequently excluded in this case. The most likely infecting organism is *Streptococcus pneumoniae*, although secondary staphylococcal chest infections often follow influenza (Chapter 31). On the basis of the vital signs alone the 'Patient at Risk' (PAR) score in this patient is >6 (at least 9), indicating the need for management in a high dependency area (Chapter 1). The CURB-65 score for assessing CAP severity was 2 (respiratory rate > 30, urea > 7 mmol/L), suggesting the need for hospital admission but not necessarily HDU. However in this case the hypoxaemia, raised white cell count and multilobar involvement on clinical examination would alert the clinician to the potential severity of the CAP (Chapter 31).

2 The A–a gradient is calculated from the difference between the alveolar oxygen partial pressure and the arterial blood oxygen partial pressure (Chapter 11).

Alveolar oxygen tension (P_AO_2) is calculated from the simplified alveolar gas equation:

$$P_AO_2 = P_IO_2 - (1.25 \times P_aCO_2)$$

where P_IO_2 is the inspired oxygen partial pressure corrected for barometric pressure and water vapour pressure:

$$P_IO_2 = F_IO_2 \times (\text{barometric pressure (kPa)}$$
$$- \text{water vapour pressure (kPa)})$$

Thus: breathing air:

$$P_IO_2 = 0.21 \times (101 - 6.2) = 19.9 \, \text{kPa}$$

Thus:

P_AO_2 (breathing air) = 19.9 − (1.25 × 5.3) =~ 13.5 kPa
The alveolar – arterial oxygen tension difference is:

$$P_{(A-a)}O_2 = P_AO_2 - P_aO_2 \text{ (in this case } P_aO_2 \text{ is 6.6 kPa at admission on air)}$$
$$=~13.5 - 6.6 = 6.9 \, \text{kPa}$$

The A–a gradient differentiates between hypoxaemia due to: (i) hypoventilation and alveolar hypercapnia (i.e. a high P_ACO_2 lowers P_AO_2); and (ii) V/Q mismatch, shunt or diffusion impairment (Chapter 11). In this case the A–a gradient is 6.9 kPa (normally <1 kPa) indicating that V/Q mismatch, shunt or diffusion impairment are the principle causes of the hypoxaemia and treatment must be aimed at these defects rather than improving ventilation.

3 This patient was admitted to the HDU with high flow oxygen therapy and physiotherapy to aid expectoration (Chapters 12, 17). As recommended by the British Thoracic Society Guidelines for the management of CAP (Chapter 31) the patient was treated with high dose intravenous antibiotics to cover *Streptococcus pneumoniae* (e.g. cefuroxime) and atypical organisms (e.g. clarithromycin). As the patient was immobile, prophylactic low molecular weight heparin (LMWH) was started as prophylaxis against venous thromboembolism. Although non-invasive ventilation can be used in patients with pneumonia it is less effective than when used in acute hypercapnic failure and some studies suggest it may be associated with a worse outcome than early mechanical ventilation (Chapter 14).

4 Although severe hypoxaemia due to V/Q mismatch can occur with pneumonia, in this case the severity of the hypoxaemia and respiratory failure appeared disproportionate to the presenting clinical features (e.g. CXR). Similarly, the failure to improve with high dose antibiotics over the first 48 hours raised the possibility of alternative diagnoses like pulmonary embolism (PE), heart failure and acute lung injury. PE should be considered in all hypoxaemic patients with a normal or near normal CXR. The air travel from New Zealand and the intermittent episodes of increased hypoxaemia and confusion also suggest PE (Chapter 30) in this case.

5 Arterial blood gas abnormalities are common after PE including hypoxaemia with widening of the alveolar–arterial (A–a) gradient, hypoxaemia and hypocapnia (despite increased dead space). In the majority of patients the ECG is not helpful and shows non-specific ST segment changes. However, ~30% of patients with large PE develop a right ventricular strain pattern with the classical changes of an S wave in lead I and a Q wave and T wave inversion in lead III ($S_1Q_3T_3$ pattern), right axis deviation and right bundle branch block. Most patients have non-specific abnormalities on CXR including atelectasis due to reduced surfactant production in areas of poorly perfused lung. The presence of a lower limb deep venous thrombosis (DVT) should be sought with a Doppler ultrasound scan (or impedance plethysmography). Echocardiography may show right ventricular dysfunction and pulmonary hypertension. A transoesophageal echocardiograph may detect PE in the main pulmonary arteries but not in lobar or segmental arteries.

Spiral CT pulmonary angiograms (CTPA) scans are increasingly the initial investigation of choice, particularly in patients with CXR abnormalities (as in this case). They have a sensitivity for PE of 70–95% (higher for more proximal emboli) and a specificity >90%. It also allows visualization of parenchymal abnormalities and is useful in patients with COPD or extensive CXR abnormalities where V/Q scanning will be indeterminate (Chapter 30). In less severe cases with a normal CXR a V/Q scan may be the initial diagnostic investigation. A negative perfusion scan rules out a PE whereas a 'high probability' scan (i.e. multiple segmental perfusion defects and associated normal ventilation) has a >85% probability of a PE. With a high clinical suspicion, a high probability V/Q scan has a positive predictive value >95%. Unfortunately, most V/Q scans are not diagnostic or are indeterminate with a 15–50% likelihood of PE, necessitating further imaging. Absence of a DVT combined with a low probability V/Q scan permits withholding treatment whereas a negative Doppler ultrasound scan with an intermediate probability V/Q scan (or underlying cardiac or pulmonary disease) necessitates further imaging. Pulmonary angiography remains the diagnostic standard but is invasive.

6 Patients with PE may present with pleuritic pain and haemoptysis in about 65% of cases, isolated dyspnoea in about 25% and circulatory collapse in ~10% of cases. Dyspnoea is not present in ~30% of patients with confirmed PE. Other non-specific features include apprehension, tachypnoea, tachycardia, cough, sweating and syncope. Following a large PE, features of right ventricular failure (e.g. hypotension, jugular venous distension) may occur.

7 Anticoagulation stops propagation of existing lower limb thrombus and allows organization of the remaining clot which reduces the risk of further PE. Immediate therapy in patients with a high suspicion of

a PE prevents further life-threatening emboli. Unfractionated heparin (UFH) or low molecular weight heparin (LMWH) for 5–7 days, is followed by warfarin for 4–6 weeks when temporary risk factors (air travel in this case) are the cause and 3–6 months in idiopathic cases. UFH and warfarin must be monitored, as subtherapeutic levels increase the risk of recurrent PE. LMWH is more bioavailable and does not require monitoring. About 20% of patients with thromboembolic disease have inherited or acquired hypercoagulation problems (e.g. antithrombin III deficiency, protein C deficiency, lupus anticoagulant) and may require lifelong therapy. If contraindications prevent anticoagulation (e.g. recent surgery, haemorrhagic stroke, CNS metastases) or PE occur whilst on therapeutic anticoagulation, an inferior vena cava filter may prevent further PE.

8 Venous admixture (Q_S/Q_T) can be calculated from the S_aO_2 (70% or 0.7) and S_vO_2 (40% or 0.4) on air and the haemoglobin concentration as illustrated in Chapter 11.

$$Q_S/Q_T = (C_cO_2 - C_aO_2)/(C_cO_2 - C_vO_2)$$
when $C_{c,a,v}O_2 = [(Hb \times S_aO_2 \times k) + (P_aO_2 \times 0.023)]$

C denotes oxygen content and c, a and v denote end capillary, arterial and venous (note that end capillary and calculated alveolar oxygen tensions are assumed to be equivalent; thus on air end capillary S_aO_2 is expected to be 0.98); Hb = haemoglobin (g/L); k = coefficient of Hb oxygen binding capacity (1.36 ml O_2/g Hb); $P_aO_2 \times 0.023$ = oxygen dissolved in plasma (usually so small as to be insignificant).

Thus:
$$Q_S/Q_T = ([100 \times 0.98 \times 1.36] - [100 \times 0.70 \times 1.36])/$$
$$([100 \times 0.98 \times 1.36] - [100 \times 0.4 \times 1.36])$$
$$= (133 - 95)/(133 - 54) = 38/79 = 0.48$$
$$= \textbf{48\% venous admixture}$$

'True shunt' (i.e. corrected for partial V/Q mismatch) is calculated from the S_aO_2 (95%) and S_vO_2 (65%) when on 100% oxygen (i.e. F_iO_2 1.0). (Note that end capillary S_aO_2 would be expected to be 100% or 1.0 on 100% oxygen).

Thus:
$$Q_S/Q_T = ([100 \times 1 \times 1.36] - [100 \times 0.95 \times 1.36])/$$
$$([100 \times 1 \times 1.36] - [100 \times 0.65 \times 1.36])$$
$$= (136 - 129)/(136 - 88) = 7/48 = 0.15$$
$$= \textbf{15\% true shunt}$$

9 The CT scan in Fig. (b) (p. 124) demonstrates consolidation consistent with pneumonia and also shows a cavitating wedge infarct following a PE in a left segmental pulmonary artery. A single, sudden, large PE with marked obstruction of pulmonary blood flow is the likely cause of the cardiac arrest. In general, circulatory collapse occurs with >50% obstruction of the pulmonary arterial bed. Smaller emboli may be fatal when pre-existing lung or heart disease co-exist. Cardiopulmonary resuscitation must be started immediately. The cardiac massage may help break up a large clot into smaller segments which travel distally and reduce the degree of pulmonary bed occlusion. Following intubation high dose oxygen must be administered. Immediate plasma expanders and inotropic support are often given in an attempt to increase right ventricular pressure and to displace clot distally but risks severe right ventricular distension and subsequent myocardial damage.

10 Thrombolytic therapy is recommended in severe life-threatening massive PE with cardiovascular collapse. Thrombolytics hasten resolution of perfusion defects and correct right ventricular dysfunction but there is limited evidence of survival benefit. Nevertheless thrombolytic therapy would be appropriate in this patient with life-threatening cardiovascular collapse. In patients without massive PE there is no survival benefit with thrombolysis and there is a substantial increase in bleeding complications, including a 0.3–1.5% risk of intracerebral haemorrhage. Consequently thrombolysis is not recommended in these patients. This patient was thrombolysed and survived.

Case 6: Diabetic emergencies

1 A bedside blood sugar (BS) level must be checked at admission in every confused, agitated or unconscious patient. The brain is dependent on glucose for its metabolism and severe hypoglycaemia results in permanent brain damage within a matter of minutes. Every year hypoglycaemic patients fail to be recognized despite protocols, education and the legal consequences.

2 The first patient is hypoglycaemic. If he were able to swallow safely he would be given a glucose drink or 'carbohydrate snack'. However, as his conscious level is severely depressed, intravenous glucose (e.g. 50 ml 20% dextrose) is given. Provided the glucose has been given before significant cerebral damage has occurred, the patient will often 'wake-up' within a few minutes. Glucagon (1 mg i.v./i.m.) or hydrocortisone therapy is occasionally required in severe or refractory hypoglycaemia, as in sulphonylurea overdoses. These patients should be admitted for blood sugar monitoring (± glucose infusions). If BS measurement is not available (e.g. sudden onset of confusion in a diabetic whilst out hill walking), glucose should be given empirically as a sugary drink. Supplemental thiamine prevents Wernicke's encephalopathy (i.e. eye movement paralysis, ataxia, confusion) in hypoglycaemic malnourished patients especially alcoholics.

3 The second patient is hyperglycaemic. An arterial blood gas (ABG) will establish that he is acidotic (in this case the ABG was pH 6.95, P_aO_2 14 kPa, P_aCO_2 3.2 kPa, bicarbonate 3 mmol/L and base excess −21), a biochemical profile confirms he is dehydrated and hyperkalaemic (urea 20 mmol/L, creatinine 140 µmol/L and K^+ 6.9 mmol/L) and a urine dipstix will demonstrate the presence of ketones. This patient is hyperventilating to blow off carbon dioxide in an attempt to correct the metabolic acidosis, consequently his P_aCO_2 is low. Similarly the bicarbonate buffer has been depleted and the base excess is high.

4 The diagnosis is diabetic ketoacidosis (DKA). The immediate threats to this patient's life are the dehydration, acidosis and rapid ion fluxes which cause haemodynamic instability, with hypotension due to hypovolaemia, and reduced myocardial contractility and cardiac arrest due to hyper- or hypokalaemia. Rapid fluid replacement with ~3–5 L normal saline (NS) in <6 hours (i.e. 1 L in 30 minutes, then 1 L over 1 hour) rapidly corrects hypovolaemia and restores initial cardiovascular stability. Total fluid deficits of ~5–10 L and sodium losses of ~400 mmol are replaced over 48 hours. Monitor CVP if pulmonary oedema is a risk. The acidosis is corrected with insulin which enables intracellular glucose uptake and metabolism. This stops intracellular lipolysis, hepatic metabolism of released fatty acids, ketone production (e.g. β-hydroxybutyrate) and reverses the metabolic acidosis (Chapter 40). Insulin is given as an initial bolus (6–10 U i.v.), followed by an infusion (~6 U/h). Hyperglycaemia is often corrected before the acidosis but insulin must be continued until the acidosis has resolved by replacing the NS with a 10% dextrose infusion to maintain BS (monitored hourly) at 6–10 mmol/L. The use of sodium bicarbonate to correct the acidosis is controversial. It may reduce oxygen delivery and cause hypokalaemia. However, in severe acidosis (pH < 7.1) with myocardial depression treatment may be unavoidable.

Potassium ion (K^+) fluxes can cause cardiac arrest during initial treatment of DKA. Initial serum K^+ levels are high due to acidosis-induced K^+ movement out of cells. Insulin therapy stimulates cellular

K+ uptake with a rapid fall in serum K+. Hourly monitoring and K+ supplements correct the K+ depletion and prevent profound hypokalaemia (± cardiac arrest). Potassium supplementation before the onset of insulin therapy may cause hyperkalaemic VF/VT arrest. Hypomagnesaemia is corrected to prevent insulin resistance and arrhythmias. Phosphate supplementation maintains tissue oxygenation.

5 Hypoglycaemia is usually related to diabetic therapy including inadequate food intake, excessive exercise, accidental or deliberate overdose of diabetic drugs (e.g. sulphonylureas), prolonged drug effect (e.g. long-acting oral hypoglycaemics) and poor clearance in renal failure (e.g. insulin). Other causes include starvation, alcohol, renal and liver disease, systemic diseases (e.g. sepsis, hypothermia), endocrine disease (e.g. hypopituitarism), poisoning or drug therapy (e.g. salicylate) and rare insulin secreting tumours (e.g. insulinomas). The first patient, a known insulin dependent diabetic, had taken his normal dose of evening insulin with his supper. The exercise of dancing at the night club had resulted in a low sugar level and faintness. He had left the nightclub for some fresh air where he had collapsed sustaining a forehead laceration during the fall.

DKA occurs in type 1 diabetes mellitus (DM) due to severe insulin deficiency. Precipitants include infection (~30%), myocardial infarction, surgery, pancreatitis and non-compliance. No cause is found in ~25%. The second patient was not known to be a diabetic but had been experiencing increasing thirst, dehydration and polyuria for several weeks following a viral illness. Whilst dancing at the night club he had felt faint and had gone outside for fresh air where he had collapsed, injuring his head during the fall. About 10% of type 1 DM presents as DKA.

6 Alternative causes of unconsciousness in a young patient include alcohol intoxication, drugs, trauma, non-convulsive epilepsy and post-ictal states, infective causes including meningitis and encephalitis. Less likely causes include cerebrovascular, metabolic (e.g. hyponatraemia), endocrine (e.g. hypopituitarism) and cardiac problems (e.g. arrhythmias).

Appendix I: Classification of antiarrhythmic drugs (based on Vaughan Williams classification)

Class/examples	Mechanisms of action	Use
Class I:	All block Na⁺ channels slowing depolarization + raising threshold for triggering impulses (AP). Drug dissociation rates from Na⁺ channels vary; Class Ia ~5 s, Ib ~500 ms, Ic ~10–20 s	Slows conduction, suppresses re-entry + automaticity
Ia: disopyramide, quinidine	↑AP duration, ↑QT interval = ↑automaticity ↑AVN conduction = ↑HR in AF	SVT + VT but must block AVN (e.g. digoxin) in AF
Ib: lidocaine (lignocaine), mexiletine	↓AP duration + greatly ↓conduction	VT especially after MI
Ic: flecainide	Greatly ↓ conduction, no effect on AP duration but ↓contractility may cause hypotension	VT + some SVT (e.g. WPW syndrome)
Class II atenolol, metoprolol	Beta-blockers act mainly on SAN: ↓spontaneous depolarization = ↓HR + ↓sympathetic drive (e.g. MI, stress) = ↓automaticity (↓latent pacemakers)	SVT + VT especially after MI
Class III amiodarone, sotalol	Block K⁺ channels. ↑AP duration by ↓ repolarization. ↑QT interval risks automaticity (e.g. torsades de pointes). Also has class Ia, II + VI actions	SVT + VT. Most effective in re-entry tachycardias
Class VI verapamil, diltiazem	Block Ca²⁺ slow channels, ↓nodal conduction + automaticity. Also ↓contractility + risks hypotension	SVT especially AVN re-entrant tachycardias
Other classes adenosine, digoxin	Adenosine acts on A₁ receptors + ↓Ca²⁺/↑K⁺ currents to ↓AVN conduction. Digoxin ↓AVN conduction by vagal stimulation	Adenosine rapidly terminates + digoxin slows (± cardioverts) SVT

AF = atrial fibrillation, AP = action potential, AVN = atrioventricular node, HR = heart rate, MI = myocardial infarction, SAN = sinoatrial node, WPW = Wolff–Parkinson–White

Appendix II: Acute injury network staging system 2008 for acute kidney injury (AKI)

AKI stage	Serum creatinine criteria	Urine output criteria
1	SCr increase ≥26.4 μmol/L (0.3 mg/dl) or SCr increase ≥150–200% (1.5–2 fold) from baseline	<0.5 ml/kg/h for >6 h
2	SCr increase >200–300% (2–3 fold) from baseline	<0.5 ml/kg/h for >12 h
3	SCr increase ≥354 μmol/L (4.0 mg/dl) with an acute rise of ≥44 μmol/L in ≤24 h or SCr increase ≥300% (3-fold) from baseline or Initiated on RRT (irrespective of stage at time of initiation)	<0.3 ml/kg/h for >24 h or anuria for 12 h

Notes: RRT = renal replacement therapy, SCr = serum creatinine, UO = urine output. Only one criterion (SCr or UO) need be fulfilled to qualify for a stage. Changes in SCr or UO should occur within <48 h.

Appendix III: Rockall risk-scoring system for GI bleeds

	Score			
	0	1	2	3
Age	<60 yr	60–79 yr	>80 yr	
Shock	SBP>100 mmHg Pulse <100/min	SBP >100 mmHg Pulse >100/min	SBP<100 mmHg	
Co-morbidity	None	CF, IHD	Renal/liver failure	Metastases
Diagnosis	No lesion, Mallory–Weiss tear	All other diagnoses	Upper GI malignancy	
Signs of recent bleeding on OGD	None or dark-red spot		Blood in upper GI tract; adherent clot; visible vessel	

Notes: Rockall score assists prediction of rebleeding risk and death after upper GI bleeding. A score >6 suggests surgery may be required, but the decision is rarely taken on the basis of the Rockall score alone
CF = cardiac failure, GI = gastrointestinal, IHD = ischaemic heart disease, OGD = oesophagogastroduodenoscopy, SBP = systolic blood pressure

Appendix IV: Child–Pugh grading: A = 5–6; B = 7–9; C = 10–15. Risk of variceal bleeding increases ≥8

	1 point	2 points	3 points
Bilirubin (µmol/L)	<34	34–51	>51
Albumin (g/L)	>35	28–35	<28
Prothrombin ratio (s>normal)	1–3	4–6	>6
Ascites	None	Minor	>Moderate
Encephalopathy (grade)	None	1–2	3–4

Appendix V: Typical criteria for liver transplantation

Paracetamol poisoning	Other pathologies (e.g. drugs, viruses)
pH < 7.3, 24 h after ingestion or INR>6.5 Creatinine >300 µmol/L Hepatic encephalopathy (grade 3–4)	INR >6.5 or any 3 of: Drug or non-A, non-B virus aetiology Age <10 or >40 years old Jaundice for > 7 days before encephalopathy INR >3.5 Bilirubin >300 µmol/L

Index

Note: page numbers in italics refer to figures

abbreviated injury scale 15
ABC(DE) system *12*, 13, *20*, 21, 33
abdomen
    acute emergencies *116*, 117
    trauma 111
absorption collapse *32*
accelerated hypertension 67
ACE inhibitors 61, *64*, 65, 67
    AKI 85
acetylcholine (ACH) 47
    receptors *102*, 103
N-acetylcysteine 95, *106*, 107
acid–base balance *44*, 45
acidosis *see* metabolic acidosis
Acinetobacter 73
activated clotting time 105
activated partial thromboplastin time (APPT)
    104, 105
activated protein 53
acute confusional state (ACS) *98*, 99
acute coronary syndrome (ACS) 58, 59, *60*,
    61
acute hypercapnia 37
acute kidney injury (AKI) *84*, 85, *86*, 87, 132
acute liver failure (ALF) *94*, 95
acute lung injury (ALI) 79
acute respiratory distress syndrome (ARDS)
    78, 79, 83
    fat embolism syndrome 115
    shock *22*, 23
Addisonian crisis *90*, 91
Addison's disease *90*, 91
adjunctive therapy for severe sepsis 53
admission guidelines 15
admission wards 15
adrenal emergencies *90*, 91
adrenal function tests 91
adrenal insufficiency *90*, 91
adrenalitis, autoimmune 91
adrenocortical excess 91
adrenocortical insufficiency *90*, 91
adrenocorticotrophic hormone (ACTH) *90*,
    91
advanced life support (ALS) *20*, 21
Advanced Trauma Life Support (ATLS)
    Programme 111
afterload, cardiac *24*, 25, *58*, *64*, 65
    reduction *64*, 65
AIDS *108*, 109
air leaks *80*, 81
airways *34*, 35, 43
    assessment *12*, 13, 39
    burns complications *120*, 121
    drainage 83
    inflammation 75, *76*, 77
    obstruction *12*, 13, *34*, 35, 82, 83, 111
    protection 83, 113
    trauma *110*, 111
alarms 17, 43
albumin *26*, 27, *28*, 105
albuterol 75

alcohol 95, *98*, 99
    overdose *106*, 107
    pancreatitis 97
aldosterone 91
alfentanil *46*, 47
alkalosis *44*, 45, 77
allergens and asthma *74*, 75
alpha-blockers 91
alpha receptors 29, 53
alveolar–arterial oxygen tension differences*30*, 31
alveolar capillaries 77
alveolar damage 77, *78*, 79
alveolar gas equation *44*
alveolar oxygen tension *30*
alveolar recruitment 33
alveolar septa 77
alveolar ventilation 17
amino acids 49
aminoglycosides 85
aminophylline 65, 75
amiodarone 21
amniotic fluid embolism *118*, 119
amphotericin 85
amylase 97
anaemia 33, 85
anaerobic pneumonia 71, 73
anaesthesia 38, 39, 75
anaesthetic masks *32*, 35
analgesia *46*, 47
    burns 121
    cholecystitis 117
    endotracheal intubation *38*, 39
    pneumonia 73
    stroke 100
anaphylactic shock *22*, 23
aneurysms 100, *116*, 117
angina 58, 59, *60*, 61, *66*
    stable 58, 59, *60*, 61
    unstable 58, 59, *60*, 61
    variant 59
angiodysplasia *92*, 93
angiography 59, 61, *82*, *92*, 93, 100
    cardiac contusion 115
    pulmonary *68*, 69
angiotensin II receptor blockers *64*
angiotensin converting enzyme (ACE) inhibitors *see*
    ACE inhibitors
anion gap *44*, 45
antepartum haemorrhage *118*, 119
antiarrhythmic drugs 63, 107
antibiotics 105
    burns 121
    cholecystitis 117
    COPD 77
    hospital-acquired infections *54*, 55
    hospital-acquired pneumonia *72*, 73
    immunocompromised patients 109
    infective endocarditis 67
    meningitis 101, 113
    pancreatitis 97
    pneumonia 71, *72*, 73
    sepsis 53
    splenectomy 109

anticholinergics 51, 77, *106*
anticholinesterase drugs 103
anticoagulation 61, 68, 69, 104, 105, 113
    AKI *86*
    stroke 100
anticonvulsants 99, 100, 113
antidiuretic hormone (ADH) 27, 41, 91
antifungal therapy 109
antihypertensives 61, 67
    pre-eclampsia 119
antineutrophil cytoplasmic antibodies (ANCA) 85
antinuclear antibodies 85
antiplatelet agents 61, 105
antipyretics 113
antithrombin III deficiency 105
antithyroid drugs 91
anuria 85
anxiolytics 47
aortic aneurysms *116*, 117
aortic dissection *114*, 115
    hypertensive emergency *66*
aortoenteric fistula 93
APACHE II (acute physiology and chronic health
    evaluation) 15, 53, 97
apnoea *36*, 37, *56*, 57
appendicitis *116*, 117
arginine 49
arrhythmias 62, 63, *64*, 65, 132
    electrical burns 121
    stroke 100
    tricyclic depressant overdose 107
    see also bradycardia; tachycardia
arterial blood gases 17, *30*, 31, *44*, 45
    analysis 45
    asthma 75
    COPD 77
    neuromuscular conditions 103
    non-invasive ventilation 37
    pneumothorax 81
    pulmonary embolism 69
arterial carbon dioxide partial pressure *44*, 45
arterial embolization 93
arterial hypoxaemia *30*, 31, *32*, 33
arterial oxygen partial pressure *44*, 45
arterial oxygen saturation 17
arterial oxygen tension *30*, 31
arteriovenous malformations 100
ascites *94*, 95
Aspergillus *70*, 109
aspiration pneumonia 48, 49, 71, 73, *82*
aspiration syndromes *82*, 83
aspirin 61, *104*
    acute pericarditis 67
    overdose *106*, 107
    stroke 100
    upper gastrointestinal bleeding 92
assessment of acutely ill patients *12*, 13
assist control ventilation 41
asthma 43, *74*, 75
atracurium *46*, 47
atrial flutter/fibrillation *62*, 63
atrial pacing, overdrive 63
atrial tachycardia *62*, 63

atrioventricular node (AVN) block 63
atrioventricular node (AVN) re-entrant
    tachycardia *62*, 63
atropine 21, 63
auscultation 25
autonomic dysfunction *102*
autonomic dysreflexia 111
autonomy, respect for 57
axonal degeneration *102*, 103
azathioprine 103, 109

bacteraemia *52*, 53, 55
bacterial overgrowth *48*
balloon tamponade *92*, 93
barbiturates 47, 99, 107, 113
barotrauma 40, 43
    ARDS *78*, 79
    pneumothorax 81
basal metabolic rate *48*, 49
base excess 45
Battle's sign 111, 113
beds, rocking 37
beneficence 57
benzodiazepines 47, 99, 113, 121
benzylpenicillin 67, 101
berry aneurysms, leaking 100
beta-agonists 63, 75, 77
beta-blockers 61, 63, *64*, 65
    oesophageal varices 93
    phaeochromocytoma 91
    thyrotoxic crisis 91
beta receptors 29
bicarbonate 27, *44*, 45
bicarbonate buffer system *44*, 45
bilevel positive pressure ventilation 37, *40*, 43
biliary drainage 117
bilirubin *94*, 95
bladder *14*
    atony 111
bleeding *104*, 105
    acute renal failure *84*, 85
    gastrointestinal *92*, 93, 133
    intra-abdominal 111
    variceal 133
    see also haemorrhage
bleeding time 105
blood 26, 27, *104*, 105
    oxygen loading *18*, 19
    tests 71
blood gases *see* arterial blood gases
blood pressure 12, 13, *24*, 25
    monitoring 17
    see also hypertension; hypotension
blood sugar level 50, *88*, 89, 113
blood transfusions 93, *104*, 105
blue bloaters 77
blunt dissection 81
B-lymphocyte disorders *108*, 109
body weight *48*
Bohr effect *18*, 19, *30*
botulism *82*, 101
bowel *116*, 117
    gangrenous 117
    ischaemia, acute 117
    obstruction *116*, 117
bradycardia 25, *62*, 63, 103
    spinal injury 111

brainstem death *56*, 57
brainstem function tests *56*, 57
breathing *see* respiration; work of breathing
bromocriptine 51
bronchial artery embolization 83
bronchitis *76*, 77
bronchoalveolar lavage 75
bronchodilators 65, 77
bronchopleural fistula 81
bronchoscopy 71, 79, 83, 115
bronchospasm 77
buffer line *44*, 45
buffers *44*, 45
burns *120*, 121
    AKI 85

caecostomy, decompressive 117
café coronary syndrome 35, 83
calcium channel antagonists (CCA) 61
calcium channel blockers 65, 100
calcium sensitizers 65
caloric testing *56*, 57
calorific requirements *48*, 49
Campylobacter jejuni 103
candidiasis 109
capillary–mitochondrial oxygen gradient 19
capillary refill time 13
capnography 17
carbamazepine 107
carbimazole 91
carbon dioxide 17
    arterial partial pressure *44*, 45
    end-tidal 17, *38*
    retention 22, *32*, 77
carbon monoxide poisoning 33, *120*, 121
cardiac arrest 12, 13, 20, 21, 99
    amniotic fluid embolism *118*, 119
cardiac catheterization 65
cardiac contusion *114*, 115
cardiac emergencies *66*, 67
cardiac enzymes 58, 59, *60*, 61, 65
cardiac failure 32, 41, *42*, *64*, 65
cardiac massage, external 20, 21
cardiac output 13, *16*, 17, *24*, 25, 29
    heart failure *64*, 65
    hypothermia *50*, 51
    low 31
    resuscitation 20, 21
    sepsis 53
    thermodilution *16*, 17
cardiac pacemakers 29, 63
cardiac tamponade 20, 21, 23, *64*, 67
cardiogenic pulmonary oedema 37
cardiogenic shock 22, 23, 29, 59, 61, 65
cardiopulmonary arrest 20, 21
cardiopulmonary resuscitation (CPR) 20, 21
    team 21
cardiorespiratory arrest 20, 21, 31
cardiorespiratory support 95
cardiovascular care *14*
cardiovascular compensatory mechanisms *64*
cardioversion 20, 21, 29, 51
    direct current 63
catecholamines 91
    sparing 29
cathartics 107
cefotaxime 101

ceftriaxone 101
central nervous system 50, 66, *82*
central venous catheter *16*
    AKI *86*, 87
    line infection 54
central venous pressure *16*, 17, *24*, 25
    AKI 87
    shock *22*, 23
cephalosporins 85
cerebral abscesses 101
cerebral angiography 57
cerebral artery vasospasm 100
cerebral blood flow *112*, 113
cerebral herniation *112*, 113
cerebral ischaemia 113
cerebral malaria 101
cerebral metabolism reduction 113
cerebral oedema 101
    head injury *112*, 113
    liver failure *94*, 95
    status epilepticus *98*, 99
cerebral oxygen saturation 113
cerebral perfusion pressure (CPP) *112*, 113
cerebral toxoplasmosis *108*
cerebrospinal fluid 101, 103
cerebrovascular accident (CVA) *82*, 100
cervical collar 111
cervical fractures *110*, 111
cervical spine trauma *110*, 111
charcoal, activated *106*, 107
chemical burns *120*, 121
chest compressions 20, 21
chest drainage 79, *80*, 81, 115
chest infections *52*, 53, *82*, 83
    immunocompromised patients *108*, 109
    see also COPD; pneumonia
chest injuries 111, *114*, 115
chest radiography 64, 65, *114*, 115
    abdominal emergencies *116*, 117
    ACS 61
    ARDS *78*, 79
    asthma 75
    COPD 77
    drug overdose 107
    pneumonia *70*, 71, *72*, 73
    pneumothorax *80*, 81
    pulmonary embolism *68*, 69
    pulmonary infiltrates *78*, 79, *108*, 109
    respiratory emergencies *82*, 83
chest trauma *114*, 115
chest wall disorders 37, *40*
Child–Pugh grading 133
chin lift 21, *34*, 35
chloride 28
cholangitis and cholecystitis *116*, 117
cholinergic crisis 103
chronic inflammatory demyelinating polyneuropathy
    (CIDP) *102*, 103
chronic kidney disease (CKD) 85, 87
chronic liver disease (CLD) 93, 95
chronic obstructive pulmonary disease (COPD) 31,
    69, *76i*, 77
    exacerbations 37, 77
    nutritional requirements *48*, 49
ciclosporin 85, 109
circulatory assessment 12, 13, *24*, 25
    trauma 111

circulatory failure 22, 23, *24*, 25, *64*, 65
circulatory support 13, 23
cirrhosis 92, 109
clopidogrel 61
Clostridium difficile 48, *54*, 55
clotting cascade *104*
clotting factor assays 105
clotting–fibrinolytic system 105
coagulation *104*, 105
   acute liver failure *94*, 95
   fat embolism syndrome 115
   genetic disorders *104*, 105
   postpartum haemorrhage *118*, 119
coagulation tests *104*, 105
cocaine 59, 100, 107
codeine 47
colloid pressure 27
colloid solutions 27, 28, 121
colonic cancer 117
colonic obstruction *116*, 117
colonoscopy 93
coma *66*, 82, *98*, 99
   diabetic emergencies 88, 89
   head injury *112*, 113
   myxoedema *90*, 91
Combitube 35
comfort for patients *14*
communication with patients and relatives *14*
community-acquired meningitis 101
community-acquired pneumonia (CAP) 70, 71, 73
compartment syndrome 111
complications of shock 23
computed tomography (CT) 69, 111
   abdominal emergencies 117
   aortic rupture 115
   ARDS *78*, 79
   cerebral toxoplasmosis *108*
   head injury *112*, 113
   meningitis 101
   pancreatitis *96*, 97
   pneumonia 72, 73
   pneumothorax *80*, 81
   pulmonary embolism *68*, 69
   stroke 100
confusional states, acute *98*, 99
congestive cardiac failure *64*, 65
connective tissue disease 109
Conn's syndrome 91
consciousness, states of *12*, 13, *98*, 99, 115
continuous positive airways pressure (CPAP) *36*, 37,
     40, 43
   heart failure 65
   weaning 43
controlled mechanical ventilation *40*, 41
cooling 51, 113
cor pulmonale *64*, 65, 77
core–peripheral temperature 17
corneal reflexes *56*, 57
coronary artery occlusion *58*, 59
coronary care units 15
coronary syndromes, acute *58*, 59, *60*, 61
corticosteroids *see* steroid therapy
cortisol *90*
costs of critical care 15
co-trimoxazole 109
cough reflex *56*, 57
cranial nerve motor responses *56*, 57

cricoid pressure *38*, 39
cricothyroidectomy 83
cricothyroidotomy, emergency 35
critical illness AKI 85
critical illness polyneuropathy 103
Crohn's disease 109, 116
crush injuries 111
cryoprecipitate 105
Cryptococcus neoformans 101, *108*, 109
crystalloid solutions 27, 28
   burns *120*, 121
cuirass ventilators 37, *40*
Cullen's sign *96*, 97
CURB-65 71
Cushing's disease 91
Cushing's syndrome 91
cyanide poisoning *120*, 121
cyanosis, central 31, 35
cyclophosphamide 109
cytomegalovirus (CMV) 101, 103, 109

daily checklist *14*
dantrolene 51
D-dimer assays 69, 105
decolonization 55
deep venous thrombosis (DVT) *68*, 69
defibrillation *20*, 21, 63
defibrillators, implantable 63
demyelination *102*, 103
dexamethasone 91, 99
dextran 27, 28
dextrose 28
diabetes insipidus 91
diabetes mellitus 88, 89, 109
diabetic emergencies 88, 89
diabetic ketoacidosis (DKA) 88, 89
dialysis *86*, 87
   gut 107
diamorphine 65
diaphragm 115
   air under *116*
diarrhoea 48, 49
   hospital-acquired infection 55
diastolic dysfunction 25, *64*, 65
diazepam 99
DiGeorge syndrome 109
digoxin 62, *64*, 65, *106*, 107
dihydrocodeine *46*, 47
diphtheria 82, 83
direct current (DC) cardioversion 63
disability assessment *12*, 13, 57
discharge guidelines 15
dislocations *110*, 111
disseminated intravascular coagulation (DIC) 22,
    104, 105
   amniotic fluid embolism *118*, 119
   sepsis 52
distributive shock 23
diuresis, forced 107
diuretics 65
   AKI 85, 87
   loop 65, 87, 113
   osmotic 99
diverticular disease 117
dobutamine 23, 29, 53
dopamine 29, 53
   low-dose renal 87

dressings *14*
Dressler's syndrome 59, 67
drugs *14*
   AKI 85, 87
   asthma 75
   COPD 77
   endocrine emergencies *90*, 91
   endotracheal intubation *38*, 39
   gastrointestinal haemorrhage 93
   hyperthermia induction *50*, 51
   identification *106*, 107
   liver failure *94*
   overdose *106*, 107
duodenal ulcers 92, 93
   perforation *116*, 117
duty of care 57

early warning scores *12*, 13
echocardiography 21, 61, *66*, 67
   asthma 75
   pulmonary embolism 69
eclampsia *66*, 91, *118*, 119
edrophonium test 103
electrical injuries *120*, 121
electrocardiogram (ECG) *16*, 17, *60*, 61, 63, 65
   asthma 75
   CPR 21
   drug overdose *106*, 107
   hypothermia *50*
   pulmonary embolism 69
electrocoagulation 93
electroencephalogram (EEG) 57, 99, 113
   acute liver failure *94*, 95
electrolyte balance *14*, 26, 27, 29, *48*, 49
   acute liver failure 95
   acute renal failure 87
   pancreatitis 97
   status epilepticus 99
electromyography 103
electrophysiology 103
embolic infarcts *66*, 67
embolic strokes 100
embolism, amniotic fluid *118*, 119
embolization, systemic 67
emergency resuscitation rooms 15
emphysema *76*, 77
   subcutaneous 81, 115
encephalitis 101
encephalopathy *98*, 99
   hepatic *94*, 95
   hypertensive emergency *66*
end of life issues *56*, 57
end-diastolic volume (EDV) *24*, 25
endocarditis, infective *66*, 67
endocrine disorders *82*
   emergencies *90*, 91
endoscopic retrograde choledochopancreatography
    (ERCP) 97
endoscopic variceal ligation 93
endoscopy 39
   drug overdose 107
   gastrointestinal haemorrhage 93
endotracheal intubation (ETI) 31, *34*, 35, *38*, 39
   coma 99
   CPR 21
   Guillain–Barré syndrome 103
   mechanical ventilation *40*

endotracheal intubation (*cont'd*)
  myasthenic crisis 103
  respiratory emergencies 83
endotracheal tubes *38, 39, 40*, 41, 43
energy requirements *48*, 49
enteral nutrition *48*, 49
environmental risk of pneumonia 71
epilepsy *98*, 99
epinephrine (adrenaline) 21, 53, 83
Epstein–Barr virus 103
Escherichia coli 73, *54*, 117
ethical principles 57
exercise testing *60*, 61
  angina *58, 59*
expiratory positive airway pressure (EPAP) 36
expiratory time *76*, 77
extension injuries *110*
extracellular fluid *26*, 27
extracorporeal membrane oxygenation (EMO) 79
extradural haematoma 100
extubation *42*, 43

faecal impaction *48*, 117
failed intubation drill (FID) 39
fat embolism syndrome 115
feeding formulas 49
feeding intolerance *48*
fentanyl *46*, 47
fever 50, 51, *52*, 71
fibreoptic endoscopy 39
fibrinogen *104*
fibrinogen degradation products 105
Fick principle *48*, 49
flail chest *114*, 115
Flenley nomogram *44*, 45
flexible stylets 3
flow-time curve in mechanical ventilation *40*
fluid aspiration 83
fluid balance *14*
fluid challenge *24, 25*, 27, 28
  AKI 87
  sepsis 53
fluid choice 27, *28*, 29
fluid management therapy 21, *24, 25, 26, 27, 28*
  AKI 87
  burns *120*, 121
  diabetic ketoacidosis *88, 89*
  enteral nutrition *48*
  pancreatitis 97
  pneumonia 71, 73
  pre-eclampsia 119
  resuscitation 23
  sepsis 53
  shock *22*, 23
  trauma 111
fluid restriction 33
fluid retention 41
flumazenil 47, 99
focal chest symptoms 71
foetal assessment 119
foetal delivery 119
forced expiratory volume (FEV) 17, *76*, 77
  asthma *74*, 75
forced vital capacity (FVC) *74*, *76*, 77
foreign body, aspirated *34, 35, 82*, 83
fractures *110*, 111
  long-bone 111, 115

rib *114*, 115
Frank–Starling curve *24, 25*
fresh frozen plasma 93, *104*, 105
fresh whole blood 105
freshwater aspiration 83
functional residual capacity (FRC) *42*
full support ventilation 41
furosemide (frusemide) 87, 113

gag reflex *56*, 57
gallstones *96, 97*, 117
ganciclovir 101
gastrectomy 93
gastric aspiration *82*
gastric dilation *36*
gastric lavage 107
gastric tonometry 17
gastric ulcers *92*, 93
  perforation *116*, 117
  stress 97
gastrin 49
gastritis *92*, 93
gastrointestinal tract *14*, 49
  abdominal emergencies *116*, 117
  haemorrhage *92*, 93, 133
  mucosal ulceration *22, 23*
  small bowel obstruction *116*, 117
gastro-oesophageal tear *92*, 93
gelatin 27, 28
Gelofusine 28
general hygiene *14, 54*, 55
general supportive care 15
general wards 15
geographical risk of pneumonia 71
Glasgow Coma Score (GCS) 17, 99, *112*
  head injury *112*, 113
  stroke 100
  trauma 111
Glasgow criteria *96*
global oxygen consumption 19
global oxygen delivery *18*, 19
glomerular disease *84*, 85
glomerular filtration rate 85
glomerulonephritis 85
glucose imbalance *14*
glutamine 49
glycaemic control 113
glycerol trinitrate 67
glycoprotein antagonists 61
goal-directed therapy 19
Goodpasture's syndrome 85
graft vs. host organ rejection 109
granulocytopenia 109
great vessel injuries *114*, 115
Grey Turner's sign *96, 97*
Guedel airways *34*, 35
Gugliemi coils 100
guiding principles *14*
Guillain–Barré syndrome *40, 82, 102*, 103
gum elastic bougies 39
gunshot wounds 115

haematemesis 83, 93
haematuria 85, 87
haemodialysis 107
haemodynamics 23
  support 23, 53

haemofiltration *86*, 87
haemoglobin *26*, 27
  buffering capacity 45
  oxygen content *18*, 19
  saturation 30, 31
haemoperfusion 107
haemophilia *104*, 105
Haemophilus influenzae 70, 71, 72, 73, *101*
haemoptysis, massive *82*, 83
haemorrhage *110*, 111
  fluids 28
  obstetric *118*, 119
  see bleeding
haemorrhagic shock *22*
haemorrhagic stroke 100
haemothorax *114*, 115
halo frame 111
haloperidol 47
halothane 75
Harris–Benedict equation 49
Hartmann's solution 28
head injury 111, *112*, 113
  fluids 28
head positioning *34, 35*, 39
health-care associated pneumonia 72, 73
heart
  acute coronary syndromes *58, 59, 60*, 61
  block 63
  failure 13, *24, 25*, *64*, 65
  hypothermia 50, 51
  injury *114*, 115
  ischaemic disease 17, 20, 29, 59, 61
  rate *12, 13, 24, 25*, *62*, 63
  see also cardiac *entries;* myocardial *entries*
heat stroke 50, 51
Heimlich manoeuvre *34, 35, 82*, 83
helium oxygen mixture 83
HELLP syndrome *118*
hemicolectomy 117
Henderson–Hasselbach equation *44*, 45
heparin 61, *68*, 69
  coagulation disorders *104*, 105
  low molecular weight 61, *68*, 69
  unfractionated 61, *68*, 69
hepatic encephalopathy *94*, 95
hepatic foetor *94*, 95
hepatic failure *see* liver failure
hepatitis *94*, 95
hepatorenal syndrome *94*, 95
herpes simplex 109
high dependency units (HDU) 15, 75
high dose supplemental oxygen 33
high-flow facemasks *32*
His–Purkinje system 63
histoplasmosis *108*, 109
HIV infection 109
Homan's sign *69*, 81
hospital-acquired meningitis 101
hospital-acquired pneumonia 71, *72*, 73
host immune response 53
hydrocephalus 101, 113
hydrocortisone 91
hydrogen ion concentration *44*, 45
hydroxyethyl starch 27, 28
hygiene, general *14, 54*, 55
hypercapnia 31, 33, 37, *98*
  chest trauma 115

head injury 113
  mechanical ventilation *40*, 41
  permissive 75, 79
hypercapnic respiratory failure 33
hyperchloraemic acidosis (HCA) 28
hypercoagulable disorders 105
hyperglycaemia, stress-induced 89
hyperkalaemia *86*, 87
hyperosmolar non-ketotic (HONK) coma 89, *98*
hypertension *66*, 67
  ACS *98*, 99
  gastrointestinal haemorrhage 92
  pregnancy-induced *66*, *118*, 119
  stroke 100
hyperthermia *50*, 51
  prevention 113
hyperthyroidism *90*, 91
hyperventilation 99, *112*, 113
hypocapnia *112*, 113
hypoglycaemia 88, 89, *94*, 95
  ACS *98*, 99
hypokalaemia 95
hypopituitary crisis 91
hypotension 31
  amniotic fluid embolism *118*, 119
  chest trauma 115
  shock 23
  trauma 111
  tricyclic antidepressant overdose 107
hypothermia *50*, 51, 111
hypothyroidism, severe 51, *90*, 91
hypoventilation 31, 33, 37
  controlled 75
hypovolaemia 111
  shock *22*, 23
hypoxaemia *30*, 31
  acute respiratory distress syndrome 79
  cardiac arrest in pregnancy 119
  chest trauma 115
  chronic bronchitis 77
  fat embolism syndrome 115
  mechanical ventilation 41
  rebound *32*
hypoxia *30*, 31, 113

ileostomy 117
immune complex deposition 67
immune response, host 53
immunity, reduced 95
immunocompromised patients *108*, 109
  meningitis 101
  pneumonia 71, *72*, 73
immunodeficiency, primary disorders 109
immunonutrition 49
immunosuppression 103, *108*, 109
  pneumonia 71, *72*, 73
impaired diffusion 31
impaired gastric emptying *48*
infections *14*, 53
  abdominal emergencies 117
  burns *120*, 121
  community-acquired *70*, 71
  hospital-acquired *54*, 55, 72
  immunosuppression *108*, 109
  neurological emergencies 101
  opportunistic 71, 109
  pancreatitis 97

respiratory emergencies *82*
  sepsis *52*, 53
  urinary tract *54*, 55
infective endocarditis *66*, 67
inferior vena cava filter 69
inflammatory bowel disease *116*, 117
in-hospital resuscitation *20*, 21
inoconstrictors 29
inodilators 29
inotropes 23, *24*, 25, 29
  acute renal failure 87
  cardiogenic shock 61, 65
  organ donation 57
  pneumonia 73
  sepsis 53
inspiratory positive airway pressure (IPAP) *36*
inspiratory time *76*, 77
inspired oxygen fraction *30*
insulin 49, *88*, 89
intensive care units (ICU) 15, 75
intermittent positive pressure ventilation *40*, 41
intra-aortic balloon pumps 65
intracellular fluid (ICF) *26*, 27
intracerebral haemorrhage 100
intracranial bleeds *118*, 119
intracranial mass lesions 111
intracranial pressure (ICP) 17, 113
  raised *98*, 99, *112*, 113
  reduction 113
intrathoracic pressure, raised 41, 115
intravenous haemoglobin 103
intubation *see* endotracheal intubation (ETI)
intussusception *116*, 117
iodine 91
ipratropium bromide 75
ischaemia, individual organ 31
ischaemic heart disease 17, 20, 29, 59, 61
isoflurane 75

jacket ventilators 37, *40*
jaundice *94*, 95
jaw thrust 21, *34*, 35
jugular vein, central venous catheter *16*
jugular venous bulb saturation 17
justice 57

kerbstone fractures *114*, 115
ketamine 121
ketogenesis 88
Klebsiella 117
  pneumoniae *70*, *72*, 73
Kussmaul's sign 67
kyphoscoliosis *37*, *82*

labetalol 67, 119
lactic acidosis 89, 99
Lambert–Eaton myasthenic syndrome *102*
laparotomy for gastrointestinal haemorrhage 93
large bowel obstruction 117
large solute loads 28
laryngeal mask ventilation *34*, 35, 39
laryngoscopes *38*, 39
laryngospasm 83
left atrial pressure (LAP) 17, 79
left ventricular afterload reduction 41
left ventricular failure *64*, 65
Legionella pneumophila *70*, 71, *72*

leptospirosis 101
lidocaine (lignocaine) 63, 107
life support, advanced *20*, 21
life-threatening organ damage 67
line care *14*
line infections *54*, 55
lipases 115
Listeria monocytogenes 101
lithium 91, *106*
liver disease *104*, 105
  chronic 93, 95
liver failure *94*, 95
  ACS *98*, 99
  fulminant *94*, 95
  nutritional requirements *48*, 49
  paracetamol overdose 107
liver flap *94*, 9
liver regeneration 95
liver transplantation 95, 107, 133
loop of Henlé *84*, *85*, 87
lorazepam 47, 99
low dose supplemental oxygen 33
low-flow facemask *32*
low inspired oxygen partial pressure 31
lower respiratory tract 71
lungs 17
  compliance 17
  injuries 79, *114*, 115
  mechanical ventilation *40*
  torsion 115
  transplantation 77
  underlying disease *12*, 13
  volume reduction 77
  see also pulmonary *entries*; respiratory *entries*

magnesium sulphate 75, 119
maintenance fluids 28
malignant hypertension 67
malignant hyperthermia *50*, 51
Mallampati's classification *38*, 39
Mallory–Weiss tear *92*, 93
malnutrition 49, 99, 105
mannitol 51, 87, 113
manual in-line stabilization (MILS) *110*, 111, 113
maternal deaths *118*, 119
maximum inspiratory pressure (MIP) 17
mean arterial pressure (MAP) *24*, 25
mediastinitis 115
medical AKI 85
Medical Emergency Team 12, 13, 21
melaena 93
meningitis 101, 113
  meningococcal *52*, 53, 101
  rash *52*, 53
mental state, altered *98*, 99, 115
  shock 23
mesenteric angiography *92*, 93
mesenteric arteries, occlusion 117
mesenteric ischaemia 117
metabolic acidosis 29, *44*, 45
  acute liver failure 95
  acute renal failure 87
  diabetic ketoacidosis *88*, 89
  hyperthermia *50*, 51
  hypothermia *50*, 51
  mechanical ventilation 41
  septic shock *52*

metabolic alkalosis *44*, 45, 77
metabolic dysfunction in liver failure *94*, 95
metabolic rate *18*, 19
methicillin-resistant *Staphylococcus aureus* (MRSA) *54*, 55, 109
methionine 107
metoprolol 61
microbiology 23, 101
   community-acquired pneumonia *70*, 71
   hospital-acquired infections 55, *72*, 73
micronutrients *48*, 49
midazolam *46*, 47
Miller–Fisher syndrome *102*, 103
milrinone 65
mini-tracheostomy *42*, 43
mitral valve endocarditis *66*
mixed venous oxygen saturation 17, 19, 31
Mobitz I and II heart block 63
moderate dose supplemental oxygen 33
monitored trends *14*, 17
   acute renal failure *84*, 85
monitoring *16*, 17, 29, *82*
   endotracheal intubation *38*, 39
   haemodynamic *16*, 17
   head injury 113
   heart failure 65
   neurological 17, *112*, 113
   non-invasive techniques 17, 65
   oxygen therapy 33
   pneumothorax 81
   respiratory 17, 103
   sepsis 53
   severe hypertension 67
   shock 23
moral principles 57
morphine *46*
motor function in ACS 99
motor neurone disease 82
mouthcare *14*
MRSA *54*, 55, 109
mucosal inflammation 76, 77, 121
mucous fistula 117
mucous hypersecretions 76, 77
multidrug-resistant (MDR) pathogens 55, *72*
multiorgan failure (MOF) 22, 23, *52*, 53
   acute liver failure *94*, 95
   pancreatitis 97
muscle relaxants *38*, 39, 51
mushroom poisoning *106*
myasthenia gravis *82*, *102*, 103
myasthenic crisis *102*, 103
Mycobacterium tuberculosis 101, *108*
Mycoplasma pneumoniae *70*, 71
myocardial contractility *24*, 25
myocardial dysfunction *58*, 59, *60*, 61, *64*, 65
myocardial infarction *58*, 59, *60*, 61
   hypertensive emergencies *66*
myocardial injury 121
myocardial ischaemia 29, *58*, 59, *60*, 61, 65
   cocaine 107
myocardial oxygen consumption 61
myocardial oxygen supply 61
myocardial perfusion scans *60*, 61
myopathies *82*
myxoedema coma *90*, 91

N-acetylcysteine 95, *106*, 107
naloxone 47, 99
narrow QRS complex tachycardia 63
nasal cannulae *32*, 33
nasal intermittent positive pressure ventilation (NIPPV) *40*
nasogastric tube *36*, *48*
nasopharyngeal airway *34*, 35
   soft (SNPA) 35
nasotracheal tubes 39
near-drowning 83
negative pressure ventilation (NPV) *36*, 37, *40*
Neisseria meningitidis 101
neomycin 95
neurogenic shock 23, 111
neuroleptic malignant syndrome *50*, 51
neurological disease *82*
neurological emergencies 100, 101
neurological examination 99
   trauma 111, *112*, 113
neurological monitoring 17, *112*, 113
neuromuscular agents 47
neuromuscular care *14*
neuromuscular conditions *102*, 103
   mechanical ventilation 41
   NIV 37
neuromuscular paralytic agents 47
New York Heart Association (NYHA) classification *64*
nifedipine 61, 67, 119
nimodipine 100
nitrates 61, 65
nitric oxide 43, 53, *78*, 79
nitrogen 49
nitrovasodilators 61
non-Hodgkin's lymphoma *108*
non-maleficence 57
non-Q wave myocardial infarction *58*, 59
non-rebreathing facemasks *32*
non-shockable ALS 21
non-steroidal anti-inflammatory drugs (NSAIDs) *46*, 47, *104*
   acute renal failure *84*, 85
   upper gastrointestinal bleeding 92
non-ST-segment elevation myocardial infarction (NSTEMI) *58*, 59, *60*, 61
noradrenaline 23
norepinephrine 53
nose bleeds 83
nursing care 15
nutrition *14*, *48*, 49, 87
   acute liver failure 95
   assessment 49
   burns patients 121
   pancreatitis 97
   route 49

obstetric emergencies *118*, 119
obstetric haemorrhage *118*, 119
obstructive shock 22, 23
obstructive sleep apnoea (OSA) 37
occupational risks of pneumonia 71
octreotide 93, 97
oculocephalic reflex *56*, 57, 99
oculovestibular reflex 99
oesophageal rupture 115
oesophageal varices 92, 93

oesophagitis 92
oesophagogastroduodenoscopy (OGD) 93
oliguria 23, *52*, 85, 87
omega-3-polyunsaturated fatty acids 49
omeprazole 93
oncotic (colloid) pressure 27
opiates *46*, 47, 61, 99
opioids 47
opportunistic infections 71, 109
organ donation 15, *56*, 57
organization of critical care medicine 15
organophosphates *106*
oropharyngeal airways 35
oropharyngeal obstruction 35
osmolarity 28
osmotic agents 113
osmotic pressure 27
out-of-hospital resuscitation *20*, 21
overdrive atrial pacing 63
oxygen *30*, 31, *32*, 33
   alveolar *18*, 19
   alveolar–arterial tension difference *30*, 31
   arterial content *18*, 19
   arterial partial pressure *44*, 45
   arterial saturation 17
   asthma 75
   cerebral saturation 113
   COPD 77
   consumption *18*, 19
   cor pulmonale *64*, 65, 77
   debt 23
   delivery *18*, 19, *32*, 33
   extraction ratio *18*, 19
   haemoglobin content *18*, 19, *30*, 31
   heart failure 65
   helium mixture 83
   home therapy 77
   hypothermia 51
   impaired tissue utilization 53
   left ventricular failure *64*, 65
   mixed venous saturation 17, 19
   myocardial consumption 61
   pneumonia 71, 73, 109
   prescription chart *32*
   supplemental 33
   tension *18*, *30*, 31
   therapy *30*, 31, *32*, 33
   transport *18*, 19, *30*, 31
oxygenation *32*, 33
   acute kidney injury 87
   failure *30*, 31
   global measures 17
   monitoring *30*, 31
   shock 23
   trauma 111
   ventilation strategies 43
oxyhaemoglobin dissociation curve *18*, 19, *30*, 31, 33

pacemakers 29, 63
packed red cells 105
pain response *56*, 57
palpation 25
pancreatic pseudocysts 97
pancreatitis *116*, 117
   acute *96*, 97
   chronic 97
   necrotizing *96*, 97

pancuronium 47
panhypopituitarism 119
papilloedema 113
paracetamol *46*, 47, 51
  liver failure *94*, 95
  overdose *106*, 107
paralysis *46*, 47
  head injury 113
  neuromuscular conditions *102*, 103
  ventilation 43
parenteral nutrition *48*, 49
partial support ventilation 41, 43
Pathology Specific Scoring Systems (PSSS) 15
Patient at Risk Team (PART) 12, 13, 21
patient at risk warning scoring system 12, 13
Paul–Bert effect *32*
peak expiratory flow rate (PEFR) 17
  asthma 75
peak inspiratory pressure (PIP) *78*
pelvic disease 117
peptic ulceration *92*, 93
  perforation *116*, 117
percutaneous coronary intervention (PCI) 61
pericardial effusion 67
  aspiration *66*
pericardial tamponade 67, 115
pericardiocentesis, needle *66*
pericarditis, acute or constrictive 67
peripheral intra-arterial lines *54*
peripheral trauma 111
peritoneal dialysis *86*, 87
peritonitis 117
  spontaneous bacterial (SBP) *94*, 95
persistent vegetative state 57
pH *44*, 45
phaeochromocytoma 91
pharyngeal airway *34*
phenothiazines 47
phenoxybenzamine 91
phenytoin 99, 107
phosphodiesterase inhibitors 65
physiotherapy 71, 73
pink puffers 77
pituitary emergencies 91
  hypoperfusion 119
placenta praevia *118*, 119
placental abruption *118*, 119
plasma 93, *104*, 105
  exchange 103
plateau pressure *74*, 75
platelets *104*, 105
pleural effusion, oesophageal rupture 115
pneumatocoele 79
pneumococcal meningitis 101
Pneumocystis jirovecii (carinii) pneumonia
  (PCP) *70*, 73, *108*, 109
pneumomediastinum 81
pneumonia 33, *70*, 71, 72, 73
  acute liver failure 95
  aspiration 71, *82*
  community-acquired *70*, 71
  hospital-acquired 71, *72*, 73
  immunocompromised patients *108*, 109
  opportunistic 71
  oxygen therapy 31
  recurrent 71
pneumopericardium 81

pneumothorax 79, *80*, 81, *114*, 115
  asthma 75
  drainage 23, *80*, 81
  oesophageal rupture 115
  primary spontaneous *80*, 81
  secondary *80*, 81
  tension 21, *80*, 81, 111
  traumatic *80*, 81, 111
poisoning 82, *106*, 107
  toxic inhalation *120*, 121
poliomyelitis *82*, 83, 101, 103
polyneuropathies 103
polyradiculoneuropathy, demyelinating 103
portal hypertension 92
positioning of patients 43, *78*, 79
  endotracheal intubation *38*, 39
  heart failure 65
  pneumonia 73
  respiratory emergencies *82*, 83
positive end-expiratory pressure (PEEP) 37, *40*,
  41, 43
  ARDS *78*, 79
  asthma *74*, 75
  COPD *76*, 77
positive pressure ventilation (PPV) *36*, 37
  asthma *74*, 75
postoperative recovery wards 15
postpartum haemorrhage *118*, 119
post-renal AKI *84*, 85 87
post-resuscitation care 21
post major surgery fluids 28
potassium (K) 28
precordial thump *20*, 21
pre-eclampsia *66*, *118*, 119
pre-excitation syndromes *62*, 63
pregnancy *118*, 119
  ectopic *116*, 119
  hypertensive emergencies *66*, 67, *118*,
  119
preload, cardiac 24, *64*, 65
preoxygenation 39
pre-renal AKI *84*, 85, 87
pressure-controlled ventilation 37
pressure overload *64*
pressure support ventilation 37, *40*, 41, 43
pressure–time curves *40*
primary axonal neuropathy *102*, 103
prion disease 101
proarrhythmias 63
professional virtue 57
prognosis after CPR 21
prokinetic agents 49
propofol *46*, 47, 99, 113
propylthiouracil 91
protective lung ventilation strategy 79, 81
protein C 53
protein requirements *48*, 49
prothrombin time (PT) 95, *104*, 105
protocolized fluid resuscitation 53
proton pump inhibitors 93
pseudocholinesterase deficiency 47
Pseudomonas aeruginosa 53, *70*, *72*, 73
pulmonary angiography *68*, 69
pulmonary artery catheter *16*, 17
  balloon-tipped *16*
  heart failure 65
pulmonary artery occlusion pressure (PAOP) *16*, 17

pulmonary artery wedge pressure (PAWP) *16*, 17
pulmonary capillary wedge pressure (PCWP) *22*,
  23
pulmonary contusions 115
pulmonary dysfunction in fat embolism
  syndrome 115
pulmonary embolism (PE) *68*, 69, 21
  thrombolysis 23
pulmonary fibrosis 31
pulmonary hypertension 77
pulmonary infarction 69
pulmonary infiltrates *78*, 79, *108*, 109
pulmonary oedema *64*, 65
  acute liver failure *94*, 95
  amniotic fluid embolism *118*, 119
  cardiogenic 37
  drug overdose 107
  hypertensive emergencies *66*
  stroke 100
pulmonary oxygen toxicity *32*
pulmonary rehabilitation 77
pulmonary thromboembolism 119
pulse oximetry 31
pulseless electrical activity (PEA) *20*, 21
pulsus paradoxus *74*, 75
papillary reflexes *56*, 57, 99, 111
pyridostigmine 103
pyrogens *50*

quality of life 57
Q-wave myocardial infarction *58*, 59

rabies 101
raccoon eyes 111, 113
radiofrequency catheter ablation 63
radioisotope scan 57
radiological percutaneous drainage 97
Ramsay's sedation score *46*, 47
ranitidine 121
Ranson's criteria *96*, 97
rapid sequence induction (RSI) *38*, 39
reassurance for patient *14*
rebound hypoxaemia *32*
rectal bleeding 93
recurrent pneumonia 71
red cells, packed 105
re-entry mechanism *62*, 63
refeeding syndrome *48*, 49
remifentanil 47
renal biopsy 85
renal blood flow (RBF) 85
renal calculi *116*, 117
renal failure
  acute confusional state *98*, 99
  acute kidney injury (AKI) *84*, 85, *86*, 87,
  132
  acute liver failure *94*, 95
  angiodysplasia 93
  management *86*, 87
  nutritional requirements *48*, 49
  shock *22*, 23
renal function *50*, 51
renal impairment in hypertensive emergencies *66*
renal ischaemia 85
renal protection during imaging 37
renal replacement therapy 85, *86*, 87
  shock 23

renin–angiotensin mechanism 27, *64*, 65, 85
respiration *12*, 13
 ARDS *78*, 79
 asthma *74*, 75
 COPD *76*, 77
 hypothermia *50*
 shock 23
 spinal cord lesions 111
 trauma 111
 see also breathing
respiratory acidosis 31, *44*, 45
 mechanical ventilation 41
respiratory alkalosis *44*, 45
respiratory care *14*, *42*, 43
respiratory centre depression *40*
respiratory emergencies *82*, 83
respiratory failure *30*, 31, 37
 COPD 69
 endotracheal intubation 35, 39
 hypercapnia 37
 mechanical ventilation *40*, 41
 neuromuscular conditions 103
 non-invasive ventilation *36*, 37
respiratory management *42*, 43
respiratory monitoring 17, 103
respiratory pattern in ACS 99
respiratory rate *12*, 13
respiratory therapy 75, 77
resuscitation *20*, 21
 burns 121
 cardiac arrest in pregnancy 119
 cholecystitis 117
 diabetic ketoacidosis *88*, 89
 drug overdoses *106*, 107
 fluids 28
 gastrointestinal haemorrhage 93
 head injury 113
 severe obstetric haemorrhage 119
 severe sepsis 53
 stroke 100
 trauma 111
retained products of conception *118*, 119
retinopathy in hypertensive emergencies *66*
retroperitoneal haematoma 117
retroperitoneal haemorrhage *96*, 97
revascularization, cardiac 61
rewarming *50*, 51
rhabdomyolysis 111
rheumatoid arthritis 109
rib fractures *114*, 115
rifampicin 101
right atrial pressure (RAP) 17
right ventricular failure *64*, 65, 69
right ventricular preload reduction 41
Ringer's solution 28
road accidents 113, *114*, 115
Rockall risk scoring system 133
rocking beds 37
rocuronium *38*, 39, *46*, 47

salbutamol 65, 75, 77
saline, normal 28
SAPS (simplified acute physiology score) 15
Schofield equation *48*, 49
sclerotherapy 93
scoring systems 15
seawater aspiration 83

secretion retention 33
sedation *46*, 47
 asthma 75
 head injury 113
 ventilation 43
sedatives overdose *106*
seizures *12*, *98*, 99, 113
 amniotic fluid embolism *118*, 119
 meningitis 101
Seldinger technique *16*, 81
self-care wards 15
self-ventilating patients 47
Sellick manoeuvre 39
Sengstaken–Blakemore tube *92*, 93
sepsis 22, *52*, 53
 ACS *98*, 99
 AKI 87
 fluids 28
 line-related *54*, 55
 pancreatitis 97
 pulmonary 121
septic shock 22, 23, 29, *52*, 53
 fluids 28
septicaemia 101
severe sepsis *52*, 53
Severity of Illness Scoring System (SISS)
 15
shear stress 115
Sheehan's syndrome 91, 119
shock 22, 23, 91
 circulatory failure 29
 mechanical ventilation *40*, 41
 spinal 23, 111
 trauma 111
 upper gastrointestinal bleeding 93
shockable ALS 21
shunt fraction *30*
shunts, true *30*, 31
sick euthyroid syndrome 91
sigmoid volvulus *116*, 117
sigmoidoscopy 93
single organ AKI 85
sinus bradycardia 63
sinus tachycardia *62*, 63
skin *14*, 107
 burns 121
 rashes *52*, 53, 115
skull fracture, basal 111, 113
small bowel obstruction *116*, 117
smoke inhalation *120*, 121
sodium (Na) 28
 loss and retention *26*, 27
sodium bicarbonate therapy 89
sodium nitroprusside 67
sodium valproate 99
somatostatin 93, 97
spinal cord lesions 111
spinal immobilization 99, *110*, 111, 113
spinal injury *110*, 111
spinal shock 23, 111
spirometry *74*, *76*, 77
spironolactone *64*
splenectomy 109
stab wounds 115
standard mortality ratio (SMR) 15
Staphylococcus 71, 73, *101*
 aureus 55, *70*, 73, *101*

infective endocarditis *66*, 67
 pneumonia *70*, 71, *72*, 73
starter feeding regime *48*, 49
starvation *48*, 49
status epilepticus *98*, 99
steroid therapy 91
 ARDS 79
 asthma 75
 COPD 77
 head injury 113
 immunosuppression 109
 meningitis 101
 myasthenia gravis 103
 sepsis 53
 spinal injury 111
 thyroid emergencies 91
Streptococcus *66*, 67
 faecalis 117
 pneumoniae *70*, 71, *72*, 73, *101*
streptokinase 61
stress ulcers 97
stroke *82*, 100
 hypertensive emergencies *66*
stroke volume *24*, 25
ST-segment elevation myocardial infarction
 (STEMI) *58*, 59, 61
subarachnoid haemorrhage 100, 119
subdural haematoma 100
succinylcholine 47
suction endotracheal intubation 39
supraventricular tachycardia (SVT) 63
surfactant *78*, 79
Surviving Sepsis Guidelines 28
suxamethonium *38*, 39, *46*, 47
synchronized intermittent mandatory ventilation
 (SIMV) *40*, 41, 43
synthetic dysfunction *94*, 95
systemic inflammatory response syndrome
 (SIRS) *52*, 53
 pancreatitis 97
systemic lupus erythematosus (SLE) 85, 109
systemic vascular resistance (SVR) 17, 23, *24*, 25
systolic dysfunction *24*, 25, *64*, 65

tachycardia 25, *62*, *63*, 64
 septic shock *52*
 shock 23
tachypnoea *52*
tank ventilators 37, *40*
technetium scans *60*
temperature 17
Tensilon test 103
tension pneumothorax 21, *80*, 81, 111
terlipressin 93
tetanus *82*, 83, 101
thallium scans *60*
theophyllines 77, *106*, 107
Therapeutic Intervention Scoring System (TISS) 15
thermal coagulation 93
thermodilution cardiac output measurement *16*, 17
thiamine 99
thrombocytopenia *104*, 105
thromboembolic infarction 100
thromboembolism 105, *118*
thrombolysis 105
 pulmonary embolism 23
 stroke 100

thrombolytic therapy *60*, 61
   contraindications *60*
   pulmonary embolism 23, *68*, 69
thromboplastin 105
thrombosis 58, 105
   deep vein (DVT) *68*, 69
thrombotic stroke 100
thymectomy 103
thymus gland abnormalities 103
thyroid emergencies *90*, 91
thyroid storm *90*, 91
thyrotoxic crisis *90*, 91
thyroxine 91
tidal ventilation 17, *40*, 41
tiotropium bromide 77
tissue factors 19
tissue hypoxaemia 23
tissue hypoxia *30*, 31
tissue oxygen delivery *18*, 19
tissue oxygenation 17
tissue plasminogen activator (tPA) 61
T-lymphocyte function *108*, 109
total parenteral nutrition (TPN) *48*, 49
toxic inhalation *120*, 121
toxic megacolon 117
toxoplasmosis *108*
trace elements *48*, 49
tracheobronchial obstruction 35
tracheobronchial tears 115
tracheostomy *40*, 41, *42*, 43, 103
   surgical 35, *42*, 43
tracheostomy tubes 43
tranexamic acid 93
transjugular intrahepatic portal stent (TIPS) 93
transplant surgery 109
trauma *110*, 111
   AKI 85
   burns *120*, 121
   chest *114*, 115
   coma 99
   electrical injuries *120*, 121
   head injury 111, *112*, 113
   mechanical ventilation *40*
   pneumothorax *80*, 81, 111
   toxic inhalation *120*, 121
trauma score, revised (RTS) 15
trauma score (TS) 15
tricyclic antidepressants *106*, 107
troponin T, cardiac *60*, 61
true shunt *30*, 31
tuberculosis (TB) *82*, 83, 109
tubular necrosis, acute (ATN) 85, 87
tubulointerstitial disease *84*, 85

ulcerative colitis 117
ultrasound *68*, 69
   dialysis *86*
   pancreatitis 97
   pneumothorax *80*
upper airways obstruction (UAO) *34*, 35
uraemic bleeding 85, 87

urinalysis 85
urinary tract infections *54*, 55
urine flow 17
urine output *12*, 13
   fluid management *26*, 27
uterine atony *118*, 119
uterine rupture *118*, 119

vagal stimulation 63
vanillyl mandelic acid 91
vascular endothelium 105
vasculitis 85
vasoactive drugs 29, 39, 121
vasoconstrictors 29
vasodilators *64*
vasopressin 53, 93
vasopressors 25, 29
   pneumonia 73
   sepsis 53
vasospasm *58*
Vaughan Williams classification *132*
venodilators *64*
venous admixture *30*
venous blood, oxygen saturation 17, *18*, 19
venous drainage 113
venous return *24*, 25
venous saturation 31
venous thromboembolism *68*, 69
venous thrombosis prophylaxis *14*
ventilation *32*, 33
   amniotic fluid embolism 119
   analgesia *46*, 47
   bag-valve mask 21
   CAP 71
   cardiogenic shock 65
   end of life issues 57
   extubation criteria *42*, 43
   failure 31
   full support modes *40*, 41
   management *42*, 43
   masks 31, *32*, 33, *34*, 35, *36*, *40*
   mechanical *40*, 41
      ARDS 79
      asthma *74*, 75
      COPD *76*, 77
      haemoptysis 83
      neuromuscular conditions 103
      pneumonia 71, 73
      pneumothorax 81
      respiratory emergencies 83
      trauma 111
   mode *40*, 41
   mouth-to-mouth *20*, 21
   negative pressure *36*, 37, *40*
   non-invasive 33, 35, *36*, 37, *40*, 41
      CAP 71
      contraindications *36*
      COPD 77
      weaning 37, 43
   paralysis 47
   partial support modes 41, 43
   positive pressure *36*, 37, *40*

   pressure controlled 37
   protective strategies *40*, 41, 43, 81
      ARDS 79
   shock management 23
   volume controlled *40*, 41
   weaning 37, *42*, 43
ventilation/perfusion (V/Q) mismatch *30*, 31, *68*, 69, *76*
   ARDS *78*, 79
ventilation/perfusion (V/Q) scanning *68*, 69
ventilator-associated pneumonia *72*, 73
ventilators *40*, 41
   dependence 43
   jacket 37, *40*
   lung damage *78*
   management 43
   set-up *40*, 41
   tank 37, *40*
   weaning 37, *42*, 43
ventricular fibrillation *62*, 63
ventricular septal defect (VSD) 29
ventricular tachycardia *62*, 63
ventriculostomy drainage 113
Venturi mask *32*, 33
vestibulo-ocular reflexes *56*, 57
video laryngoscopes 39
vigabatrin 99
Virchow's triad 68
visiting hours *14*
vital signs in shock 23
vitamin K deficiency *104*, 105
vitamin requirements *48*, 49
volume controlled ventilation *40*, 41
volume overload *64*
volutrauma *40*, 43, *78*, 79, 81
vomiting, induced 107
von Willebrand's disease *104*, 105

Wallace's rule of 9s *120*, 121
warfarin 69, *104*, 105
water
   distribution in body *26*
   loss and retention *26*
   requirements *48*, 49
weaning from ventilation 37, *42*, 43
wedge pressure *16*
Weil's disease 101
Wernicke's encephalopathy *98*, 99
white blood cell count 91
   septic shock *52*, 53
WHO analgesic ladder *46*, 47
whole blood 105
wide QRS complex tachycardia 63
Wilson's disease *94*
withdrawal of treatment 57
work of breathing (WoB) 31, *42*
   asthma 75
   COPD *76*, 77
   mechanical ventilation 41, 77
   non-invasive ventilation 37
   shock 23
wound care *14*, 121